Issues in Public Health

Second edition

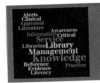

Understanding Public Health Series

Series editors: Ros Plowman and Nicki Thorogood, London School of Hygiene & Tropical Medicine.

Throughout the world, there is growing recognition of the importance of public health to sustainable, safe and healthy societies. The achievements of public health in nineteenth-century Europe were for much of the twentieth century overshadowed by advances in personal care, in particular in hospital care. Now, as we move into the new century, there is increasing understanding of the inevitable limits of individual health care and of the need to complement such services with effective public health strategies. Major improvements in people's health will come from controlling communicable diseases, eradicating environmental hazards, improving people's diets and enhancing the availability and quality of effective health care. To achieve this, every country needs a cadre of knowledgeable public health practitioners with social, political and organizational skills to lead and bring about changes at international, national and local levels.

This is one of a series of books that provides a foundation for those wishing to join in and contribute to the twenty-first-century regeneration of public health, helping to put the concerns and perspectives of public health at the heart of policy-making and service provision. While each book stands alone, together they provide a comprehensive account of the three main aims of public health: protecting the public from environmental hazards, improving the health of the public and ensuring high quality health services are available to all. Some of the books focus on methods, others on key topics. They have been written by staff at the London School of Hygiene & Tropical Medicine with considerable experience of teaching public health to students from low, middle and high income countries. Much of the material has been developed and tested with postgraduate students both in face-to-face teaching and through distance learning.

The books are designed for self-directed learning. Each chapter has explicit learning objectives, key terms are highlighted and the text contains many activities to enable the reader to test their own understanding of the ideas and material covered. Written in a clear and accessible style, the series is essential reading for students taking postgraduate courses in public health and will also be of interest to public health practitioners and policy-makers.

Titles in the series

Analytical models for decision making: Colin Sanderson and Reinhold Gruen
Controlling communicable disease: Norman Noah
Economic analysis for management and policy: Stephen Jan, Lilani Kumaranayake, Jenny Roberts, Kara Hanson and Kate Archibald
Economic evaluation: Julia Fox-Rushby and John Cairns (eds)
Environmental epidemiology: Paul Wilkinson (ed.)
Environmental health policy: Megan Landon and Tony Fletcher
Financial management in health services: Reinhold Gruen and Anne Howarth
Global change and health: Kelley Lee and Jeff Collin (eds)
Health care evaluation: Sarah Smith, Don Sinclair, Rosalind Raine and Barnaby Reeves
Health promotion practice: Maggie Davies, Wendy Macdowall and Chris Bonell (eds)
Health promotion theory: Maggie Davies and Wendy Macdowall (eds)
Introduction to epidemiology, Second Edition: Ilona Carneiro and Natasha Howard
Introduction to health economics, Second Edition: Lorna Guinness and Virginia Wiseman (eds)
Issues in public health, Second Edition: Fiona Sim and Martin McKee (eds)
Managing health services: Nick Goodwin, Reinhold Gruen and Valerie Iles
Medical anthropology: Robert Pool and Wenzel Geissler
Principles of social research: Judith Green and John Browne (eds)
Public Health in History: Virginia Berridge, Martin Gorsky and Alex Mold
Understanding health services: Nick Black and Reinhold Gruen

Forthcoming titles

Sexual health: a public health perspective: Kaye Wellings, Martine Collumbien, Wendy Macdowall and Kirstin Mitchell
Conflict and health: Egbert Sondorp and Annemarie ter Veen (eds)
Making health policy, Second Edition: Kent Buse, Nicholas Mays and Gill Walt
Environment, health and sustainable development, second edition: Emma Hutchinson and Megan Landon (eds)

Issues in Public Health

Second edition

Edited by Fiona Sim and
Martin McKee

 Open University Press

Open University Press
McGraw-Hill Education
McGraw-Hill House
Shoppenhangers Road
Maidenhead
Berkshire
England
SL6 2QL

email: enquiries@openup.co.uk
world wide web: www.openup.co.uk

and Two Penn Plaza, New York, NY 10121-2289, USA

First published 2005
Reprinted 2008, 2009
First published in this second edition 2011

A catalogue record of this book is available from the British Library

ISBN-13: 978-0-33-524422-5
ISBN-10: 0-33-524422-X
eISBN: 978-0-33-524423-2

Library of Congress Cataloging-in-Publication Data
CIP data applied for

Typesetting and e-book compilations by
RefineCatch Limited, Bungay, Suffolk
Printed and bound by CPI Group (UK) Ltd, Croydon, CR0 4YY

Fictitious names of companies, products, people, characters and/or data that may be used herein (in case studies or in examples) are not intended to represent any real individual, company, product or event.

The McGraw·Hill Companies

Dedication

This book is dedicated to the memory of Professor Jerry Morris CBE, a giant of public health and Emeritus Professor at the London School of Hygiene and Tropical Medicine, who died in 2009, a few months short of his 100th birthday.

Contents

List of figures

List of tables

Disclaimer

Every effort has been made to obtain permission from copyright holders to reproduce material in this book and acknowledge these sources correctly. Any omissions brought to our attention will be remedied in future editions.

Overview of the book

Introduction

This book is designed for students who want to answer the question 'What is public health?'. It thus focuses on those things that societies do collectively to enhance the health of populations. This, as you will see by going through the book, includes a lot of different things, many of which you may never have thought of as public health. For one thing, it includes health care. However, you will not learn here about the interaction between the health professional and the individual patient. Instead, the book looks at how societies organize health care to make it accessible to all, and it discusses the nature of the care that is provided to ensure that the health system actually does things that will benefit people.

The book also discusses big issues. Take smoking, for example. Of course societies want to make sure that children are taught that smoking is bad for them. But you should not be so naïve as to think this is enough. Much of modern public health is about tackling strong vested interests head on – in this case the transnational tobacco industries, but in other cases the food or alcohol industries. So if you want to be serious about reducing smoking, you need to know your enemy and know what it is they don't want us to do.

The book also discusses the importance of empowering people, so they can make healthy decisions. Public health actions should bring opportunities and, as importantly, hope.

Finally, the book confronts explicitly the political nature of public health. Much disease has its origins in the way that we organize our society, in deciding how much income to redistribute, how resources such as education, transport and housing should be provided, and who pays for what. Anyone who doubts the association between deprivation and ill health should read Charles Dickens' accounts of the working classes in nineteenth-century England. The political question is what to do about the situation we find ourselves in.

Why study public health?

If a society is to achieve these things, it needs skills and vision. Skills, so that it can make problems that are invisible visible, and skills to design interventions that work, not just for the average person, but also for those who are far from average, especially those who are at the bottom of the pile. Many of those who are worst off in society are effectively invisible. They are the people who clean the streets before we wake, the people who labour in sweat shops to allow us to eat low-cost junk food and to wear cheap clothes. Society does not see them, nor does it see their health needs. But rather like looking at the dots on an impressionist painting, health professionals may be too close to see the big picture. Unless you look at the level of a population, you may miss a large rise or fall in deaths from a particular disease.

Skills are also needed to know what works, and in what circumstances. It is important to understand the often complex determinants of disease. Take alcohol and deaths from injuries, for example. We may need to know why people drink, why they get drunk, why they injure themselves when they are drunk, why no-one helps them, and why, when they get to a health care facility, it is unable to provide them with effective care. Which of these is most important will depend on the circumstances, as will how we intervene to reduce deaths, but understanding what has gone wrong is a first, essential, step.

But skills are not enough. One also needs a vision of what the future can be. Effective public health practitioners cannot be complacent. Just because things have always been the way they are does not mean that they cannot change. This means that it is important to think laterally, understanding why things are as they are, who benefits from the status quo and who might benefit from change, what are the power structures on which our societies are based and the mechanisms by which they might change, who is really in charge and what can we do to influence them.

Public health is often seen as unexciting, even boring; in many places it is done by people who do not get out of their offices enough and who, as a consequence, are largely irrelevant to events in the real world. In some places this is a fair reflection of what happens. But it is hoped that this book will convince you that this is not the case everywhere and where public health is working it is exciting, challenging, controversial and certainly never boring!

Structure of the book

This book follows the conceptual outline of the 'Issues in Public Health' unit at the London School of Hygiene and Tropical Medicine (LSHTM). It is based on the materials presented in the lectures and seminars of the taught course, which have been adapted for distance learning.

The book is divided into two sections. The first section looks at the foundation of public health and at a series of themes that underpin public health. The second section turns to a series of specific determinants of health among the most important causes of avoidable disease globally. Inevitably, choices had to be made as it is not possible to cover everything in the time available. For example, apart from reference to firearms injuries in the first chapter and armed conflict in the ninth, injuries and violence are not covered. Illicit drugs and sexual health are not covered either. All of these, and many others, are important, but it is hoped that the basic concepts that will be drawn on will provide you with the tools to understand how you might intervene to reduce the burden of disease caused by these and other factors.

The two sections, and the 12 chapters within them, are shown on the book's contents page. Each chapter includes:

- an overview
- a list of learning objectives
- a list of key terms
- a range of activities
- feedback on the activities
- a summary.

It is important to point out that most examples in this book are drawn from industrialized and middle-income countries, but the principles involved apply more generally and some examples are also chosen from developing countries.

The following description of the book will give you an idea of what you will be studying.

Foundation of modern public health

This section discusses what modern public health is. The first chapter traces the historical evolution of the public health movement and how it influences our current perception of public health and its goals. Chapters 2 to 5 then look at a series of themes that underpin public health. These include the use of basic data on populations and mortality (Chapter 2), the methods used to estimate the burden of disease and to assess the factors that contribute to it (Chapter 3), the extent to which health care contributes, or fails to contribute, to population health (Chapter 5), and how to determine the effects on health of policies in other sectors such as transport or the environment (Chapter 6). The final theme involves looking beyond average levels of health in a population to understand how they differ within populations. In particular, you will explore inequalities in health: why are some people, most often the poor, less healthy than others, and what can we do about it (Chapter 4)?

Major determinants of health

The second part of the book turns to a series of specific determinants of health. Chapter 7 discusses the evolution of infectious diseases and of their control, and describes the burden of disease attributable to infectious diseases and the factors that can affect it. Tobacco use, as a major public health issue worldwide, is then explored in Chapter 8. The health impact of tobacco use and the four-stage model of the smoking epidemic are described. Then, current debates around tobacco control policies and options for these policies are examined, as well as how globalization represents a new challenge for tobacco control. Chapter 9 introduces three issues rather more recently highlighted as significant in population health, namely human rights, genetics and armed conflict. Chapter 10 discusses the relationships between food and health, including the relevance of industry and other influences on healthy public policy. Next, the health and environmental impacts of waste disposal activities, including landfill and incineration, are discussed in Chapter 11, as well as the potential health effects of indoor air pollution. Finally, in Chapter 12, the subjects of sustainable development and climate change are explored as critical global public health issues.

A variety of activities are employed to help your understanding and learning of the topics and ideas covered. These include:

- reflection on your own knowledge and experience
- questions based on reading key articles or relevant research papers
- outlining short policy papers.

Introduction to the Second Edition

The first edition of this book was well received and seemed to work for students and teachers alike, whether participating in face to face or distant learning courses. So, on the principle of not trying to fix something that is not broken, this second edition of *Issues in Public Health* follows the same structure as the first edition. We have, however, taken heed of comments received about the first edition by making efforts to make changes in response to those comments, as well as updating the content where appropriate. This second edition introduces two new chapters in Section 2, to reflect the expanding role of public health, covering the issues of sustainability and climate change, human rights, genetics and armed conflict, all of which were only cursorily mentioned in the first edition. We have tried to address known gaps in the first edition, by increasing reference and cross reference to other books in the series, concerning health promotion and mental health, for example, and by ensuring plenty of examples from the UK and Europe, where many of our readers are based.

Acknowledgement

The editors would like to acknowledge the contributions of Allison Thorpe, Ros Plowman, Francesco Checchi and Nicki Thorogood, for their help in reviewing this second edition.

SECTION I

Foundation of modern public health

The emergence of public health and the centrality of values

Martin McKee, Fiona Sim and Joceline Pomerleau

Overview

In this chapter you will learn about the historical development of the **public health** movement. You will be introduced to some key documents that paved the way of the current public health movement and learn that public health scientists do not all share the same views about where public health should go.

Learning objectives

After completing this chapter you will be able to:

- describe the development of ideas on the role of public health
- discuss the arguments for and against societal interventions to promote health
- describe the scope to use advocacy to promote health and the limitations in doing so

Key terms

Intersectoral action for health   The promotion of health through the involvement of actors in other sectors, such as transport, housing, or education.

Libertarianism   Philosophical approach that favours individualism, with a free-market economic policy and non-intervention by government.

Public health   The science and art of promoting health and preventing disease through the organized efforts of society.

Historical development of public health

The development of public health started in the eighteenth century with the *sanitary movement*. The concept of contagion was key to this early development, whether from disease (cholera) or ideas (communism). Then, as now, policies were often motivated as

much by self-interest as by altruism. The very unsanitary conditions in the newly industrializing cities demanded a response but there was intense debate about what to do.
Many of the discussions at the time resonate with contemporary ones about the balance between the role of the individual, with those who were regarded as 'the feckless
poor' having only themselves to blame, and that of the state in protecting the population
from a range of hazards and enabling them to make healthy choices. Again, the contemporary relevance of the debates will become apparent, in particular when we reflect on
the concerns voiced by the employers of the time about the unfairness of the burdens
being placed upon them to improve the conditions of their workers.

We then move on to the rise of what was called *preventive medicine*. This emerged in
many developed countries in the middle of the twentieth century, coinciding with the
rise of scientific medicine and optimism about its potential achievements. It was characterized by its focus on the concept of hygiene. This was not just in relation to infectious diseases but, in some countries in the 1930s, taking a rather less innocuous form
with its emphasis on genetic or racial hygiene. The legacy of that period has had profound implications until the present day for the ability to undertake collective health
interventions in the countries concerned. In this period health professionals assumed
they knew best and played a key role. Education (especially when undertaken by doctors or nurses) was thought sufficient to change behaviour and much disease was
avoidable by means of mass activities such as screening.

Later in the twentieth century, new ideas began to emerge, rejecting the dominance
of the medical model. In 1974 the Canadian Government published the 'Lalonde
Report', which proposed the *health field concept* (Figure 1.1).

This report signalled the beginning of a move away from the medicalization of public
health towards one that emphasized the building of *healthy public policy*. In 1978, WHO
expressed 'the need for urgent action by all governments, all health and development

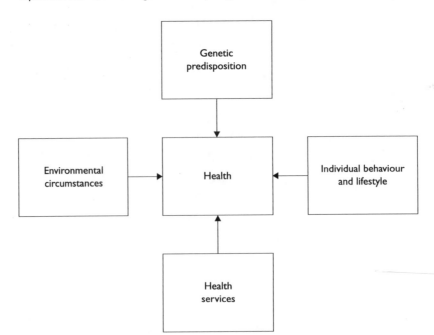

Figure 1.1 The health field concept

workers, and the world community to protect and promote the health of all the people of the world' in its Declaration of Alma Ata (World Health Organization 1978). Subsequently, there was a growing focus on intersectoral action, working with sectors such as housing, transport, education and others, enshrined in the World Health Organization's 'Health for All by the Year 2000' (HFA) movement and eponymous declaration (World Health Organization Regional Office for Europe 1985). These principles were reinforced in the Ottawa Charter in 1986, which called for the following approaches to promote population health:

- building healthy public policy
- creating supportive environments
- strengthening community actions
- developing personal skills
- reorienting health services
- demonstrating commitment to health promotion

The HFA programme emphasized intersectoral action and, somewhat controversially at the time, the importance of certain prerequisites for health, such as peace and equity. In Europe it was developed into a set of 38 targets (World Health Organization Regional Office for Europe 1985). However, many of these were rather vague and unquantified, and of those that were quantified, some countries had already achieved them by the time they were published, while others had little chance of reaching them before the end of the century. In addition, while all European governments signed up to the idea of HFA, few went any further towards actually doing anything about it. Even when they did initiate healthy public policies, there was rarely any reference to HFA.

Yet internationally, HFA was effective patchily in catalysing action at local level, because public health advocates used the fact that their governments had endorsed it in order to support initiatives such as the 'Healthy Cities' movement, in which local administrations developed wide-ranging programmes to improve health, through setting and implementing local policies on transport, housing and education.

By the mid-1990s, when it became clear that 'health for all' would not be achieved by the year 2000, the World Health Organization policy strategy was renewed, leading to 'Health 21'. This has a more limited set of targets but, like HFA, it has received relatively little attention by national governments (World Health Organization Regional Office for Europe 1999). It is currently being updated as 'Health 2020'.

At the same time, however, a new issue had emerged that was seen, by many but by no means by everyone, to link closely with issues of health. Concerns about the global environment had forced governments to come together at the Rio Earth Summit. One of the outcomes of that meeting was 'Agenda 21', a plan for sustainable development. Many people who had been working to improve health locally, implementing intersectoral responses, saw this as a process that they could link with. As a consequence, in many localities there is now a close association between those seeking to enhance health and those working for a sustainable environment.

In contrast, the commitment by national governments to improving health is less obvious. Some countries have developed health strategies but many are aspirational, providing little basis for concrete policies. We also have to take account of the facts that different countries have different models of public health delivery that reflect their politics, the evolution of their health care systems, their economic situations, and above all their histories.

Since the early 2000s it has become more widely recognized that the physical health of a population is not all that contributes to its productivity and success. Mental health and wellbeing have begun to feature more prominently in national policy, both in terms of promoting better mental health of the population and in improving access to effective services for people with mental health problems. Internationally, WHO recognized that public mental health had been neglected and aimed to rectify this in its 2001 World Health Report, which emphasized the importance of mental health as being 'crucial to the overall well-being of individuals, societies and countries' (World Health Organization 2001).

In the UK, for example, the latest Mental Health Strategy for England is entitled 'No Health Without Mental Health' (DH 2011) and focuses on both services for people with mental illness and on promoting better public mental health. The workplace is a key environment for promotion of mental health and there is growing evidence that interventions in the workplace can improve or maintain an individual's mental health. Interventions to enhance the amount of control people have over their work can be effective, and more so with those in lower paid, lower grade jobs. However, there is even greater evidence of effectiveness for interventions that address the culture and practices of the organization as a whole, as well as working with individual employees (Raine et al. 2010). Government policies that aim to improve mental health are not simply altruistic, of course. In the UK, mental illness accounts for over 20 per cent of the total **burden of disease**; as well as the costs of health care, productivity is lost and people unable to work due to mental illness are eligible for state benefits, so that the annual wider economic costs of mental health problems in the UK are estimated by government to be £110 billion a year (NHS Public Mental Health & Wellbeing website 2011).

There is evidence that cohesive communities and the presence of social capital are associated with better mental health than those lacking these characteristics. Perhaps not surprisingly, communities affected by adverse circumstances, such as war or following natural disaster (such as an earthquake or volcano eruption) have a higher prevalence of poor mental health, often for lengthy periods after the event has passed. Understanding these consequences of adverse events allows for effective interventions to be planned and implemented for protection of public mental health alongside interventions to protect the physical health of vulnerable populations.

There are two main reasons that the historial development of public health is relevant today. One is that, in many countries, what is called public health has still to emerge from the model adopted until the 1950s, telling people what they should and should not do, with little understanding of why they do things that will harm them. A second is that it helps us to understand that public health has always had an important political dimension. It is quite explicitly not value free. Its commonly used definitions talk about the organized actions of society. This assumes an acceptance that society, and not just a collection of individuals, actually exists and has identifiable responsibilities; and it assumes that it is justifiable to constrain the freedom of one individual to benefit the population as a whole. Indeed, a public health intervention may mean more than constraining someone's freedom to do something. It may mean actively doing something to them, such as immunizing them against disease, fortifying their food with vitamins, or adding fluoride to drinking water.

Activity 1.1

Some people object to this vision of public health. Briefly describe the reasons why this might be the case.

Feedback

Some people take a very different view for various reasons. For example, Peter Skrabanek, who worked in an academic department of public health in Dublin, argued vehemently in the 1980s that many public health interventions were unjustified because we simply did not know enough about the determinants of disease and whether what we were proposing would work (Skrabanek and McCormick 1989). A refugee from then communist Czechoslovakia, he rejected what he saw as an over powerful role of the state. He described a whole range of activities, such as advocating a low-fat diet or cancer screening as 'gratuitous intervention'. In particular, he argued that much of our apparent understanding of risk factors for common diseases stems from an inappropriate use of epidemiology, in which we seize on chance associations between risk factors and disease as signifying that the risk factor actually causes the outcome in question.

Bruce Charlton, writing from a libertarian perspective, argued that many public health policies amounted to 'health fascism', imposing a particular lifestyle on others whether they like it or not (Charlton 2001). This idea resonates in some countries in Europe where totalitarian regimes in the 1930s were extremely active in, for example, promoting exercise and opposing smoking. George Davey Smith has provided a detailed account of the anti-smoking policies pursued by the Nazis in pre-war Germany (Davey Smith and collaborators 1994), although this has subsequently been exaggerated by the tobacco industry (Bachinger et al. 2008), who have coined the term 'nico-nazis' to attack anti-smoking campaigners. In the UK the concept of the 'nanny state', using the analogy of a nanny telling children what to do, is often invoked by the tabloid press to oppose public health interventions and in recent times successive governments across the political spectrum have shied away from acquiring this image.

Another criticism is that the intersectoral approach that is now a feature of public health is a form of 'health imperialism', with 'health' being equated with 'happiness' or 'wellbeing'. Criticism focuses in particular on the WHO definition of health as 'a state of complete physical, mental, and social well-being and not merely the absence of disease or infirmity' (World Health Organization 2003), which is seen as allowing public health professionals to justify their involvement in many issues where they really have no right to be.

Then there is the charge that some forms of public health intervention are patronizing and do not respect the autonomy of the individual. This is especially likely to be levelled in relation to activities such as social marketing, in which techniques traditionally associated with commercial advertising are used to promote healthy messages.

Finally, public health may on rare occasions involve depriving someone of their liberty. In the past this was much more frequent, typically in relation to psychiatric illness or contagious disease. Indeed, in some countries the threshold for detention in a health facility remains low and, in others, such as the USA, the emphasis on a criminal justice rather than a health response to illicit drugs, means that very large numbers of people (predominantly young male African-Americans) serve long periods in jail. This raises even more profound issues. A variant on detention is compulsory treatment in a non-custodial setting, as is commonly used for treatment of TB (DOT: directly observed treatment) and for people with severe, enduring mental ill health.

We cannot assume that everyone sees the world in the same way – indeed, some of you may have very different views. And even if we agree on an approach in broad terms we may still have many questions of detail.

Who provides the voice of society? Is it the government? What if they have been bought by powerful vested interests, such as the tobacco or oil industry? Is it our local community leaders, who may understand our concerns better than politicians who only visit us when they need our votes, showing little interest at other times?

What freedoms are we willing to give up for the collective benefit? The right to bear arms? The right to travel at speed on open roads, free from the threat of speed cameras? The right to smoke in public places? The right to feed ourselves and our children a daily diet of junk food? What do you think?

You will now read extracts from two papers that address some of these questions. The first is by Beaglehole and Bonita (1998) and the second by Rothman and colleagues (1998). These papers set out a quite different vision of the role of epidemiologists in public health and where public health should be going.

Read the extracts and summarize briefly the arguments of both of them. Then, decide which vision you identify with most closely and say why.

Extract from Beaglehole and Bonita (1998)

The discipline of public health

Epidemiology is flourishing, especially clinical epidemiology, but there is a shortage of epidemiologists and the workforce is not representative of the population worldwide served. Epidemiologists have collaborated with laboratory scientists to explore the mechanisms of disease and gene-environment interactions, although the danger is that such collaboration could reduce epidemiology to a mere tool of molecular biology which requires DNA samples from human populations. More importantly, epidemiology focuses on the fundamental social, economic, and cultural determinants of health status. Ecological variations are under investigation and multidisciplinary studies of the effect of the socioeconomic environment on the health of populations may yet inform social policy.

The other disciplines of public health are less well developed. For example, it is difficult to implement the powerful rhetoric of the Ottawa Charter on health promotion, and much health-promotion practice uses an outdated model of health education. Health promotion is further hampered by the privatisation of health care services and the division of 'purchaser' and 'provider' functions. This organisational model diverts attention from the powerful intersectoral determinants of health and discourages cooperation between health sectors. Only a few useful insights are available from attempts to develop intersectoral public health policy, such as work on food and nutrition.

The practice of public health

The key themes in public health practice are recurrent and must be readdressed by each new generation of public health professionals in a dialogue with the populations they serve. Most importantly, the scope and purpose of public health is unresolved. What are the current limits of public health? Should public health professionals be concerned with the fundamentals of health such as employment, housing, transport, food and nutrition, and global trade imperatives, or should attention be restricted to individual risk factors for diseases? A broad focus inevitably leads to involvement in the political process, an arena which is not emphasised in current training; the intersection between public health and democracy demands exploration.

No country has implemented the full range of public health functions. Public health in the USA was described in 1988 as being in 'disarray' in a report by the Institute of Medicine (IOM). The report stimulated programmes to link academic and practising public health communities and to upgrade public health leadership. There has also been progress in the organisation of state health agencies and the public health infrastructure, but there is still little focus on policy development at the state level. Lack of resources at the local level is the main reason for failure to implement the IOM recommendations, and public health agencies remain crippled by the need to provide last-resort medical care. In the UK, the emphasis has been on strengthening public health medicine which is increasingly concerned with the purchase of health services. The rest of the public health workforce is professionally and institutionally fragmented and there is no national focus for public health outside of communicable disease. Academic public health is dominated by public health physicians and is not integrated with operational public health services; there is also a lack of co-ordinated infrastructure for public health functions. Although the Labour government promises to target **health inequalities**, it will be hard to produce measurable results while continuing to stress the merits of a meagre public purse.

Public health: the way forward

The central challenge for public health practitioners is to articulate and act upon a broad definition of public health which incorporates a multidisciplinary and inter-sectoral approach to the underlying causes of premature death and disability. Since the value system of public health professionals tends to be egalitarian and supports collective action, it is important to affirm and make explicit these values and to seek public support for them.

A broad focus easily leads to accusations of 'woolly breadth', but this breadth is exactly what public health should be about. The challenge for public health practitioners is to justify and promote global concerns and at the same time proceed with evidence-based, public health programmes that deal with disease-specific factors and more general issues such as health inequalities. By contrast, the competing pathway, and one which increasingly characterises modern public health, is narrowly focused on health services research, evidence-based health care, and the search for new risk factors at the individual level. This activity will improve the effectiveness and efficiency of medical services, but clinical medicine is only a small part of the total public health endeavour.

An initial challenge is to improve worldwide health statistics. Sample sentinel populations are adequate to monitor trends in mortality and morbidity rates and risk factors. WHO should develop basic monitoring systems with electronic communication methods. A fundamental organisational challenge is the relationship between public health and medical-care policy. Public health is the poor cousin to medical care, both in terms of budget and status. Typically, the public health sector receives less than 5 per cent of the total health care budget and, from a policy perspective, is overshadowed by the demands of acute medical-care services and the power of the pharmaceutical industry.

Ideally, the public health sector rather than the medical care sector, should be responsible for population health status and for informing and monitoring all government policy initiatives that affect population-health status. Perhaps a more feasible option is for equality between the interests of public health and medical care through a Minister of Public Health supported by an independent Ministry.

WHO is the obvious focal point for worldwide public health leadership, and for the first decades of its existence it has fulfilled this role. The question now is whether WHO can be reformed, after more than a decade of decline, to articulate a broad vision with a focused set of priorities and withstand the increasing encroachment of vested commercial interests in the guise of collaboration. As WHO's leadership has declined, other agencies, particularly the World Bank, have taken up this role often with even less explicit public health imperatives.

At the local level there is much to be gained by a closer relationship between the practitioners of public health and the society they serve. The ideology of individual responsibility and reliance on market forces must be challenged to develop strong and enduring partnerships between public health practitioners and communities, and to rekindle a commitment to sharing the benefits of national wealth. A global deregulated economy is unlikely to provide the appropriate basis for a fair and ecologically sustainable world.

There is justification for optimism. The opportunity exists for public health considerations to become central to the role of the World Trade Organisation. The revision of the health-for-all strategy includes a firm commitment to reduce poverty and its effects on health. The World Bank has recognised the need for a strong and effective state in the process of social and economic development. The next important step is to reduce Third World debt and reverse the negative effects of structural readjustment programmes. There is potential for the development of a constructive partnership between the World Bank and WHO.

Although the past 20 years have seen a stagnation in income growth in many regions, the eradication of absolute poverty, the most important priority for human development, is a feasible goal. Health professionals have a particular responsibility to exert pressure on national governments and the World Bank to support policies to reduce poverty and oppose those that increase it. Public health education for much of the world is a welcome development and public health-leadership pro-grammes are under development. The positive impact of environmental activists on the health of communities and positive connections between academic and practical public health are promising. These developments will encourage the empowerment of local communities, a necessary step in the rejuvenation of public health. If public health becomes more broadly focused, the health outlook will be better for all.

Extract from Rothman and colleagues (1998)

Accusation 1: epidemiology is too individualistic
As with other biomedical sciences, epidemiology yields practical knowledge. Many applications can be carried out directly by individuals. For example, information about the risks of having unprotected sex can persuade people to change their sexual behaviour, and information about the risks of smoking can motivate smokers to give up their habit. These actions are, to some extent at least, personal choices, which public health programmes can influence through educational materials, as they have done through campaigns on smoking and health.

Other epidemiological knowledge, however, cannot be easily applied without actions at societal level. Thus, smallpox could not have been eradicated without a clever, global strategy to contain it, and malnutrition rooted in poverty cannot be prevented without societal interventions that ease the burden of poverty or that address malnutrition directly.

The distinction between individual and societal applications of epidemiological knowledge are at the core of the new wave of criticism. The central complaint is that epidemiologists have focused on individual risk factors to the exclusion of broader societal causes of disease.

Pearce, one of the harshest critics of epidemiologists, portrays this slant as a personal and political choice (Pearce 1996). In his view, it is not so much the lure of science as an end in itself that has swivelled epidemiologists to a biomedical orientation; rather it is a tide of political conservatism and a personal indifference to the health problems of others that account for the new direction in epidemiology. According to Pearce, epidemiologists are so self-indulgent that they prefer to study 'decontextualised individual risk factors' instead of 'upstream' causes of health problems, such as poverty ...

Accusation 2: epidemiologists need more moral and political fibre

Critics contend that epidemiologists have a greater responsibility than merely to study the causal role in human health of factors such as poverty or tobacco consumption. In their view, epidemiologists must also strive to eradicate the upstream causes of health problems. For example, if epidemiological research indicates that poverty causes malnutrition, which in turn causes infant death, the epidemiologist's responsibility is to work towards the elimination of poverty. This activity requires the lumbering apparatus of social and political forces to be set in motion – something that most epidemiologists have been loath to attempt. Critics claim that today's epidemiologists lack the moral resolve and political fire to complete their professional mission.

In short, some critics believe that epidemiologists of today lack a firm commitment to public health. Instead, claim the critics, they fritter away their professional time by studying scientific minutiae at the expense of urgent public health problems.

Knowledge before action, or 'Ready, Fire, Aim'?

There is no denying that epidemiologists have progressively concentrated on the details of causal mechanisms. The only surprise to us is that anyone would regard this preoccupation with causal mechanisms as a problem. In past decades, epidemiologists could be criticised for studying mostly superficial relations between exposure and disease occurrence. Now the field is maturing, along with other biological sciences, and such superficiality is gradually being replaced with clearer insights into causal pathways. Whereas epidemiologists once studied factors such as dietary-fat consumption and total serum cholesterol, they have now progressed to classifying dietary fat by chemical structure – by comparison of low to high lipoprotein ratios – and are moving on to assessing the protective effect of antioxidants on fat-induced endothelial impairment.

Is the preoccupation with causal mechanisms as detrimental as critics allege? – Not if reasonable knowledge of causation is deemed a sensible antecedent to intervention. If the moral purpose of epidemiology is to alleviate the human burden of disease, the primary task of epidemiologists should be to acquire insight into the causal chain, starting from root causes and continuing up through the beginnings of the disease itself. True, we do not necessarily need to know every detail about the pathway between intervention point and outcome; we can infer the effects of interventions even with gaps in understanding. Knowledge is never perfect, and action is often indicated in the face of substantial uncertainty. Public health professionals, however, do not have a license to tinker promiscuously with society. Public health programmes may be conceived and implemented with great hope and yet turn out to be useless, or even damaging. One and a half centuries after Snow's work on cholera, the public health threat from the disease lingers, as research continues into how pathogenicity of the *Vibrio* organism depends on the El Niño Southern Oscillation, and how cholera may spread between continents through ocean currents. For cholera, as for other diseases, the more knowledge we acquire of causal pathways at all points – from the most 'fundamental' or 'ultimate' social, political, and economic determinants to the molecular and biochemical determinants most proximal to disease occurrence – the better the foundation we lay for any effective public health action.

To observe, for example, that in regions where poverty is rife, a given disease occurs at a greater rate than in areas not affected by poverty, is surely not enough. Epidemiologists have been preoccupied with methodology mainly because they understand that such comparisons are often affected by innumerable biases that can lead to false inferences. Their preoccupation with methods is the inevitable evolutionary consequence of their drive to understand the causes of disease in the natural human environment – rather than in the laboratory cage or the petri dish. The same kind of concern that makes epidemiologists wary of ecological comparisons impels them to carry out randomised trials when experiments are ethical and feasible.

When is intervention most effective?

Generally, the further upstream we move from the occurence of disease towards root causes, the less secure our inferences about the causal path to disease become. Even if our inference is correct, moreover, intervention with respect to upstream causes may be less efficient and therefore less effective than intervention closer to disease occurrence. Consider the causal path: poverty to malnutrition to infection to death. Control of infection at the level of the human individual may be the most efficient way to prevent death in this causal chain. True, if control of infection does not address the malnutrition underlying the infection, the infection is likely to recur; one might therefore reasonably look upstream to address the malnutrition problem. Nevertheless, if we attempt to combat malnutrition without also dealing with the concomitant infections, many people will die needlessly. Furthermore, there may be little that an epidemiologist can do in the short term to overcome malnutrition as a population problem. To awaken the public or political authorities to the problem of malnutrition and to redirect societal resources may eventually do the trick, but public health accomplishments mediated through social changes are won slowly. In the meantime, through their study of risk factors at the individual level and by the use of randomised trials, epidemiologists have discovered that vitamin-A supplements can prevent serious morbidity and many deaths in malnourished children. This knowledge will save lives, despite the fact that it does not alleviate gross malnutrition, does not require manipulation of any upstream cause, and is obtained from the type of epidemiological work that critics of epidemiology disparage.

What is the public health solution to the poverty problem?

The ultimate step in the preceding intervention scenario is to eliminate the poverty that causes the malnutrition. The critics urge that we take this step. It requires deep societal involvement in a laudable public health end – one that any humane person would embrace. Yet, it is only fair to ask whether epidemiologists have the means to eradicate poverty. Is poverty eradication a public health programme? How exactly should it be accomplished? Economists would seem the most likely candidates to supply the answer, which might go something like – 'Let markets be free to expand without guiding them too firmly'. But other economists might give a different answer. Do the critics of epidemiology suggest that epidemiologists should lobby against **international** trade barriers, or in favour of them, in the pursuit of their public health objectives? Perhaps the critics believe that epidemiologists should second-guess economists and attempt to eradicate poverty using their own epidemiological model.

All poverty is unacceptable

We agree wholeheartedly that the study of the social causes of disease is an important epidemiological goal, and that societal causes can explain much of the variation in disease occurrence. We abhor tobacco promotion and production. We would like to see the eradication of poverty, and agree that epidemiologists should be well educated with regard to their public health role.

Nevertheless, the importance of societal causes of disease does not mean that biological pathways to disease should be ignored, or that epidemiologists who choose to study causal mechanisms have been neglecting their mission. Furthermore, as with any public health professionals who share humanist values, epidemiologists do not need to establish the health effects of poverty to know that society should aim to eliminate it. Today's critics of epidemiology use health as an argument for social ends – such as the eradication of poverty – the desirability of which is obvious and quite independent of their public health consequences.

Perhaps the most valuable message in this new criticism of epidemiology is simply that those who wish to ease the burden of disease should not forget that the people of the world often bear larger burdens than those we sometimes choose to study. Nevertheless, epidemiologists cannot be expected to solve every problem, especially not those beyond our expertise.

Epidemiologists are not social engineers; they are public health scientists who have a right to specialise as they see fit. They should be free to choose the subject of their inquiries, whether it be social causes or molecular causes of disease.

It is remarkable that epidemiologists are now chastised for their scientific accomplishments, which include such victories as the elaboration of the effects of tobacco smoking on many diseases, and the effect of folic acid on neural-tube defects. Countless other fragments of useful epidemiological knowledge, such as the benefits of breast milk over infant formula, have enabled many people to improve their health even if they could not avoid poverty and repression. If an astrophysicist can study the origin of the universe without apology, should an epidemiologist have to apologise for work that is so practical?

Feedback

Summary of the arguments of both papers:

Beaglehole and Bonita argue that public health should take a multidisciplinary and intersectoral approach to dealing with health problems worldwide and that this would involve public health scientists becoming increasingly concerned with the political process. They suggest that public health measures should be global in perspective, and that epidemiology should focus on the fundamental social, economic and cultural forces affecting individual behaviour and health status. They argue that public health should proceed with evidence-based, public health programmes that deal with disease-specific factors and more general issues such as health inequalities, rather than adopting a narrow focus on activities such as health services research and evidence-based health care, or – a main criticism of epidemiology – on the search for new risk factors at the individual level. They suggest that the public health sector rather than the medical care sector should be responsible for population health, and that there should be a closer relationship between public health practitioners and the society they serve.

Although Rothman and colleagues agree that the study of the social causes of disease is an important epidemiological goal and that social inequalities should be eliminated within and between countries, they believe that the work of epidemiology in acquiring insight into the specific causes of diseases is essential to lay a good foundation for effective public health actions. They argue that epidemiologists are not social engineers or economists, but public health scientists who have the right to specialize. They also suggest that because public health accomplishments mediated through social changes are won slowly, epidemiologists help in the meantime to gain significant knowledge that can save lives (for example, vitamin A supplementation to save the lives of malnourished children) although not resolving global upstream causes such as malnutrition or poverty.

Factors that might have influenced your choice:

There is, of course, no good or wrong answer in this exercise and various factors might have influenced your choice in deciding which vision you identify most closely with. One of them is probably the type of work that you are doing. For example, if you are involved in more methodological epidemiological work investigating disease causation, you probably identify more closely to the views of Rothman and colleagues. Conversely, if you are closely involved in public health policy and political processes, your views might then be closer to those of Beaglehole and Bonita. Undoubtedly, both visions offer advantages and are important to the future of improved public health and better health worldwide.

Activity 1.3

This activity relates to gun control as a public health issue.

In March 1996 a man walked into a school in Dunblane, Scotland, armed with an assortment of high power handguns. He made his way to the gym hall and opened fire on a class full of 4- and 5-year-old children, killing 16 children and their teacher. Then he turned one of his own weapons on himself. One year later the British government imposed a comprehensive ban on the private ownership of handguns.

Also in 1996, in Port Arthur, Tasmania, a man armed with semi-automatic weapons walked into a café and killed 35 people. Soon afterwards, the Australian government introduced a ban on semi-automatic rifles and pump action shotguns, a national gun registration scheme, and a buy-back programme to reduce the number of weapons in circulation.

In April 1999 two pupils in Columbine, Colorado, walked into their school armed with a sawn-off shotgun, a semi-automatic rifle, a handgun and a selection of grenades. Within a few minutes they had killed 13 of their fellow students and teachers before shooting themselves. Although there had been four other multiple shootings in American schools in the preceding two years, the legislative response was essentially limited to additional funding for ballistics testing and media campaigns. Controls on gun ownership were seen as a non-starter.

In 1998, handguns were used to murder 51 people in New Zealand, 54 people in Australia, 19 in Japan, 54 in Great Britain, 151 in Canada, 373 in Germany and 11,215 in the United States.

Use the following resources to acquaint yourself with the background to the three events and the arguments for and against gun control in the USA.

- You can read about the Columbine shooting and the responses to it on various web-sites including: http://news.bbc.co.uk/1/hi/world/americas/324995.stm
- Details of the Dunblane shooting and responses to it can also be found on several websites including: http://www.dvc.org.uk/~johnny/dunblane/ (Dunblane massacre resource page 2005).
- You can read about the Port Arthur shooting in an Internet article from Bellamy (2005) and on different websites.
- For further reading on the issues surrounding gun control in the US see documents from the National Rifle Association (2005), a powerful and well financed organization lobbying against gun control in any form, and from The Brady Campaign to Prevent Gun Violence (2005), an organization dedicated to gun control and named after Jim Brady, press secretary to President Ronald Reagan, who was shot and seriously wounded during an assassination attempt on President Reagan.
- For another perspective on advocacy in relation to gun control, you may want to view the film *Bowling for Columbine*, directed by Michael Moore (2002).

Now answer the following questions:

1 In your opinion, should gun control be a public health issue? Why do you take this view?
2 The US Centers for Disease Control (CDC) has been criticized by some American politicians for becoming involved in this issue, especially when there are much more important matters to deal with. What criteria might an organization such as CDC adopt when deciding what to focus its efforts on?

Feedback

1 This is a matter for you as an individual. The purpose of this exercise is to allow you to reflect on why you hold the view you do, and to consider why others may take a different view.
2 Criteria that might be considered include:
   - the current burden of disease attributable to the issue in question: how much death and disability does easy availability of guns cause?;
   - the scope for preventing this burden: will gun control be effective in reducing deaths and disability?;

- the future consequences of failing to act: this is especially relevant with infectious disease where the current burden may be small but the scope for spread great, for example, the early stages of the AIDS epidemic;
- the cost of acting: in many areas of life states decide that the cost of intervening to save a life is too high, although the implied value of a life varies widely – for example being prepared to spend enormous sums to reduce a death in a plane or train crash but much less to prevent a death on the road;
- the feasibility of acting: this is something to consider. What are the obstacles to action and what are the opportunities? Who are the stakeholders, what are their positions, and how might they be influenced?;
- where you sit in the spectrum between extreme **libertarianism** (the role of the state should be as small as possible) and collective action.

Activity 1.4

This activity relates to alcohol consumption as a public health issue.

The harm to physical and mental health caused by alcohol is a major global public health problem. The problem of alcohol misuse continues to grow throughout the EU and in other developed countries. The EU is the heaviest drinking region of the world, with on average 11 litres of pure alcohol being consumed per adult each year. Alcohol is associated with scores of medical conditions from those affecting the unborn child to chronic diseases of adulthood, as well as many social harms including domestic and stranger violence and road traffic accidents: it causes an estimated 115,000 deaths in people up to the age of 70 each year across the EU, even after allowing for prevention of some deaths attributable to moderate consumption (Anderson and Baumberg 2006). More men than women drink and most people consume alcohol within low levels of risk. The disease burden of alcohol is massive and should include consideration of the impact on health and wellbeing of relatives of dependent drinkers and the victims of alcohol related crime and injury, as well as the harmful effects on drinkers themselves. Alcohol causes proportionately more harm in younger people: in Western European countries an estimated 25 per cent of male mortality and over 10 per cent of female mortality in those aged 15–29 years is alcohol related.

There is evidence that demonstrates an association between harmful drinking (i.e. drinking associated with harmful outcomes) of both total quantity consumed and patterns of consumption. The riskiest pattern for short-term harmful outcomes is so-called 'binge' drinking. Whereas the volume of consumption is associated primarily with long-term consequences, risky patterns of drinking are mainly associated with acute consequences. In summary:

- the higher the total volume of alcohol consumption, the greater the risk of harm; and
- the more alcohol consumed on one occasion, the more serious the injury or crime.

So, national alcohol policies must address both total consumption and risky drinking. Policies can be directed at the population or at individuals. With the exception of brief intervention with risky drinkers in primary care, the most effective interventions are usually population based and influence supply, availability and access to alcohol, with particular need to consider young people.

What policies are most likely to be effective in the EU (or in your country or region) in reducing the health and social burden of alcohol?

Feedback

Alcohol policy measures should combine *both* policies directed at the whole drinking population and measures directed at more risky drinkers with more detrimental drinking patterns (Allamani et al. 2001; Babor 2002; Edwards, 2001). This is because alcohol-related harms stem mainly from alcohol consumption in the general population, rather than from alcohol consumption by a specific group of risky drinkers. Reducing total alcohol consumption in a population will result in a reduction in alcohol-related public health problems, while implementing interventions focused on high-risk drinking, like interventions to reduce drink-driving, will result in a reduction of specific types of harm, such as accidents. Interventions directed at drinkers in general will however also affect heavy and risky drinkers.

Policy interventions can be categorized as follows (EUPHIX):

- policies that reduce drinking and driving;
- policies that support education, communication, training and public awareness;
- policies that regulate the alcohol market (regulating physical availability; taxation and pricing; regulating alcohol promotion);
- policies that support the reduction of harm in drinking and surrounding environments;
- policies that support interventions for individuals (treatment and early intervention).

Regulating the market through taxation is an effective policy. In regions with high-risk alcohol use, such as most European countries, taxation has the greatest and most cost-effective impact on reducing the average burden of high-risk alcohol use. This has led to calls for minimum alcohol pricing as a means to reducing overall consumption. In many countries, including the UK, large retailers can and frequently do choose to sell alcohol at minimal profit, so undermining the effect of high taxation. This has led some experts, including England's former Chief Medical Officer and the National Institute for Health & Clinical Excellence (NICE 2010), to call for a minimum price per unit of alcohol, so that the consumer cannot purchase legally at a lower price. Voluntary agreements with the retail trade or manufacturers have so far been shown to be ineffective, but no Western government has yet imposed a minimum pricing policy, although at the time of writing the Scottish government is proposing to do so. Indeed, in the UK, the Treasury has not yet closed the loophole whereby supermarkets reclaim Value Added Tax (VAT) (a sales tax) when discounted alcohol is a 'promotion' (Chick et al. 2010). While the average price of alcohol was about £1.10 (€0.96; $0.69) per unit in 2010, researchers found that a sample of people with alcohol related illness were paying an average of £0.43 (€0.38; $0.27) per unit, mainly by buying in shops and not in drinking settings (bars, pubs, etc.). In addition to a minimum price, per se, the possibility of variation in VAT in different alcohol sales settings and changes in duty on alcohol are other possible policy options (Sheron 2010).

You may also be interested in the first EU Strategy on alcohol, which was adopted by the European Commission in October 2006 (EC 2006). It identifies five priorities, which are to:

- protect young people, children and the unborn child;
- reduce injuries and deaths from alcohol-related road accidents;
- prevent alcohol-related harm among adults and reduce the negative impact on the workplace;

- inform, educate and raise awareness on the impact of harmful and hazardous alcohol consumption, and on appropriate consumption patterns; and
- develop, support and maintain a common evidence base.

Activity 1.5

Imagine that you are a political adviser to the health minister of a country of your choice in which guns are widely available *or* there are no controls on access to alcoholic beverages. Your minister thinks that a stance on either issue should be taken, on grounds of public health, but his/her colleagues believe they have nothing to do with him/her. Describe the arguments that you would use in a briefing, putting the case for these being legitimate health concerns.

Feedback

The main arguments you might make centre around the *burden of disease* (access to guns and alcohol are both important causes of avoidable death and disability), the *scope for prevention*, and that these are *legitimate areas for the state* to get involved.

Summary

This chapter discussed the historical development of public health. It described how ideas on the role of public health have changed since the eighteenth century, and described some key international documents on the role of public health. It also discussed the arguments for and against societal interventions to promote health.

References

Allamani A, Hope A, Byrne S and Room B (2001) Lessons from the ECAS study: comments and policy implications, in T Norström (ed.) *Alcohol in Postwar Europe: Consumption, Drinking Patterns, Consequences and Policy Responses in 15 European Countries*. Luxemburg: European Commission.

Anderson P and Baumberg B (2006) *Alcohol in Europe: A Public Health Perspective*. London: Institute of Alcohol Studies.

Babor T (2002) Linking science to policy: the role of international collaborative research. *Alc Res Health* **26**(1).

Bachinger E, McKee M and Gilmore A (2008) Tobacco policies in Nazi Germany: not as simple as it seems. *Public Health* **122**: 497–505.

Beaglehole R and Bonita R (1998) Public health at the crossroads: which way forward? *The Lancet* **351**: 590–2.

Bellamy P (2005) The Port Arthur massacre: a killer among us. New York: Crime Library (available at http://www.crimelibrary.com/notorious_murders/mass/bryant/index_1.html).

Brady Campaign to Prevent Gun Violence (2005) *Fact sheets*. Washington, DC: The Brady Campaign to Prevent Gun Violence.

Charlton B (2001) Personal freedom or public health? in M Marinker (ed.) *Medicine and Humanity*. London: King's Fund, pp. 55–69.

Chick J, Jonathan D, Gill JS and Black H (2010) Ways to control alcohol price. *BMJ* **341**: c7007.

Davey Smith G, Strobele SA and Egger M (1994) Smoking and health promotion in Nazi Germany. *J Epidemiol Community Health* **48**: 220–3.

Dunblane massacre resource page (2005) (available at http://www.dvc.org.uk/~johnny/dunblane/).

EC (2006) *An EU Strategy to Support Member States in Reducing Alcohol Related Harm*. COM (2006) 625. Brussels: European Commission.

Edwards G (2001) Alcohol policy: securing a positive impact on health, in N Rehn, R Room and G Edwards (eds) *Alcohol in the European Region: Consumption, Harm and Policies*. Copenhagen: WHO Regional Office for Europe.

EUPHIX (2011) *European Public Health Information System. Alcohol Use* (available at http://www.euphix.org/object_class/euph_health_behaviours_alcohol_use.html).

Moore M (director) (2002) *Bowling for Columbine*. Film produced by Moore M, Glynn K, Czarnecki J, Bishop C (II), Donovan M, Bishop C.

National Rifle Association (2005) *Fables, Myths and Other Tall Tales about Gun Laws, Crime and Constitutional Rights*. Fairfax, Virginia: National Rifle Association Institute for Legislative Action (available at http://www.nraila.org/media/misc/fables.htm, last visited 2 February 2005).

NHS Public Mental Health and Well-being website (available at http://www.dh.gov.uk/en/Healthcare/Mentalhealth/Publicmentalhealthandwellbeing/index.htm).

NICE (National Institute for Health & Clinical Excellence) (2010) Guidance on prevention of alcohol use disorders, June (available at http://guidance.nice.org.uk/PH24).

Pearce N (1996) Traditional epidemiology, modern epidemiology, and public health. *Am J Public Health* **86**: 678–83.

Raine G, Robinson M and South J (2010) Mental health and employment: evidence summary. Leeds: Centre for Health Promotion Research (available at http://www.apho.org.uk/resource/view.aspx?RID=96683).

Rothman KJ, Adami HO and Trichopoulos D (1998) Should the mission of epidemiology include the eradication of poverty? *The Lancet* **352**, 810–13.

Sheron N (2010) Vary VAT on alcohol: *BMJ* 2010; 341:c6573 doi: 10.1136/bmj.c6573 (17 November 2010).

Skrabanek P and McCormick J (1989) *Follies and Fallacies in Medicine*. Glasgow: Tarragon Press.

World Health Organization (1978) Declaration of Alma Ata (available at http://www.who.int/hpr/NPH/docs/declaration_almaata.pdf).

World Health Organization (2001) The World Health Report 2001 – Mental Health: New Understanding, New Hope (available at http://www.who.int/whr/2001/en/whr01_en.pdf).

World Health Organization (2003) WHO definition of health from the Preamble to the Constitution of the World Health Organization as adopted by the International Health Conference, New York, 19–22 June, 1946; signed on 22 July 1946 by the representatives of 61 States (Official Records of the World Health Organization, no. 2, p. 100) and entered into force on 7 April 1948. Geneva: World Health Organization.

World Health Organization Regional Office for Europe (1985) *Targets for Health for All*. Copenhagen: WHO.

World Health Organization Regional Office for Europe (1999) *Health 21 Health for All in the 21st Century*. Copenhagen: WHO.

📖 Further reading

McKee M, Colagiuri R (2007) What are governments for? *Med J Australia* **187**: 654–5. This paper asks what governments are for if not to protect the health of their populations.

Marinker M (ed.) (2002) *Health Targets in Europe: Polity, Progress and Promise*. London: BMJ Publications. In this book, Marshall Marinker has brought together a group of writers from across Europe to review the experience of national and regional health strategies. Chapter 13, entitled 'Values, beliefs and implications', provides an overview of the values underpinning **health systems** in Europe, contrasting them with those in the USA.

National Mental Health Development Unit: http://www.nmhdu.org.uk/nmhdu/ (Unit operational 2009–11; website maintained afterwards)

Nuffield Council on Bioethics – Public Health pages: http://www.nuffieldbioethics.org/public-health

Reynolds L, McKee M (2010) Organised crime and the efforts to combat it: a concern for public health. *Globalization & Health* **6**: 21. This paper argues that an area not normally seen as being the concern of the public health community actually should be, because of its many consequences for population health.

Data on populations and mortality 2

Martin McKee, Joceline Pomerleau,
Marina Karanikolos and Fiona Sim

Overview

This chapter discusses the building blocks of public health, that is, the data on populations and mortality. You will learn about where you can find such data and how you can combine them to describe a population's health and compare it with the health of other populations. You will also become familiar with different international sources of information on health.

Learning objectives

By the end of this chapter you should be able to:

- describe the main sources of data on populations and mortality, and discuss their strengths and weaknesses
- know where to obtain data on populations and mortality
- interpret commonly used indicators of population health, such as age-standardized death rates, life expectancy and survival

Key terms

Age-standardization A way of controlling for age so that we can compare rates of deaths or disease in populations with different age structures.

Life expectancy The average number of years a person can expect to live in a given population. It can be expressed as life expectancy at birth or at a particular age. It is based on current patterns of mortality so, technically, it is not a measure of how long a child born today can expect to live as we cannot yet know the death rates that will apply at different ages in the future. It is, however, the most widely used summary measure of mortality in a population.

Survival rate The proportion of population who survives a disease for a specified period of time (typically 5 years).

Understanding the health of a population

In public health, we want to understand what is happening to a population's health over time. There are several potential sources of information that can be used to do this. In this chapter we will be exploring some of the basic building blocks of public health – the data on populations and mortality and what you can do with them. In essence, to understand what is happening to a population over time we need to know about three things: births, deaths and migration. To begin with we will be focusing on deaths.

Mortality data are a fundamental source of information on the health of a population. Because of their generally widespread availability and timeliness, they are widely used to describe and monitor major public health issues, including the progression (and decline) of chronic diseases, the emergence of recent threats to health such as HIV/AIDS, or the evaluation of public health interventions. In order to be able to interpret mortality data you need two types of information. First, and most obviously, you need to know how many deaths have occurred, among whom, and from what. Second, and often forgotten, you need to know the composition of the population.

How many people?

We will look first at the population. The most common method used to find out how many people there are in a population is the census. Censuses have been conducted throughout recorded history, often for military or tax purposes. However, systematic modern censuses have their origins in Western Europe in the nineteenth century. Typically undertaken every ten years, they now usually include information on age, sex, marital status, employment and a varying selection of other factors (see Box 2.1).

Box 2.1 Census in England and Wales

The last census in England and Wales was held in 2011. The previous one was in 2001. The most recent detailed census data, from 2001, including demographic, social and health characteristics of the population, are available through the Office of National Statistics (www.statistics.gov.uk) or through the Neighbourhood Statistics website (www.neighbourhood.statistics.gov.uk).

Carrying out a census is an enormous undertaking. For this reason, there are still many countries throughout the world where there have been no censuses, or ones covering only urban populations, for several decades. The only country never to have conducted a census is Chad. In a few cases there may be even political sensitivity to holding a census, such as countries divided among different ethnic groups. The last census in Lebanon was in 1932. However, a few advanced industrialized countries, including the Netherlands and Germany, have abandoned censuses, because they now have population registers (for example, requiring everyone to register with local government when they move house). These countries obtain information about their population from the continually updated population and other registers rather than from censuses.

In an increasingly mobile world, the challenges of undertaking censuses are growing and censuses can rapidly become out of date. In some cases, certain population sub-groups are especially difficult to reach. For example, in the 2001 British census it was estimated that over 900,000 people, mostly men in their twenties or people over 85, were missed. In some parts of the country, such as inner London, the under-reporting is thought to be especially high. The British government has signalled its intention to abandon the census after the 2011 census, instead relying on other sources of data. Controversially, the Canadian government has reduced the amount of data it collects in its census.

Censuses are also susceptible to misreporting by respondents. In particular, the elderly tend to overstate their age, divorced men tend to report that they are single (i.e. never married), and all people tend to inflate their socioeconomic status. In addition, especially at older ages, and in some countries, especially those where people may not have records of their precise birth date, there is a tendency to give one's age to the nearest five years, causing the phenomenon known as 'heaping' (Figure 2.1). For these reasons, especially when undertaking analyses involving small populations, it is necessary to take care when interpreting results.

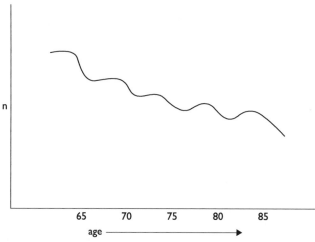

Figure 2.1 Heaping

Knowing population age structure is crucial in describing population mortality and health. Thus, two populations of the same size, but different age composition may have different patterns of mortality and morbidity. Population estimates allow us to know the size of specific population groups in the years between censuses, and are back-adjusted when the next census data becomes available. They are usually produced by a country's central statistical office. Population projections estimate the future changes in population numbers by age. Figure 2.2 illustrates population structure of Kazakhstan and England and Wales in 2007 using population pyramids.

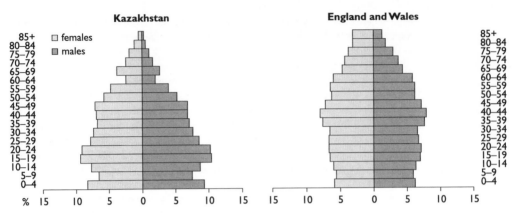

Figure 2.2 Population pyramids of Kazakhstan and England and Wales in 2007

Source: WHO population files, July 2010

What are people dying of?

Vital registration of death exists in about seventy countries worldwide. In a few others, such as India and China, there are sentinel surveillance systems covering some parts of the population. Mainly in Africa, but extending to some other parts of the world, the IN-DEPTH network (www.indepth-network.org) has established a number of sentinel sites to provide some, albeit limited, information. Death certification is often based on a standard certificate on which the age, sex and cause(s) of death of the deceased is recorded along with various other pieces of information (which may include some or all of: gender, age, marital status, occupation, educational achievement, income, address, and so on) and vary from country to country. In some countries, the section describing the cause of death has to be completed by a doctor, or, if the death happened as a result of an accident, suicide or homicide, by the police or a coroner. In England, the General Register Office records deaths and issues death certificates. Public Health Mortality Files, available through the Office of National Statistics for restricted use, provide timely individual-level information, including demographic characteristics, occupation and causes of death.

Cause of death is recorded using a classification developed by WHO, the International Classification of Diseases (ICD). This classification is updated intermittently to take account of changing patterns of disease, such as the emergence of AIDS. Most countries changed to the tenth (most recent) revision of the ICD in the late 1990s, having used the ninth revision from about 1979.

The ICD is divided into a series of chapters, such as II for 'Neoplasms' or IV for 'Endocrine, nutritional and metabolic diseases'. In the tenth revision each individual disease is given a unique alpha numeric code. For example, cancer of the stomach is C16, which can be subdivided to give more precise localization (C16.2 is cancer of the body of the stomach).

Clearly, many people die from a combination of disease processes and death certificates generally provide space for multiple causes (this is particularly important for older people who are more likely to have multiple conditions contributing to death). However, summary statistics usually report a single cause, which is selected according to standardized procedures that aim to identify the 'underlying cause of death'. In those countries where it is possible to obtain data with multiple causes of death, the scope for analysis is clearly increased, although the analytic methods also become more complex.

While death registration data are generally more complete and reliable than many routine sources of morbidity data, several issues need to be taken into account when interpreting cause of death data. Diagnosis is inevitably an inexact science and comparisons of causes of death certificated by clinicians with those determined by autopsy often find disagreements. One reason is that, especially in patients presenting with advanced disease, it may not be considered appropriate to undertake invasive investigation just to confirm a diagnosis when there is no prospect of cure. Another issue is the variable effort put into attributing cause of death by the certifying doctor. Systematic differences have also been noted in the choice of diagnosis given by a physician depending on the social class of the patient or the gender of patient and doctor. A further problem arises when deaths are compared between countries, or compared over time where they may span more than one revision of the ICD. There are, however, bridging tables to inform comparisons over time, although there may also be changes in coding rules between revisions in some countries.

In developing and middle-income countries, where vital registration systems are often poorly developed, it may be possible to get information from surveys. The most widely used example is the series of Demography and Health Surveys (DHS) that are conducted every few years in many countries. They are, however, limited in their coverage to childhood and maternal events. Although cross-sectional, they can be used to estimate mortality in the preceding years using the 'sisterhood' method, in which women are asked about any deaths among siblings and, in particular, whether they are pregnancy related. 'Verbal Autopsy' can be used to collect information on symptoms before death and assign an appropriate ICD code. This method is based on recall by relatives of symptoms prior to death and has been used mainly for infant and maternal deaths, as well as deaths due to injuries, as it requires identification of clearly distinguishable symptom complexes for each cause of interest. Other methods for estimating mortality in a population include modelling, for example by applying data from surveys of childhood mortality to standard life tables, or developing equations using available data, such as economic measures, to predict mortality using information from a large number of countries. The major centre undertaking this work is the Institute for Health Metrics and Evaluation, based in Seattle, whose website contains a wealth of useful resources (see the further reading section at p. 41).

From numbers to rates

Numbers of deaths have limited value in isolation. They become more useful when divided by the number of people in the population to give a rate. In calculating a rate it is essential that the numerator (the top line – the events or conditions of concern) and the denominator (the bottom line – the population at risk) match. In other words, anyone who could be included in the numerator should also appear in the denominator. But this creates more problems than you might at first think. For example, death rates in a town could be inflated by deaths of people who come from surrounding areas to die in hospital, unless their death is traced back to their area of residence, where they would normally have been recorded in the last census.

Now, let us assume that you have gathered information both on the numbers of deaths (overall and by cause) and on the population at risk. It is then possible to combine them to obtain rates. Table 2.1 gives several standard definitions used when reporting mortality data – you should become familiar with them.

Table 2.1 Standard definitions used to report mortality data

$$\text{Crude death rate} = \frac{\text{number of deaths}}{\text{mid year population}} \times 1000$$

$$\text{Cause specific mortality rate} = \frac{\text{deaths by cause x}}{\text{mid year population}} \times 1000$$

$$\text{Age specific mortality rate} = \frac{\text{deaths to persons aged x}}{\text{mid year population of persons aged x}} \times 1000$$

$$\text{Infant mortality rate} = \frac{\text{number of deaths to infants aged} < 1 \text{ year in year x}}{\text{number of live births in year x}} \times 1000$$

*

$$\text{Perinatal mortality rate} = \frac{\text{stillbirths} + \text{deaths under 1 week}}{\text{stillbirths and live births}} \times 1000$$

*The infant mortality rate can also be subdivided into neonatal mortality (deaths of live born infants in the first 4 weeks) and post neonatal mortality (from 4 to 52 weeks).

The scope for analysis of death rates is almost limitless. You can analyse them for all causes combined or for specific causes, for males and females separately, for people living in different parts of a country, and for different age groups. If you are able to break down the data on population and deaths in the same way, for example by social class or ethnicity, you can explore inequalities in health (although caution is needed – see Chapter 4). Imaginative use of data, for example tracking changes in age-specific death rates, can provide many valuable insights into the health of populations (for example, the dramatic changes in mortality rates that occurred in Russia since the mid-1980s affecting predominantly young and middle-aged men and driven by deaths from injuries and cardiovascular disease).

Activity 2.1

You can find in Table 2.2 the number of deaths from cancer of the lung and bronchus that occurred in England and Wales in 2009 in individuals aged 15 and over. Data are stratified by gender and 10-year age group. Table 2.3 gives the mid-year population estimates for England and Wales, as at 30 June 2009, by sex and age. Look at the data carefully and then answer the two questions that follow.

Table 2.2 Number of deaths from cancer of the lung and bronchus by sex and age in England and Wales, 2009

	Age (years)							
	15–24	25–34	35–44	45–54	55–64	65–74	75–84	85+
Males	1	10	128	673	2913	5398	5753	2167
Females	1	6	94	588	2152	3704	4382	2029

Source: ONS vital statistics

Table 2.3 Estimated resident population (in thousands) for England and Wales, 2009

	Age (years)							
	15–24	25–34	35–44	45–54	55–64	65–74	75–84	85+
Males	3729.4	3603.5	3981.9	3635.5	3178.2	2228	1317.6	399.2
Females	3548.5	3505.6	4029.2	3722	3304.3	2441.1	1758.9	837.9

Source: ONS population estimates

1 Using data from Table 2.2, comment on the sex and age distribution of deaths from this cause.
2 Using data from Tables 2.2 and 2.3, calculate age-specific mortality rates from lung and bronchus cancer. Comment on the sex differences in mortality rates from this cause.

Feedback

1 In each sex, we can see that the number of lung/bronchus cancer deaths increases with age up to ages 75 to 84, decreasing in over 85 year olds. There were more lung cancer deaths in men than in women in each of the age groups. However, nothing can be said about sex and age differences in mortality from this cancer without taking into account the number of persons at risk in each sex and age group.
2 Using the formula described in Table 2.1, we can calculate sex- and age-specific death rates for cancer of the lung and bronchus. Let's calculate, for example, death rate for males aged 45 to 54 years:

Number of deaths in males aged 45–54 in 2009 = 673
Estimated population of males aged 45–54
    at mid-2009   = 3,635,500
Death rate in males aged 45–54   = 673/3,635,500
     = 0.0001851 per person-year
Death rate per 100,000 males aged 45–54   = 18.51 per 100,000 person-year

You should have obtained the following rates for each sex- and age-group (Table 2.4).

Table 2.4 Sex- and age-specific death rates (per 100,000) from cancer of the lung and bronchus in England and Wales, 2009

	Age (years)							
	15–24	25–34	35–44	45–54	55–64	65–74	75–84	85+
Males	0.03	0.28	3.21	18.51	91.66	242.28	436.63	542.84
Females	0.03	0.17	2.33	15.80	65.13	151.73	249.13	242.15

The results confirm a general increase in risk with age. However, in males there was no decline in risk in over 85-year-olds. This means that the decline in the number of deaths in males at these ages was just a reflection of the decrease in the number of persons at risk.

Death rates were higher in males than in females in all age groups. The sex differences might be due to differences in survival or differences in incidence between males and females.

Age-standardized rates

Most rates, including the death or disease rates, are strongly age dependent. For example, the probability of death falls after the first year of life, and then increases relatively steeply with age, especially from middle age onwards. If we need to compare mortality rates in two different populations or changes in mortality in the same population over the years, using the crude mortality rate may be quite misleading. In order to account for underlying age structure differences in these populations, it is more appropriate to use a measure that takes into account the age distribution. This can be achieved by applying age-adjustment or **age-standardization**.

Figure 2.3 illustrates this problem. On the left you can see crude (unstandardized) mortality rates per 100,000 for males and females in the Netherlands. The graph suggests that rates are quite similar for the two sexes and while those for men seemed to have fallen slightly over time, those for women showed a slight increase in the middle of the period and remained relatively stable in recent years. On the graph on the right hand side you can see the same data, now adjusted for differences in the age structure. This shows that not only have death rates declined for both men and women but, importantly, for women rates have consistently been much lower than those for men. This is because the female population has a higher proportion of elderly people than the male population and consequently a higher number of deaths.

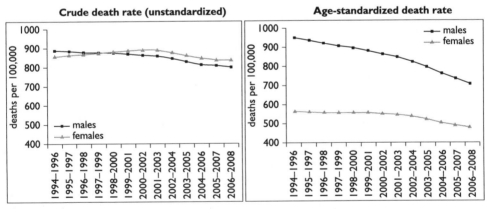

Figure 2.3 The effect of age-standardization – crude and directly standardized death rates in males and females in the Netherlands (3-year rolling average)

Source: WHO Health for All database, updated July 2010

There are several techniques to control for age, but the two most common ones are direct and indirect standardization. Both are described below.

Direct age-standardization

For the *direct* method of age-standardization, you need two sources of information. First, you need age-specific mortality rates from the population you are interested in. Second, you need a defined standard population with a known age structure (number of persons in each age category). The direct method relates the observed age-specific mortality rates to the standard population by means of weighing the age-specific mortality rates according to the age structure of the standard population. This gives you the so-called age-standardized mortality or death rate (SDR), which is also known as a directly standardized rate (DSR). It represents what the crude death rate would have been if the population under study had the same age distribution as the standard population. In Table 2.5 you can find an example of how the direct method of standardization can be used to compare mortality rates between two countries that have different age structures.

Table 2.5 Direct method of standardization – worked example*

Year	Age-specific rates (per 1,000)		Standard population	Expected no. of deaths in standard population	
	Czech Republic	Finland		Czech Republic	Finland
<1	2.88	2.69	1600	= 2.88 × 1600/1000 = 4.61	= 2.69 × 1600/1000 = 4.30
1–4	0.17	0.18	6400	= 0.17 × 6400/1000 = 1.10	= 0.18 × 6400/1000 = 1.15
5–9	0.09	0.12	7000	= ... = 0.63	= ... = 0.81
10–14	0.14	0.10	7000	= ... = 1.01	= ... = 0.69
15–19	0.40	0.41	7000	= ... = 2.78	= ... = 2.90
20–24	0.55	0.67	7000	= ... = 3.83	= ... = 4.72
25–29	0.62	0.68	7000	= ... = 4.31	= ... = 4.77
30–34	0.74	0.83	7000	= ... = 5.16	= ... = 5.79
35–39	1.02	1.22	7000	= ... = 7.11	= ... = 8.52
40–44	1.84	1.85	7000	= ... = 12.88	= ... = 12.97
45–49	3.03	2.68	7000	= ... = 21.18	= ... = 18.79
50–54	5.29	4.50	7000	= ... = 37.04	= ... = 31.52
55–59	8.67	6.86	6000	= ... = 52.05	= ... = 41.19
60–64	13.23	9.51	5000	= ... = 66.15	= ... = 47.53
65–69	19.06	13.31	4000	= ... = 76.24	= ... = 53.24
70–74	29.69	20.74	3000	= ... = 89.06	= ... = 62.21
75–79	49.09	35.78	2000	= ... = 98.18	= ... = 71.56
80–84	87.46	63.11	1000	= ... = 87.46	= ... = 63.11
85+	175.44	151.02	1000	= ... = 175.44	= ... = 151.02
			100,000	= Σ (all age groups) = 746.21	= Σ (all age groups) = 586.78

* Based on WHO global mortality database data for Czech Republic and Finland (2008); European Standard Population is used as the standard population.

Table 2.5 shows that if we apply age-specific rates from the two countries to the Standard Population, the age-adjusted mortality rates in the Czech Republic and Finland will be 746.2 and 586.7 per 100,000, respectively.

The calculations are as follows:

1 Apply the age-specific death rates from population(s) of interest to standard population
2 Add up all deaths expected in the standard population over the same period of time
3 Express this as a rate (typically per 100,000 or per 1,000)

In international comparisons the most frequently used (hypothetical) standard populations are the Segi 'world' population and the 'European' standard population (see Table 2.6). The European standard was developed based on the experience of Scandinavian populations, which contained a relatively high proportion of elderly and was judged particularly suitable for comparison within Western Europe. The Segi was based on the experience of 46 countries to represent an intermediate 'world' standard between the European standard and a standard with a high proportion of young people (considered appropriate for making comparisons with populations in Africa). A newer WHO standard population aims to reflect the world's population structure for the period 2000–2025. Mortality rates as given in the WHO Health for All database – which you will be using later in this chapter – are generally standardized to the European standard.

Table 2.6 Standard populations commonly used

Age group	Segi world population	European standard population	WHO world standard*
0–4	12 000	8 000	8 860
5–9	10 000	7 000	8 690
10–14	9 000	7 000	8 600
15–19	9 000	7 000	8 470
20–24	8 000	7 000	8 220
25–29	8 000	7 000	7 930
30–34	6 000	7 000	7 610
35–39	6 000	7 000	7 150
40–44	6 000	7 000	6 590
45–49	6 000	7 000	6 040
50–54	5 000	7 000	5 370
55–59	4 000	6 000	4 550
60–64	4 000	5 000	3 720
65–69	3 000	4 000	2 960
70–74	2 000	3 000	2 210
75–79	1 000	2 000	1 520
80–84	500	1 000	910
85+	500	1 000	630
Sum	100 000	100 000	100 000

* For purposes of comparisons, the WHO world standard age group 85+ is an aggregate of the age groups 85–89, 90–94, 95–99, 100+.

Source: Ahmad and collaborators (2001)

Indirect method of age-standardization

When there is no information on age-specific mortality rates of the population under study, we have to use the *indirect* approach, which applies the age-specific death rates of a standard population to the age structure of the population under study, thus just the reverse of the direct method. This method also allows you to calculate the so-called *standardized mortality ratio (SMR)*. The SMR is the ratio ($\times 100$) of observed to expected deaths in a study population. Standardized mortality ratio is also often used when looking at district data or specific population groups. Smaller geographical areas or certain populations can have small numbers of deaths in each of the age groups, so their age-specific death rates are more likely to be subject to variation due to chance. SMRs use the standard or national population's deaths rates based on a larger sample, and therefore are more stable. Say, for example, you wish to compare mortality in a region with that in the entire country. The expected deaths are estimated by applying the age-specific death rates in the whole country to the population divided into age bands in the local population, and then adding together the expected deaths in each age band to get the total for the population. You can find a worked example in Table 2.7.

Table 2.7 Indirect method of standardization (SMR) – worked example*

Year	England			South-East England		
	Population	Deaths	Rate per 1,000	Population	Deaths observed	Deaths expected
Under 1	667400	3184	4.77	103900	417	= 4.77 * 103900 = 495.68
1–4	2462000	515	0.21	393500	81	= 0.21 * 393500 = 82.31
5–14	5900900	594	0.10	984200	...	= ... = 99.07
15–24	6869600	2633	0.38	1059300	...	= ... = 406.01
25–34	6707400	4210	0.63	1005300	...	= ... = 630.99
35–44	7715000	9578	1.24	1263200	...	= ... = 1568.23
45–54	6793100	19099	2.81	1136600	...	= ... = 3195.58
55–64	6060900	42113	6.95	1018900	...	= ... = 7079.63
65–74	4275700	75969	17.77	705900	...	= ... = 12542.16
75–84	2878000	147315	51.19	489000	...	= ... = 25030.24
85 and over	1134600	170553	150.32	208800	...	= ... = 31386.80
						= Σ (all age groups)
Total (all ages)					75917	= 82516.7

* Based on the ONS mid-year estimates 2008 for England and South-East and ONS mortality statistics 2008

$$ SMR = \frac{observed\ deaths}{expected\ deaths} = \frac{75,917}{82,517} = 0.92 \times 100 = 92\% $$

Table 2.7 shows that allowing for the difference in age distribution in the two populations, the death rate in the South-East is lower than in the country as a whole.

Activity 2.2

Table 2.8 gives population sizes (in thousands) and numbers of deaths from all causes by age group in two countries in 2007.

Table 2.8 Population sizes and number of deaths in two countries

Age group	Country A		Country B	
	Population	No. of deaths	Population	No. of deaths
0–14	1,545,664	424	1,476,506	
15–44	3,619,591	2,161	4,511,353	
45–54	1,168,586	2,798	1,403,399	
55–64	1,219,336	7,597	1,435,761	
65–74	794,836	12,657	827,929	
75–84	561,724	27,858	548,771	
85+	238,369	38,325	118,970	
Total	9,148,106	91,820	10,322,689	104,636

Source: WHO mortality database, updated July 2010

1 Calculate and compare the all-cause crude death rates for Country A and Country B.
2 Calculate a ratio to compare the observed number of deaths in Country B with the number of deaths that would be expected if the age-specific death rates of Country A were applicable.
3 How do you interpret this ratio?

Feedback

1 Crude death rate = total number of deaths/total no. of persons × 1,000 (per 1,000 population)
   All-cause crude death rate for Country A = 91,820/9,148,106 = 10.04 per 1,000 population
   All-cause crude death rate for Country B = 104,636/10,322,689 = 10.14 per 1,000 population
   The crude rates are relatively similar. However, because we have no information on the deaths distribution by age in Country B (and thus whether there are differences in the age structure in the two countries which could lead to confounding), it will be important to calculate age-standardized death rates.
2 To be able to calculate this ratio, we need the following information:
   a) The total number of observed deaths in Country B (n = 104,363)
   b) The age-specific death rates in Country A (used here as the set of standard rates) – these need to be calculated for each age group as follows:
      Number of deaths in Country A (column I in Table 2.9) in each age group divided by the number of persons for the selected age group in Country A (column II in Table 2.9).
      The age-specific death rates are expressed as death rate per 1,000 person-years in Country A (standard) (column III in Table 2.9)
   c) The population distribution by age groups in Country B (column IV in the table below in Table 2.9)

As a result, the total number of expected deaths in Country B, using the age-specific death rates of Country A, is equal to the sum over all age categories (column V in Table 2.9).

Table 2.9 Calculation of the number of expected deaths in Country B using age-specific death rates in Country A as the standard rates

Age group	I No. of deaths in Country A	II Population in Country A	III Age-specific death rate (per 1,000 population) in Country A	IV Population in Country B	V No. of deaths expected in Country B
0–14	424	1,545,664	= 424/1545664*1000 = 0.27	1,476,506	= 0.27*1476506*1000 = 405.03
15–44	2,161	3,619,591	= ... = 0.60	4,511,353	= ... = 2693.41
45–54	2,798	1,168,586	= ... = 2.39	1,403,399	= ... = 3360.22
55–64	7,597	1,219,336	= ... = 6.23	1,435,761	= ... = 8945.42
65–74	12,657	794,836	= ... = 15.92	827,929	= ... = 13183.97
75–84	27,858	561,724	= ... = 49.59	548,771	= ... = 27215.61
85+	38,325	238,369	= ... = 160.78	118,970	= ... = 19128.01
All ages (Σ)	91,820	9,148,106		10,322,689	74,931.68

$$\text{The standardized mortality ratio (SMR)} = \frac{\text{observed number of deaths in Country B}}{\text{expected number of deaths in Country B}}$$

$$= \frac{104,636}{74,932} = 1.40 = 140\%$$

3 The number of observed deaths is equal to 140 per cent of the number of deaths that would be expected if, in Country B, the population had experienced the same mortality rates as in Country A; in other words, adjusted for age structure, Country B has 1.4 times more deaths. Unfortunately, this ratio could hide differences in age-specific death rates between the countries.

Life expectancy

Another way of looking at the health of a population is to ask how long people can expect to live. Life expectancy, usually reported as life expectancy at birth (although you may come across life expectancy at, for example, age 15, 45 or 60) is a commonly used summary measure based on death rates at a single point in time. Life expectancy is calculated using life tables. You should become familiar with their basic principles, described below.

The basic information used in life tables are age-specific mortality rates. These are applied to a theoretical population of some multiple of 100 (typically 100,000). Starting at birth, the probability of dying in each period is applied to the number of people surviving to the beginning of the period, so that the initial figure slowly reduces to zero. Most of you will never have to calculate a life table, so we will not confuse you by explaining the mathematics involved. If you find that you do need to calculate one, then you can download from the Internet a spreadsheet that will calculate life tables (and which will also allow you to see the calculations involved: Simple Interactive Statistical Analysis can be found at: http://www.quantitativeskills.com/sisa/).

An example of a life table is illustrated in Table 2.10. But to interpret the table you need to know certain standard notations:

l_x = number of survivors at age x
$_nq_x$ = probability of dying between age x and x + n
$_nD_x$ = number of deaths between age x and x + n
$_nL_x$ = number of person-years lived between age x and x + n
T_x = total number of person-years lived after age x
e_x = life expectancy at age x.

Table 2.10 Example of a life table for a fictitious country

Age	l_x	$_nq_x$	$_nD_x$	$_nL_x$	T_x	e_x
0–1	100000	0.02623	2623.38	97638.96	6966171	69.66171
1–4	97377	0.00436	424.13	388471.6	6868532	70.53573
5–9	96952	0.00245	237.74	484120.6	6480060	66.83748
10–14	96715	0.00219	211.84	483086.5	5995939	61.99612
15–19	96503	0.00458	441.61	481565.1	5512853	57.12628
20–24	96061	0.00616	591.59	478798	5031288	52.3758
25–29	95470	0.00652	622.14	475793.2	4552490	47.68517
30–34	94848	0.00800	758.92	472416.5	4076697	42.98156
35–39	94089	0.01159	1090.91	467934.2	3604280	38.30728
40–44	92998	0.01840	1711.60	461052	3136346	33.72497
45–49	91286	0.02902	2648.86	450338.3	2675294	29.30668
50–54	88637	0.04571	4051.67	433665	2224956	25.1018
55–59	84586	0.06577	5563.01	409576.8	1791291	21.17725
60–64	79023	0.10257	8105.13	375660.7	1381714	17.48505
65–69	70917	0.14763	10469.69	329460.1	1006053	14.18625
70–74	60448	0.21472	12979.48	270439.2	676593	11.19302
75–79	47468	0.31103	14764.02	201169.6	406153.8	8.556318
80–84	32704	0.46312	15146.08	124141.6	204984.2	6.267811
85–89	17558	0.61437	10787.24	58126.06	80842.65	4.604269
90–95	6771	0.78812	5336.34	18112.55	22716.59	3.355007
95+	1435		1434.61	4604.041	4604.041	3.209264

Thus, in this example, life expectancy at birth is 69.66 years. You should also note that life expectancy at age 1 is slightly longer, at 70.5 years. This reflects the relatively high mortality in the first year of life.

Obviously, a full life table can only be calculated where comprehensive data exist. However, there are a number of model life tables that can be used to fill in gaps where data are incomplete. These are based on what has been observed in countries with different characteristics. Clearly this must be done with caution but it is a commonly used approach in developing countries.

Finally, the principles underlying life tables can also be used in any circumstances where you want to follow up outcomes over time, such as survival after a diagnosis of cancer. It is also possible to undertake more complex analysis. For example, it can be used to identify the causes of and ages at death that account for differences in life expectancy between two populations or within a population at two points in time, or to ask what would happen if a particular cause of death was eliminated. But this is beyond the scope of this unit (and is covered in standard demography texts).

Activity 2.3

Why is life expectancy a hypothetical measure?

Feedback

This is because, except in the rare circumstances when a cohort life table is used (which can only be done once everyone in it is dead!) this is based on *current* age-specific death rates in each age group ('period life table'). Thus, it is not a measure of how long someone born now can expect to live.

Beyond mortality

Survival

In those cases where there are data on incidence and mortality it is possible to calculate disease-specific survival. Similarly to life tables, survival analysis looks at the time from an event (disease onset, diagnosis) to a certain endpoint (death, re-admission). It is frequently applied in cancer as the average length of time that individuals survive following diagnosis. Cancer survival rates have frequently been used in comparing quality of care within and between countries and in different time periods. However, when interpreting cancer survival rates it is important to keep in mind that coverage by cancer registries is limited in many countries. In addition, survival rates are dependent on diagnostic practices, existence of screening programmes, stage of the disease at presentation, incidence and mortality rates. Nonetheless, cancer survival data provide useful insights into access to and quality of care.

Measuring morbidity

Existing measures of morbidity allow better understanding about the current physical and mental state of a population. Population health surveys collect mostly self-reported data on perceived health status from representative population samples. Examples of these include the World Health Survey, European Core Health Interview Survey and various national surveys such as the Health Survey for England or US National Health Interview Survey. These typically contain data on self-rated health and selected lifestyle and socioeconomic indicators.

Hospital data, such as inpatient admissions, provides information about health service utilization. However, these data tell us very little about disease burden. Instead, they tell us about those who have a disease and then, for whatever reason, use health care facilities. Specifically they tell us nothing about those people who may have disease or disability but do not access care.

WHO: the main worldwide source of summary statistics on mortality and populations

International data

WHO is a very important source of information on the health of populations world-wide. The numerous WHO publications (most of which are directly available from the Internet, at www.who.int) supply health service providers, researchers, public health scientists, policy-makers, and members of the general population with detailed information on many aspects of health and diseases. In addition, useful comparative summary statistics are also readily available in tabular graph or map formats just a 'click' away on the WHO website. For example, it allows you to choose from the list of 192 WHO member states and obtain basic demographic and health statistics for that country. These include estimates of total population size, gross domestic product (GDP), life expectancy at birth, healthy life expectancy at birth and at age 60, child and adult death rates, and per capita health expenditure. Tables presenting data for all countries or for countries within a region are also directly available. This is particularly useful for international comparisons.

Activity 2.4

Go to the WHO website (http://www.who.int, World Health Organization) and select 'Countries' (top left corner of the screen). Then find the following information for the latest year available:

1 Total population Russian Federation, the United Kingdom, Kyrgyzstan and San Marino.
2 Total expenditures on health as a proportion of national gross domestic product (GDP) in Uzbekistan, Czech Republic, and Sweden.
3 Healthy life expectancy at birth in Spain.

Feedback

1 By clicking in turn on the name of each of these countries you will find their total population easily. The Russian Federation is the most populated country in the WHO European Region with over 143 million inhabitants in 2006. In comparison there are only approximately 60.5 million persons in the UK, 5 million in Kyrgyzstan, and 31,000 in San Marino (2006).

2 The total expenditures on health represent 4.7 per cent of the gross domestic product (GDP) in Uzbekistan, 6.8 per cent in the Czech Republic, and 8.9 per cent in Sweden (2006).

3 The healthy life expectancy at birth in Spain is 70 years for males and 75 years for females (2003). Health life expectancy is equivalent to the number of years in full health that a newborn can expect to live based on current rates of ill health and mortality. We will talk about this indicator in Chapter 3.

European data: the WHO Health for All Database

If you are looking for easy and rapid access to basic health statistics for the 53 member states of the WHO European Region, you can use the WHO Health For All (HFA) database. It was developed in the mid-1980s to support the monitoring of health trends in the region (HFA strategy). It is a key tool for international comparisons in Europe (including central Asia). It is regularly updated (twice per year) and freely available online (for direct access to the data using the Internet) or offline (to be downloaded for use on a PC). You can find both versions on the WHO Euro website (www.euro.who.int, World Health Organization Regional Office for Europe – select 'What we do', then 'Data and evidence', then 'Databases' and then 'European Health for All Database – HFA-DB'). The offline version is recommended for frequent users and also offers several different output options not available online. The database is easy to interrogate. You simply need to click on the health indicators, countries, and years you are interested in (see Figure 2.4).

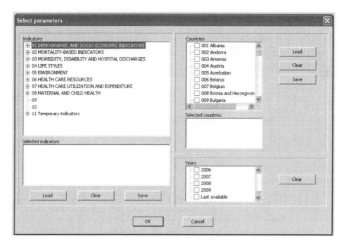

Figure 2.4 Illustration of the Health For All Database worksheet

Source: World Health Organization Regional Office for Europe (2010)

Indicators

The indicators that can be studied include demographic and socioeconomic statistics (18); mortality (58); morbidity, disability and hospital discharges (48); lifestyles (12); environment (14); health care resources (22); health care utilization and costs (29); maternal and child health (23).

Countries covered

The database covers all 53 WHO member states in the European region and allows you to select certain pre-specified groups: European Average (53 WHO European member states); EU average (27 EU member states); EU members before May 2004 average; EU members since 2004 or 2007 average; CIS average ('Commonwealth of Independent States'); CARK average (5 Central Asian republics and Kazakhstan); Eur-A: 27 countries in the WHO European Region with very low child and adult mortality; Eur-B & C: 26 countries in the Region with higher levels of mortality.

Years

Data are available from 1970 to present (or latest available).

Presentation of the results

The database allows you to use several predefined table and graph formats, such as trends over time, with an option to adjust scales on both axes. You can also create scatter-plots, comparing two indicators, ranked bar charts and maps.

Data sources

The data have been obtained from focal points for health statistics in member states, WHO technical units and collaborating centres, and other international sources, such as the Organization for Economic Cooperation and Development (OECD).

Data availability and quality

There are differences in recording practices for health data between countries, with the most complete data being for mortality-related indicators and incidence of infectious diseases.

Problems

There is incomplete registration of births and deaths in some countries, a lack of accurate populations estimates – for example, in Tajikistan, Georgia (Badurashvili and collaborators 2001), Albania and Bosnia and Herzegovina – and no mortality data in suitable detail for Andorra, Monaco, and Turkey. For further details please see the HFA-DB 'Help' section, Notes on data availability and quality.

Activity 2.5

You will now get information on time trends for the average life expectancy in Europe by using the HFA database. In order to do this, you simply need to follow these steps:

1 Go to the WHO Euro website (www.euro.who.int World Health Organization Regional Office for Europe). Select 'What we do', then 'Data and evidence', then 'Databases' and then 'European Health for All Database – HFA-DB' to reach the HFA database website. Download and launch the offline version of the database.

2 In Parameters section, click 'Select parameters', indicator group: Select 'Mortality based indicators'

3 Indicator: Select 'Life expectancy at birth in years' for both genders
4 Start year: Select 'First available'
5 End year: Select 'Last available'
6 Countries: Select Lithuania, Greece, Sweden, Poland
7 Submit query: Click on 'Ok'
8 Output selection screen: Select 'Line chart'

Use the 'temporary indicators' function to create a new variable (option only available in offline version): male/female birth ratio. The formula to use is C*(I1/I2) where I1 is the number of male births and I2 the number of female births. Plot the ratio of male to female births each year since 1985 in the following countries: Georgia, Armenia, Russia, Sweden, United Kingdom. What do you see? What might explain these appearances?

Now describe the graph you have obtained.

Feedback

The graph you obtained should look like Figure 2.5.

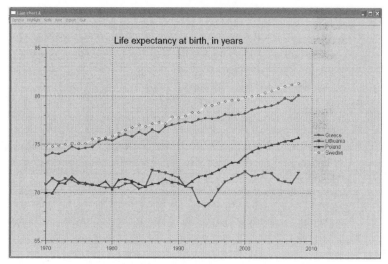

Figure 2.5 Life expectancy at birth (in years) in selected European countries
Source: World Health Organization Regional Office for Europe (2010)

This graph shows that life expectancy has been increasing steadily in Sweden since at least the 1970s. In Greece, there was a sustained steady increase. However, there was a decrease in 2007, which is likely to indicate that the high smoking prevalence and westernized diets high in energy-dense foods are impacting upon ischaemic heart disease mortality rates (Hirte et al. 2008). In Poland life expectancy stagnated during the 1970s and 1980s, only increasing following the early 1990s when the country introduced market reforms. Similarly, in Lithuania, life expectancy did not change much in the 1970s and early 1980s. However, in the mid-1980s there was a dramatic improvement (this was at the time that Mikhail Gorbachev launched a wide-ranging anti-alcohol campaign), but it then started falling back again at the end of the 1980s (when the USSR was in a period of rapid transition), accelerating during the early 1990s. After an improvement during 1995–2000, stagnation and decline followed during the 2000s, which is likely to reflect the liberalization of alcohol control policy (Grabauskas et al. 2009). In 2008 (the latest year available) a further improvement is seen.

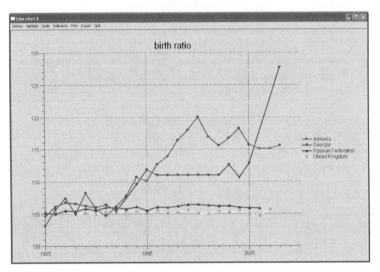

Figure 2.6 Male/female birth ratio in selected countries

Source: World Health Organization Regional Office for Europe (2010)

The most obvious finding is that of a marked increase in male/female births in the 1990s in Georgia and Armenia. This coincides with the introduction of ultrasound scanners following the break up of the USSR. The years of the late 1990s are remarkably flat in Georgia: this was because at that time the authorities realized that there were problems with data collection and estimated figures.

Take some time to browse through the different health indicators, countries and group of countries and types of graphs you can obtain. You will see that such information can be extremely useful for international comparisons across Europe.

Summary

This chapter described the usefulness of population, mortality and morbidity data in public health and discussed their strengths and weaknesses. It looked into the different sources of such data and described how they can be employed to obtain commonly used indicators of population health, such as age-standardized death rates and life expectancy. Finally, it allowed you to examine different types of basic health indicators that can be obtained from the WHO websites.

References

Ahmad OB, Boschi-Pinto C, Lopez AD, Murray CJD, Lozano R and Inoue M (2001) *Age Standardization of Rates: A New WHO Standard. GPE Discussion Series: No. 31.* EIP/GPE/EBD/ World Health Organization.

Badurashvili I, McKee M, Tsuladez G, Meslé F, Vallin J and Shkolnikov V (2001) Where there are no data: what has happened to the life expectancy of Georgia since 1990? *Public Health* **115**: 394–400.

Grabauskas V, Prochorskas R, Veryga A (2009) Associations between mortality and alcohol consumption in Lithuanian population. *Medicina (Kaunas)* **45**(12):1000–12.

Hirte L, Nolte E, Mossialos E and McKee M (2008) The changing regional pattern of ischaemic heart disease mortality in southern Europe: still healthy but uneven progress. *J Epidemiol Community Health* **62**: e4.

Neighbourhood Statistics (2010) (available at www.neighbourhood.statistics.gov.uk).

Office of National Statistics (2010) (available at www.statistics.gov.uk).

World Health Organization (2010) Home page. Geneva: World Health Organization (available at http://www.who.int/).

World Health Organization Regional Office for Europe (2010) *World Health Organization Regional Office for Europe website.* Copenhagen (available at www.euro.who.int).

 Further reading

ICD Homepage: (www.who.int/classifications/icd/en/)

Institute of Health Metrics and Evaluation Homepage: (http://www.healthmetricsandevaluation.org/)

Leon DA, Chenet L, Shkolnikov VM, Zakharov S, Shapiro J, Rakhmanova G, Vassin S and McKee M (1997) Huge variation in Russian mortality rates 1984–94: artefact, alcohol, or what? *The Lancet* **350**: 383–8. This paper discusses the dramatic changes in mortality rates that occurred in Russia since the mid-1980s.

Shkolnikov V, McKee M and Leon DA (2001) Changes in life expectancy in Russia in the mid-1990s, *The Lancet* **357**: 917–21. This is a second paper that could provide you more details of the observed gap in life expectancy and health between Western and Eastern Europe.

World Health Organization (2010) *International Statistical Classification of Diseases and Related Health Problems, tenth revision.* Version for 2007. (http://apps.who.int/classifications/apps/icd/icd10online/)

WHO World Standard Population: (http://www.who.int/whosis/indicators/compendium/2008/1mst/en/index.html).

Understanding the burden of disease: using the available data

Martin McKee, Marina Karanikolos, Fiona Sim and Joceline Pomerleau

Overview

In Chapter 2, you learned about a simple and widely used health statistic, that is, population-level standardized mortality rates. This and various estimates of morbidity and health states are useful measures for numerous public health purposes ranging from the monitoring of new health problems to evaluating progress in reducing old ones for which disease control programmes are already in place. However, these approaches rapidly become unwieldy when several health problems and conditions are being monitored over time across numerous population sub-groups. In that case, **summary measures of population health** (SMPH) become useful tools that combine information on mortality and non-fatal health outcomes to represent a population's health in a single number. This chapter will introduce you to SMPH, with a particular emphasis on estimates of disease burden within the context of the Global Burden of Disease (GBD) study.

Learning objectives

By the end of this chapter you should be able to:

- describe the uses of SMPH
- discuss some limitations of SMPH
- discuss the methods used to assess burden of disease in a population and the major contributors to it
- discuss results from the GBD and Global Health Risks studies

Key terms

Burden of disease   A measure of the physical, emotional, social and financial impact that a particular disease has on the health and functioning of the population.

Disability Adjusted Life Year (DALY)   estimates the equivalent years of 'healthy' life lost by being in a state of poor health or disability.

Health Adjusted Life Expectancy (HALE)   estimates the equivalent of 'healthy' expected number of years of life for a newborn in a given population, if current disability and mortality conditions in that population continue to apply.

Health expectancy   Summary measure of population health that estimates the expectation of years of life lived in various health states.

Health gap   Summary measure of population health that estimates the gap between the current population health and a normative goal for population health.

Summary measures of population health   Indicators that combine information about mortality and health to summarize the health of a population in a single number.

Summary measures of population health (SMPH)

Chapter 2 discussed data on mortality and populations. The use of mortality data as a fundamental component of the public policy process is related in part to their widespread availability and timeliness. Statistics on causes of death are undoubtedly useful for public health surveillance, providing overall pictures of mortality. Inevitably, however, they say much less about those who are still alive. In particular, although they have formed the basis of comparisons of the health of nations for many decades, they have been criticized because they disregard the importance of widely prevalent conditions that are less likely to kill you but still create considerable disability or use of health care resources. This has led to attempts to bring together morbidity and mortality. An ideal health metric is therefore one that simultaneously measures and contrasts both fatal and non-fatal health outcomes. Indeed, such a measure is needed to assess the benefits of health interventions which may reduce both mortality *and* the period of life lived in a disabled state.

In this chapter we will discuss indicators that combine information on mortality and non-fatal health outcomes to give information on a population's health in a single number, that is, SMPH. Interest in and work on SMPH indicators has grown during the last decades and, although there has also been increasing debate about their application, their use has become routine in a number of settings.

SMPH fall into two broad categories: health expectancies and health gaps. Health expectancy is a generic term to describe SMPH that estimate the average time that a person could expect to live in various states of health. Health gaps quantify the difference between the actual health of a population and some stated norm or goal for population health. Both types of indicators include weights that account for time lived in health states worse than ideal health.

Activity 3.1

Think of potential uses of SMPH in the public health policy process. Give a few examples.

Feedback

There are several potential uses of SMPH in public health policy. These include:

- comparing the health of one population with that of another
- monitoring time trends in the health of a given population
- assessing overall health inequalities within populations
- providing appropriate and balanced attention to the effects of non-fatal health outcomes on overall population health
- informing debates on priorities for health service delivery and planning
- informing debates on priorities for research and development
- improving curricula for professional training in public health
- analysing the benefits of health interventions for use in cost-effectiveness analyses

Healthy life expectancy – more than simply life and death

The most widely used SMPH example among health expectancy measures is *Health Adjusted Life Expectancy*, or HALE. Data on HALE is available for over 190 WHO member states. HALE estimates the average equivalent 'healthy' expected number of years of life for a newborn in a given population, if current disability and mortality conditions continue to apply in this population. It is calculated by subtracting from the life expectancy a figure which is the number of years lived with disability multiplied by a weighting to represent the effect of the various disabilities. This is illustrated in Figure 3.1.

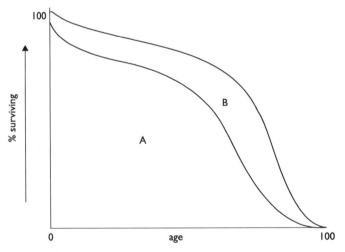

A = healthy life expectancy; B = period with disability; life expectancy = A + B; health adjusted life expectancy = A + fB (where f is a weighting to reflect disability level). For example, if the area A = 50 and B = 20, and the average weight of the disabilities is 0.5 (so that a year with disability is considered equivalent to 6 months in good health), then health adjusted life expectancy = 50 + (20 × 0.5) = 60 years.

Figure 3.1 Health-adjusted life expectancy

Activity 3.2

1 Figure 3.2 shows the probability of being healthy by age and sex in Western Europe, Eastern Europe, and the Russian Federation. Examine the figure and describe how this probability varies among regions.

2   Now examine Figure 3.3, in which data on health and mortality are combined to give years of healthy life expectancy by age, sex, and region, and answer the following questions.

   a) How does total survival (sum of survival in good or poor health) vary among regions and genders?
   b) How does survival in poor health vary among regions and gender?

3   Figure 3.4 shows the contribution of ill health and increased mortality to the gap in health expectancy between the Russian Federation and Western Europe.

   a) Find the difference in health expectancy (in years) between the Russian Federation and Western Europe, in men and women aged 50 to 54 years.
   b) Describe how the contribution of ill health and death to this gap varies between genders. Try to explain the differences observed.
   c) In this study the authors used survey data on self-reported health for the calculation of healthy life expectancy. Why do you think this might be a problem?

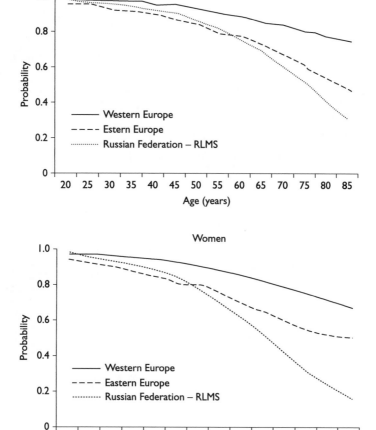

Figure 3.2 Probability of being healthy, by age and sex in Western Europe, Eastern Europe, and the Russian Federation (RLMS: Russian Longitudinal Monitoring Survey)

Source: Andreev and collaborators (2003)

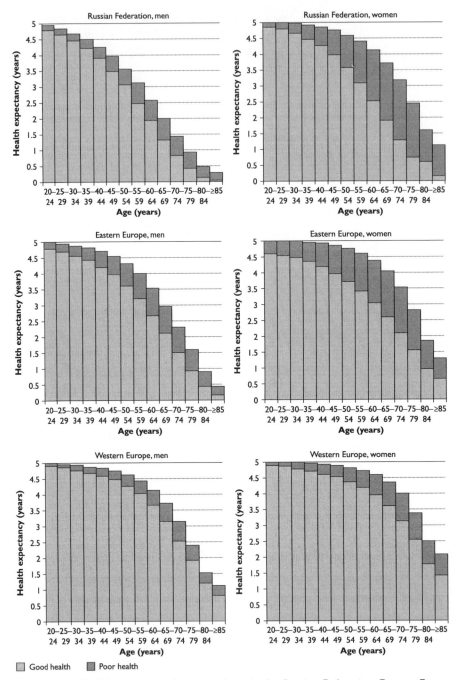

Figure 3.3 Years of health expectancy, by age and sex in the Russian Federation, Eastern Europe, and Western Europe

Source: Andreev and collaborators (2003)

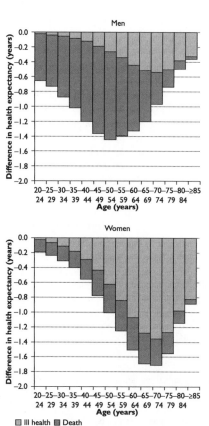

Figure 3.4 Contribution of ill health and increased deaths to the gap in health expectancy between the Russian Federation and Western Europe

Source: Andreev and collaborators (2003)

Feedback

1 As expected, we can see that the probability of being healthy decreases with age in both genders and in all three regions. However, this decrease is steeper in Eastern Europe and the Russian Federation than in Western Europe. When comparing Eastern Europe and the Russian Federation, we can see that the probabilities are generally similar until about the age of 50 but after 50, the trends diverge with a more rapid decline in health in the Russian Federation.

2 Survival tends to be highest in Western Europe, intermediate in Eastern Europe, and lowest in the Russian Federation. Regional differences are particularly important in men. In all regions survival is better in women than in men. The decline in survival is particularly steep in males from the Russian Federation than in females from the Russian Federation or in males from other regions.

3 In women we can see a clear gradation in the likelihood of surviving in poor health. Western European women not only are more likely to survive into old age compared with those from Eastern Europe or the Russian Federation, but they are also more

likely to survive in good health (thus less likely to survive in poor health). Intermediate results are found in Eastern Europe and the worst scenario is observed in women from the Russian Federation where few appear to survive in good health. In men, survival in poor health also tends to be lowest in Western Europe but the difference between Eastern Europe and the Russian Federation is less striking than in women.

Differences in males and females are most important in the Russian Federation. Indeed, there appears to be a major burden of ill health afflicting women from the Russian Federation that is not apparent from analysing mortality data (total survival considerably higher compared to Russian Federation men). A similar but less marked pattern can be seen in Eastern Europe.

4   The gap in health expectancy is approximately 1.4 years in men and 1.0 years in women.

5   In men, the majority of the difference is due to death while in women it is largely due to poor health. This suggests that the responses of men and women to adversity differ, leading to premature death in men and survival in poor state of health in women.

6   There are many limitations associated with the use of self-reported health for the estimation of healthy life expectancy. For example, it is possible that self-reported health does not measure the same thing in different population sub-groups and may not be interpreted in the same way by different groups (for example, the ability of self-rated health to predict mortality varies among countries, and the perception of health varies between genders). As well it may not be the most appropriate measure of health.

In order to learn more about this issue, read the following extract from a commentary by Mathers (2003).

Extract from Mathers (2003)

Towards valid and comparable measurement of population health

Women generally report worse health than men. Thus, the large male–female gap in life expectancy in the Russian Federation is offset by worse reported health status in women.

The reporting by women of worse health, generally, than men has been seen in health surveys across many developed countries. Can we conclude that the health status of Russian Federation women is worse than that of Russian Federation men? Several paradoxical findings have been reported in analyses of population health surveys, suggesting that self-reported health measures may give misleading results if differences in the way people use question responses are not taken into account. This evidence has been ignored by many who use self-report-survey measures of health status to report on population health, health inequalities, or intervention outcomes. Indeed, there is substantial literature arguing that within-group correlations of self-reported health measures with other observed or measured health indicators, or with mortality risk, show the validity and comparability of such measures across groups.

Although there are, undoubtedly, correlations between self-reported health status measures and other health indicators, and there is no doubt that health status influences self-report, this does not ensure comparability of self-report measures across groups. Several studies have reported significant correlations between perceived health (with response categories such as excellent, good, fair, poor) and mortality risk within groups such as men and women, or groups defined by socioeconomic or ethnic characteristics, and argued that these correlations provide evidence that self-perceived health is a valid measure of health status. Similar arguments are made for within group correlations with observed or measured functional indicators, with morbidity and health service utilization.

However, it is possible to have consistent associations of perceived health with survival within groups without such associations holding across groups. This is illustrated in Fig. 3.5, where survival is lower for worse perceived health in both men and women, while at the same time the survival of women with worst perceived health is better than that of men with excellent perceived health. Suppose that a population survey found most women reporting worse health than men for a population with the associations shown in Fig. 3.5. It would clearly be fallacious to deduce that women have worse survival (or health) than men: the indicator is not comparable across groups because women are using the response categories differently to men.

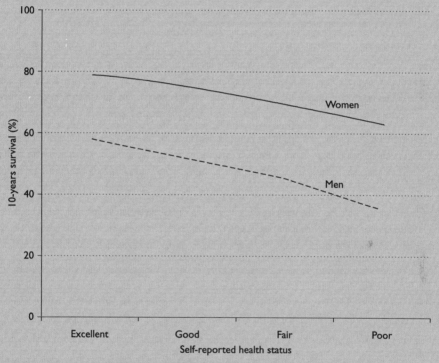

Figure 3.5 Plots showing that within group correlation of self-reported health status with other health indicators does not provide evidence for cross-group correlations

Source: Mathers (2003)

Survey developers have emphasized the importance of establishing the validity of instruments and their reliability, but until recently, little attention had been paid to the issue of cross-population comparability. The latter relates fundamentally to unmeasured differences in expectations and norms for health, so that the meaning that different populations attach to the labels used for response categories in self-reported questions, such as mild, moderate, or severe, can vary greatly. Recent developments in survey methodology using measured tests and anchoring vignettes to calibrate self-report health questions hold considerable promise in addressing this problem.

Health gaps and disease burden

Health gaps are particularly useful measures as they allow for the quantification of the burden of disease and injury in terms of absolute numbers of life years. The burden of disease can be seen as a measurement of the gap between the current health of a population and an ideal situation where everyone in the population lives to old age in full health. It is usually expressed in disability-adjusted life years (DALY) which represent one lost year of 'healthy' life.

The GBD programme is a major undertaking to estimate the worldwide burden of disease from major disease and injuries by geographical region. You can read more about this programme on the WHO website (http://www.who.int/healthinfo/global_burden_disease/en/). We will discuss some GBD findings later in this chapter.

Key issues in using summary measures of population health (SMPH)

Clearly the use of SMPH raises many technical and, by implication, ethical complexities. Many of the technical arguments are beyond the scope of this chapter but some will be discussed below. A key issue is how to define and measure disability and then select the weights to apply to particular health states. Obviously, the choices made in respect to particular conditions will be important. There are several ways in which this can be done. Each method involves asking groups of people for their preferences. The methods used in the GBD programme will be used as an example.

In the first round of the GBD study (estimates of disease burden were for 1990, small groups of participants (medical and public health experts) were asked to make a value judgement about the severity of given health conditions and the preference for time spent in each severity level for these conditions. To a large extent, this was necessitated by the lack of population information on the severity distribution of most conditions at global and regional levels. For each condition, this assessment was based on a detailed case. For example, angina, in this exercise, was defined as reproducible chest pain when walking for 50 minutes or more, which the individual would rate as measuring five on a subjective pain scale from zero to ten. The effect of disability weighting is that conditions which, while disabling, rarely cause death (in particular mental illness and chronic, non-lethal conditions) are ranked as more important than they would be using mortality alone.

The second round of the GBD project calculated disease burden estimates for the year 2000 and for subsequent years (revised versions have provided estimates for 2001, 2002 and 2004). It adopted a similar approach to health state valuation, using a standard health state description based on eight core domains of health (mobility, self care, pain and discomfort, cognition, interpersonal activities, vision, sleep and energy, affect) (Prüss-Üstün et al. 2003). In order to address the limitations of the methods used, WHO, in collaboration with its member states, initiated a two-tiered data collection strategy involving general population surveys, combined with more detailed surveys among people with higher education qualifications (Ustun et al. 2000). The experience gained in eliciting health state valuations from general population samples was then used in designing the health status and health state valuation modules for the World Health Survey, which was carried out in 73 member states in 2003. The disability weights used in the GBD 2004 update study are still based largely on the GBD 1990 disability weights, although some the weights have been revised for a number of causes in the latest version (examples are provided in Table 3.1). A new round of the Global Burden of Disease (GBD 2010) study is underway. It has greatly expanded the volume and quality of data available and includes a

Table 3.1 Disability weights used in the GBD study[a]

Disability class	Severity weights	Conditions[b]
I	0.00–0.02	Stunting due to malnutrition, schistosomiasis infection, long-term scarring due to burns (less than 20% of body)
II	0.02–0.12	Amputated finger, asthma case, edentulism, mastectomy, severe anaemia, stress incontinence
III	0.12–0.24	Angina, HIV not progressed to AIDS, infertility, alcohol dependence and problem use, low vision (<6/18, >3/60), rheumatoid arthritis
IV	0.24–0.36	Amputated arm, congestive heart failure, deafness, drug dependence, Parkinson disease, tuberculosis
V	0.36–0.50	Bipolar affective disorder, mild mental retardation, neurological sequelae of malaria, recto-vaginal fistula
VI	0.50–0.70	AIDS cases not on antiretroviral drugs, Alzheimer and other, dementias, blindness, Down syndrome
VII	0.70–1.00	Active psychosis, severe depression, severe migraine, quadriplegia, terminal stage cancer

Source: World Health Organization (2008)

Notes:

a Based on average severity weight globally for both sexes and all ages in the GBD 2004 update.

b Conditions are listed in the disability class for their global average weight. Most conditions will have distributions of severity spanning more than one disability class, potentially up to all seven.

comprehensive revision of disability weights, based on large scale household surveys in specific countries and, in its online version, worldwide (World Health Organization 2010). These results are expected to be published during 2011.

The effect of disability weighting can be seen in Figure 3.6. Conditions which, while disabling, rarely cause death, in particular mental illness, are ranked as more important than they would be using mortality alone (note, the figure uses Disability Adjusted Life Years (DALY), which is equivalent to one year of healthy life, and which is derived in a similar way to HALE).

A second issue is the value placed on a life at different stages in life. This is extremely controversial. Is a year of life worth as much when it is a new born infant as it is when it is an adult responsible for a family? The authors of the GBD study decided there was a difference and placed more weight on a year of life of a young adult. The weightings they used are shown in Figure 3.7. This has the effect of reducing the burden of disease arising from deaths in childhood.

A third issue is how to obtain SMPH in countries from which data are unavailable. This is somewhat controversial and has been done using estimates. For example, data that exist (usually on childhood mortality) have been applied to model life tables or, where no data exist, as with a number of specific causes of death, they have been modelled using equations that include a range of variables believed to correlate with them (such as national income or levels of female education) derived from analyses of data from those countries where data exist.

The book by Murray and collaborators published in 2002 provides a good description of the debates as they stood in 1999 (see list of suggested reading at the end of

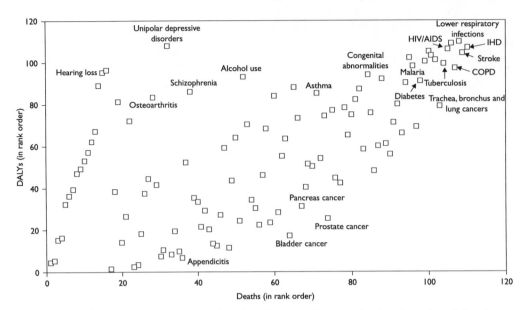

Figure 3.6 Relationship between rank order of conditions[a] using mortality (number of deaths) and total disease burden (DALYs)

Source: adapted from World Health Organization (2008)

a Ranking of causes from 1 (lowest number of deaths/DALYs) to 110 (highest number of deaths/DALYs)

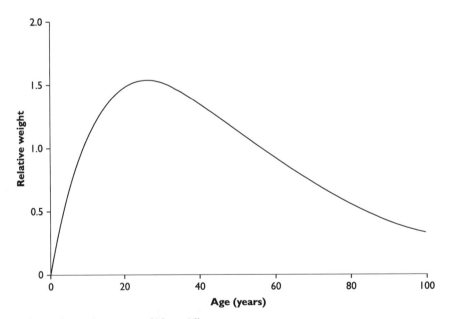

Figure 3.7 Weighting allocated to a year of life at different ages

Source: Lopez et al. (2006)

this chapter). Additional material can be obtained from the website of the Institute of Health Metrics and Evaluation (www.healthmetricsandevaluation.org/)

Results from the Global Burden of Disease (GBD) programme

The most recent results (at the time of writing) from the second round of the GBD Study were published in the Global Burden of Disease: 2004 update report (World Health Organization 2008). For the presentation of results, countries were grouped as high and medium or low income, depending on their gross national income per capita in 2004. Regional and income groups are defined in Table 3.2. Detailed tables for a range of regional groupings by age and sex are available on the WHO website (http://www.who.int/health-info/global_burden_disease/estimates_regional/en/index.html). However, it is expected that revised and updated results will be available shortly after this book is published.

Overall burden of disease

It is possible to estimate the contribution of different conditions to the overall disease burden. As expected, this varies greatly by gender and by region. The ten worldwide leading causes of disease burden in 2004 in males and females are described in Table 3.2.

Table 3.2 Leading causes of disease burden (DALYs) for males and females, worldwide, 2004

Males	% DALYs	Females	% DALYs
Perinatal conditions	8.1	Perinatal conditions	8.5
Lower respiratory infections	6.2	Lower respiratory infections	6.2
Diarrhoeal diseases	4.8	Unipolar depressive disorders	5.6
Ischaemic heart disease	4.7	Maternal conditions	5.4
Road traffic accidents	3.7	Diarrhoeal diseases	4.8
HIV/AIDS	3.6	HIV/AIDS	4.1
Unipolar depressive disorders	3.1	Ischaemic heart disease	3.5
Cerebrovascular disease	3.0	Cerebrovascular disease	3.1
Tuberculosis	2.7	Malaria	2.3
Alcohol use disorders	2.7	Childhood diseases	1.9

Source: Adapted from World Health Organization (2008)

Activity 3.3

Now take a close look at Table 3.3.

1 Identify which regions bear the greatest burden of disease.
2 Describe differences in the causes of disease burden between developed and developing regions.

Table 3.3 Burden of disease in disability-adjusted life years (DALYs) by cause in WHO sub-regions, estimates for 2004

	Africa	South-East Asia	The Americas		Eastern Mediterranean		Europe		Western Pacific	
	Low and middle income	Low and middle income	High income	Low and middle income	High income	Low and middle income	High income	Low and middle income	High income	Low and middle income
Population (millions)	738	1,672	329	545	31	489	407	476	204	1,534
Total number of DALYs (000)	376,525	442,979	45,116	98,116	4,379	137,614	49,331	102,130	22,305	242,466
Infectious and parasitic diseases	159,817	82,900	1,102	8,548	241	23,450	838	5,203	490	19,272
Respiratory infections	43,058	29,078	365	3,512	110	12,311	488	2,419	390	5,973
Maternal conditions	14,906	12,892	290	1,962	99	4,982	171	691	95	2,805
Perinatal conditions	38,191	46,503	794	5,677	258	16,699	515	3,173	170	14,293
Nutritional deficiencies	11,753	13,503	155	2,139	82	4,207	285	1,608	237	4,683
Neoplasms	6,231	14,482	5,772	5,958	181	4,412	8,453	8,916	3,713	21,520
Diabetes and nutritional endocrine disorders	5,188	5,781	2,326	4,287	256	1,991	2,029	1,898	882	5,424
Neuropsychiatric disorders	19,403	52,279	12,846	20,914	811	15,155	12,590	16,342	5,115	43,446
Cardiovascular diseases	14,243	42,061	6,291	8,926	548	12,547	7,915	26,845	2,984	28,776
Respiratory diseases	7,169	16,270	2,966	4,792	119	3,615	2,918	2,992	1,214	16,899
Digestive diseases	5,523	12,874	1,495	3,665	91	3,348	2,190	4,755	899	7,592
Other non-communicable conditions, congenital abnormalities	21,384	51,538	6,220	12,426	773	14,705	7,391	10,865	3,868	40,038
Injuries	29,658	62,818	4,493	15,311	810	20,192	3,550	16,424	2,248	31,744

Source: Adapted from World Health Organization (2008)

Feedback

1 A disproportionate disease burden is borne by developing sub-regions with 70 per cent of the worldwide total burden of disease originating from the low and middle income countries of South-East Asia (29 per cent), Africa (25 per cent) and Western Pacific (16 per cent) regions representing 61 per cent of the world population.

2 The results also showed marked differences in disease patterns among sub-regions. In high income sub-regions, communicable diseases and maternal, perinatal and nutritional conditions represent only low proportion of the total disease burden while in low and middle income sub-regions this figure rises considerably, reaching for example more than 70 per cent in the African sub-regions. In contrast, non-communicable diseases account for a large proportion of DALYs in high-income countries (for example, 84 per cent in America and Western Pacific, and 88 per cent in Europe).

Underlying causes of disease burden

The next step is to look at the underlying causes of the burden of disease. This is done by combining information on the distribution of specified risk factors in the population, the relative risk of different deaths and disabilities associated with exposure to them, and the overall burden of the deaths and disabilities in question. This immediately poses a challenge because clearly very few diseases (if any) are caused by a single risk factor. For example, while smoking is clearly the immediate (or proximate) cause of the vast majority of cases of lung cancer, the risk can be modified by other factors such as diet and, almost certainly, genetics. However, there are also distal factors, which influence why people smoke. So, for example, poverty and homelessness might be considered, at this level, as another risk factor for lung cancer.

Once again, the calculations are complicated (but clearly described in the supporting documentation for the Global Health Risks report (World Health Organization 2009) for those who are interested). The report provides estimates for the 24 global health risk factors for the year 2004 (it takes some years for mortality data to be collated in many countries). You will become more familiar with the contents of the report from the extracts cited below.

Activity 3.4

If you had been in charge of the study, what risk factors would you have selected for study?

Feedback

You probably included factors such as malnutrition, tobacco, alcohol consumption, hypertension, unsafe sex, air pollution, and so on. But have you also thought about indoor smoke from solid fuels (you will read about this in Chapter 11), physical workload in the working environment that could lead to low back pain, noise, childhood sexual abuse, or exposure to lead? In the Global Risk Factor study (World Health Organization 2009), a total of 24 risk factors covering a wide range of physiological, behavioural, environmental, and socioeconomic factors were examined. You will be introduced to these in Activity 3.5.

Activity 3.5

Read the following extracts from the Global Health Risks report (World Health Organization 2009) and an editorial by Stevens et al. 2009 (Box 3.1). These will give you an overview of the methods used to estimate the contributions of the 24 risk factors to global and regional burden of disease in the GBD study and the main results found. Then answer the following questions:

1 Using data from Figure 3.9, describe what the authors mean by risk factor transition.
2 Some say that nutritional diseases create a dual burden. What does this mean?
3 List the main limitations of the methods used to obtain the results presented in the report.

Extract from World Health Organization (2009)

Understanding the nature of health risks
To prevent disease and injury, it is necessary to identify and deal with their causes – the health risks that underlie them. Each risk has its own causes too, and many have their roots in a complex chain of events over time, consisting of socioeconomic factors, environmental and community conditions, and individual behaviour. The causal chain offers many entry points for intervention. As can be seen from the example of ischaemic heart disease (Figure 3.8), some elements in the chain, such as high blood

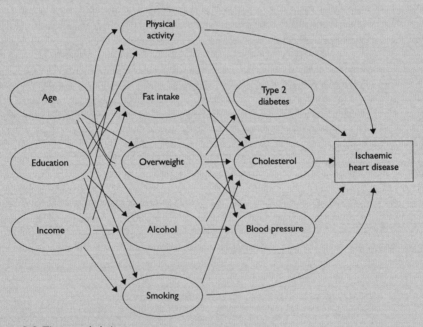

Figure 3.8 The causal chain

Source: WHO

Note: Major causes of ischaemic heart disease are shown. Arrows indicate some (but not all) of the pathways by which these causes interact.

pressure or cholesterol, act as a relatively direct cause of the disease. Some risks located further back in the causal chain act indirectly through intermediary factors. These risks include physical inactivity, alcohol, smoking or fat intake. For the most distal risk factors, such as education and income, less causal certainty can be attributed to each risk. However, modifying these background causes is more likely to have amplifying effects, by influencing multiple proximal causes; such modifications therefore have the potential to yield fundamental and sustained improvements to health.

The risk transition

As a country develops, the types of diseases that affect a population shift from primarily infectious, such as diarrhoea and pneumonia, to primarily non-communicable, such as cardiovascular disease and cancers. This shift is known as the 'epidemiological transition' (Omran, 1971) and is caused by:

- improvements in medical care, which mean that children no longer die from easily curable conditions such as diarrhoea
- the ageing of the population, because non-communicable diseases affect older adults at the highest rates
- public health interventions such as vaccinations and the provision of clean water and sanitation, which reduce the incidence of infectious diseases.

This pattern can be observed across many countries, with wealthy countries further advanced along this transition. Similarly, the risks that affect a population also shift over time, from those for infectious disease to those that increase non-communicable disease (Figure 3.9). Low-income populations are most affected by risks associated with poverty, such as undernutrition, unsafe sex, unsafe water, poor sanitation and hygiene, and indoor smoke from solid fuels; these are the so-called 'traditional risks'. As life expectancies increase and the major causes of death and disability shift to the chronic and non-communicable, populations are increasingly facing modern risks due to physical inactivity; overweight and obesity, and other diet-related factors; and tobacco and alcohol-related risks. As a result, many low- and middle-income countries now face a growing burden from the modern risks to health, while still fighting an unfinished battle with the traditional risks to health. The impact of these modern risks varies at different levels of socioeconomic development. For example, urban air pollution is a greater risk factor in middle-income countries than in high-income countries because of substantial progress by the latter in controlling this risk through public-health policies (Figure 3.9). Increasing exposure to these emerging risks is not inevitable: it is amenable to public health intervention. For example, by enacting strong tobacco-control policies, low- and middle-income countries can learn from the tobacco-control successes in high-income countries [see Chapter 8]. By enacting such policies early on, they can avoid the high levels of disease caused by tobacco currently found in high-income countries.

Regional estimates for 2004

This report presents estimates for regional groupings of countries (including the six WHO regions) and income groupings, with the countries grouped as high, medium or low income, depending on their gross national income per capita in 2004. The classification of countries most commonly used here is seven groups, comprising the six WHO regions plus the high-income countries in all regions forming a

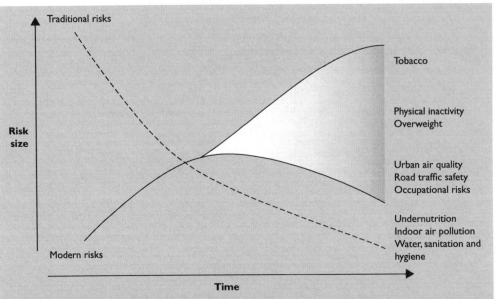

Figure 3.9 The risk transition

Note: Over time, major risks to health shift from traditional risks (e.g. inadequate nutrition or unsafe water and sanitation) to modern risks (e.g. overweight and obesity). Modern risks may take different trajectories in different countries, depending on the risk and the context.

seventh group. Lists of countries in each regional and income group are available in Table 3.4.

High-income countries represent 15% of the world population, middle-income countries about 47% and low-income countries about 37%. The distribution of deaths is similar to that of population across the country income groups, despite

Table 3.4 Countries grouped by WHO region and income per capita[a] in 2004

African Region	Low and middle	Algeria, Angola, Benin, Botswana, Burkina Faso, Burundi, Cameroon, Cape Verde, Central African Republic, Chad, Comoros, Congo, Côte d'Ivoire, Democratic Republic of the Congo, Equatorial Guinea, Eritrea, Ethiopia, Gabon, Gambia, Ghana, Guinea, Guinea-Bissau, Kenya, Lesotho, Liberia, Madagascar, Malawi, Mali, Mauritania, Mauritius, Mozambique, Namibia, Niger, Nigeria, Rwanda, Sao Tome and Principe, Senegal, Seychelles, Sierra Leone, South Africa, Swaziland, Togo, Uganda, United Republic of Tanzania, Zambia, Zimbabwe
Region of the Americas	High	Bahamas, Canada, United States of America
	Low and middle	Antigua and Barbuda, Argentina, Barbados, Belize, Bolivia, Brazil, Chile, Colombia, Costa Rica, Dominica, Dominican Republic, Ecuador, El Salvador, Grenada, Guatemala, Guyana, Haiti, Honduras, Jamaica, Mexico, Nicaragua, Panama, Paraguay, Peru, Saint Kitts and Nevis, Saint Lucia, Saint Vincent and the Grenadines, Suriname, Trinidad and Tobago, Uruguay, Venezuela (Bolivarian Republic of)

Eastern Mediterranean Region	High	Bahrain, Kuwait, Qatar, Saudi Arabia, United Arab Emirates
	Low and middle	Afghanistan, Djibouti, Egypt, Iran (Islamic Republic of), Iraq, Jordan, Lebanon, Libyan Arab Jamahiriya, Morocco, Oman, Pakistan, Somalia, Sudan, Syrian Arab Republic, Tunisia, Yemen
European Region	High	Andorra, Austria, Belgium, Cyprus, Denmark, Finland, France, Germany, Greece, Iceland, Ireland, Israel, Italy, Luxembourg, Malta, Monaco, Netherlands, Norway, Portugal, San Marino, Slovenia, Spain, Sweden, Switzerland, United Kingdom
	Low and middle	Albania, Armenia, Azerbaijan, Belarus, Bosnia and Herzegovina, Bulgaria, Croatia, Czech Republic, Estonia, Georgia, Hungary, Kazakhstan, Kyrgyzstan, Latvia, Lithuania, Poland, Moldova, Romania, Russian Federation, Serbia and Montenegro, Slovakia, Tajikistan, The former Yugoslav Republic of Macedonia, Turkey, Turkmenistan, Uzbekistan, Ukraine
South-East Asia Region	Low and middle	Bangladesh, Bhutan, Democratic People's Republic of Korea, India, Indonesia, Maldives, Myanmar, Nepal, Sri Lanka, Thailand, Timor-Leste
Western Pacific Region	High	Australia, Brunei Darussalam, Japan, New Zealand, Republic of Korea, Singapore
	Low and middle	Cambodia, China, Cook Islands, Fiji, Kiribati, Lao People's Democratic Republic, Malaysia, Marshall Islands, Micronesia (Federated States of), Mongolia, Nauru, Niue, Palau, Papua New Guinea, Philippines, Samoa, Solomon Islands, Tonga, Tuvalu, Vanuatu, Viet Nam
Non-Member States or territories		American Samoa, Anguilla, Aruba, Bermuda, British Virgin Islands, Cayman Islands, Channel Islands, Faeroe Islands, Falkland Islands (Malvinas), French Guiana, French Polynesia, Gibraltar, Greenland, Guadeloupe, Guam, Holy See, Isle of Man, Liechtenstein, Martinique, Montserrat, Netherlands Antilles, New Caledonia, Northern Mariana Islands, West Bank and Gaza Strip, Pitcairn, Puerto Rico, Réunion, Saint Helena, Saint Pierre et Miquelon, Tokelau, Turks and Caicos Islands, United States Virgin Islands, Wallis and Futuna Islands, Western Sahara

[a] WHO Member States are classified as low and middle income if their 2004 gross national income per capita is less than US$ 10 066, and as high income if their 2004 gross national income per capita is US$ 10 066 or more, as estimated by the World Bank.

the comparatively young populations in the middle-income countries, and the even younger populations in the low-income countries. In contrast, more than half of DALYs occur in low-income countries. A further 38% occur in middle-income countries, while only 8% occur in high-income countries.

Global patterns of health risk
More than one third of the world's deaths can be attributed to a small number of risk factors. The 24 risk factors described in this report are responsible for 44% of global deaths and 34% of DALYs; the 10 leading risk factors account for 33% of deaths. Understanding the role of these risk factors is key to developing a clear and effective strategy for improving global health.

The five leading global risks for mortality in the world are high blood pressure, tobacco use, high blood glucose, physical inactivity, and overweight and obesity. They are responsible for raising the risk of chronic diseases, such as heart disease and cancers. They affect countries across all income groups: high, middle and low (Figure 3.10).

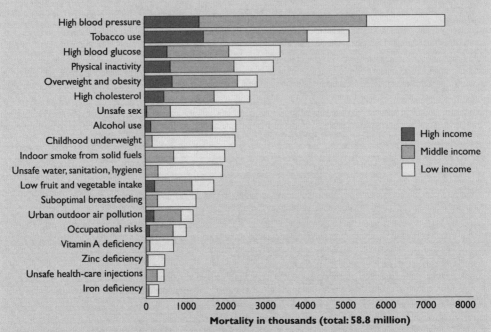

Figure 3.10 Deaths attributed to 19 leading risk factors, by country income level, 2004

This report measures the burden of disease, or lost years of healthy life, using the DALY: a measure that gives more weight to non-fatal loss of health and deaths at younger ages. The leading global risks for burden of disease in the world are underweight and unsafe sex, followed by alcohol use and unsafe water, sanitation and hygiene (Figure 3.11). Three of the four leading risks for DALYs – underweight, unsafe sex, and unsafe water, sanitation and hygiene – increase the number and severity of new cases of infectious diseases, and particularly affect populations in low-income countries, especially in the regions of South-East Asia and sub-Saharan Africa (Table 3.5). Alcohol use has a unique geographic and sex pattern: it exacts the largest toll on men in Africa, in middle-income countries in the Americas, and in some high-income countries.

Geographical patterns
Substantially different disease patterns exist between high-, middle- and low-income countries. For high and middle-income countries, the most important risk factors are those associated with chronic diseases such as heart diseases and cancer. Tobacco is one of the leading risks for both: accounting for 11% of the disease burden and 18% of deaths in high-income countries. For high-income countries,

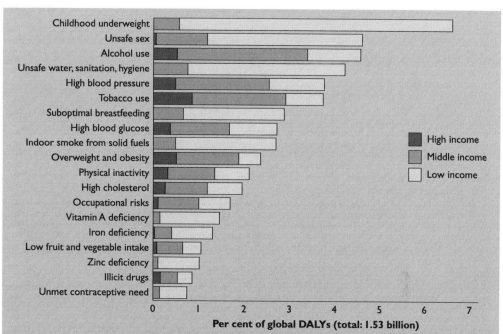

Figure 3.11 Percentage of disability-adjusted life years (DALYs) attributed to 19 leading risk factors, by country income level, 2004

alcohol, overweight and blood pressure are also leading causes of healthy life years lost: each being responsible for 6–7% of the total. In middle-income countries, risks for chronic diseases also cause the largest share of deaths and DALYs, although risks such as unsafe sex and unsafe water and sanitation also cause a larger share of burden of disease than in high-income countries (Tables 3.5 and 3.6).

Table 3.5 Ranking of selected risk factors: 10 leading risk factor causes of death by income group, 2004

	Risk factor	Deaths (millions)	Percentage of total
	World		
1	High blood pressure	7.5	12.8
2	Tobacco use	5.1	8.7
3	High blood glucose	3.4	5.8
4	Physical inactivity	3.2	5.5
5	Overweight and obesity	2.8	4.8
6	High cholesterol	2.6	4.5
7	Unsafe sex	2.4	4.0
8	Alcohol use	2.3	3.8

(Continued overleaf)

Table 3.5 Continued

	Risk factor	Deaths (millions)	Percentage of total
9	Childhood underweight	2.2	3.8
10	Indoor smoke from solid fuels	2.0	3.3
	Low-income countries[a]		
1	Childhood underweight	2.0	7.8
2	High blood pressure	2.0	7.5
3	Unsafe sex	1.7	6.6
4	Unsafe water, sanitation, hygiene	1.6	6.1
5	High blood glucose	1.3	4.9
6	Indoor smoke from solid fuels	1.3	4.8
7	Tobacco use	1.0	3.9
8	Physical inactivity	1.0	3.8
9	Suboptimal breastfeeding	1.0	3.7
10	High cholesterol	0.9	3.4
	Middle-income countries[a]		
1	High blood pressure	4.2	17.2
2	Tobacco use	2.6	10.8
3	Overweight and obesity	1.6	6.7
4	Physical inactivity	1.6	6.6
5	Alcohol use	1.6	6.4
6	High blood glucose	1.5	6.3
7	High cholesterol	1.3	5.2
8	Low fruit and vegetable intake	0.9	3.9
9	Indoor smoke from solid fuels	0.7	2.8
10	Urban outdoor air pollution	0.7	2.8
	High-income countries[a]		
1	Tobacco use	1.5	17.9
2	High blood pressure	1.4	16.8
3	Overweight and obesity	0.7	8.4
4	Physical inactivity	0.6	7.7
5	High blood glucose	0.6	7.0
6	High cholesterol	0.5	5.8
7	Low fruit and vegetable intake	0.2	2.5
8	Urban outdoor air pollution	0.2	2.5
9	Alcohol use	0.1	1.6
10	Occupational risks	0.1	1.1

[a] Countries grouped by gross national income per capita – low income (US$ 825 or less), high income (US$ 10 066 or more).

Table 3.6 Ranking of selected risk factors: 10 leading risk factor causes of DALYs by income group, 2004

	Risk factor	DALYs (millions)	Percentage of total
	World		
1	Childhood underweight	91.0	5.9
2	Unsafe sex	70.0	4.6
3	Alcohol use	69.0	4.5
4	Unsafe water, sanitation, hygiene	64.0	4.2
5	High blood pressure	57.0	3.7
6	Tobacco use	57.0	3.7
7	Suboptimal breastfeeding	44.0	2.9
8	High blood glucose	41.0	2.7
9	Indoor smoke from solid fuels	41.0	2.7
10	Overweight and obesity	36.0	2.3
	Low-income countries[a]		
1	Childhood underweight	82.0	9.9
2	Unsafe water, sanitation, hygiene	53.0	6.3
3	Unsafe sex	52.0	6.2
4	Suboptimal breastfeeding	34.0	4.1
5	Indoor smoke from solid fuels	33.0	4.0
6	Vitamin A deficiency	20.0	2.4
7	High blood pressure	18.0	2.2
8	Alcohol use	18.0	2.1
9	High blood glucose	16.0	1.9
10	Zinc deficiency	14.0	1.7
	Middle-income countries[a]		
1	Alcohol use	44.0	7.6
2	High blood pressure	31.0	5.4
3	Tobacco use	31.0	5.4
4	Overweight and obesity	21.0	3.6
5	High blood glucose	20.0	3.4
6	Unsafe sex	17.0	3.0
7	Physical inactivity	16.0	2.7
8	High cholesterol	14.0	2.5
9	Occupational risks	14.0	2.3
10	Unsafe water, sanitation, hygiene	11.0	2.0
	High-income countries[a]		
1	Tobacco use	13.0	10.7
2	Alcohol use	8.0	6.7
3	Overweight and obesity	8.0	6.5
4	High blood pressure	7.0	6.1

(Continued overleaf)

Table 3.6 Continued

	Risk factor	Deaths (millions)	Percentage of total
5	High blood glucose	6.0	4.9
6	Physical inactivity	5.0	4.1
7	High cholesterol	4.0	3.4
8	Illicit drugs	3.0	2.1
9	Occupational risks	2.0	1.5
10	Low fruit and vegetable intake	2.0	1.3

[a] Countries grouped by 2004 gross national income per capita – low income (US$ 825 or less), high income (US$ 10 066 or more).

In low-income countries, relatively few risks are responsible for a large percentage of the high number of deaths and loss of healthy years. These risks generally act by increasing the incidence or severity of infectious diseases. The leading risk factor for low-income countries is underweight, which represents about 10% of the total disease burden.

In combination, childhood underweight, micronutrient deficiencies (iron, vitamin A and zinc) and suboptimal breastfeeding cause 7% of deaths and 10% of total disease burden. The combined burden from these nutritional risks is almost equivalent to the entire disease and injury burden of high-income countries.

Demographic patterns
The profile of risk changes considerably by age. Some risks affect children almost exclusively: underweight, undernutrition (apart from iron deficiency), unsafe water, smoke from household use of solid fuels and climate change. Few of the risk factors examined in this report affect adolescent health *per se*, although risk behaviours starting in adolescence do have a considerable effect on health at later ages. For adults, there are considerable differences depending on age. Most of the health burden from addictive substances, unsafe sex, lack of contraception, iron deficiency and child sex abuse occurs in younger adults. Most of the health burden from risk factors for chronic diseases such as cardiovascular disease and cancers occurs at older adult ages.

Men and women are affected about equally from risks associated with diet, the environment and unsafe sex. Men suffer more than 75% of the burden from addictive substances and most of the burden from occupational risks. Women suffer all of the burden from lack of contraception, 80% of the deaths caused by iron deficiency, and about two thirds of the burden caused by child sexual abuse.

Joint contribution of risk factors to specific diseases
Many diseases are caused by more than one risk factor, and thus may be prevented by reducing any of the risk factors responsible for them. As a result, the sum of the mortality or burden of disease attributable to each of the risk factors separately is often more than the combined mortality and burden of disease attributable to the groups of these risk factors (Table 3.7).

For example, of all infectious and parasitic child deaths (including those caused by acute lower respiratory infections), 34% can be attributed to underweight; 26% to

Table 3.7 Definitions, theoretical minima, disease outcomes and data sources for the selected global risk factors

Risk factor	Exposure variable	Theoretical minimum	Outcomes[a]	Exposure estimates	Hazard estimates
Childhood and maternal undernutrition					
Underweight	Children < –1 SD weight-for-age compared with the new WHO standards in 1 SD increments (37, 38); maternal body mass index <20 kg/m²	Same proportion of children below – 1 SD weight-for-age as the international reference group; all women of childbearing age with body mass index ≥20 kg/m²	Mortality and acute morbidity from diarrhoeal diseases, malaria, measles, pneumonia and selected other infectious diseases and protein-energy malnutrition for children <5; perinatal conditions from maternal underweight	Updated estimates of childhood underweight prevalence in 2005 according to new WHO standards (35–38). Updated estimates of maternal underweight for WHO Member States (39)	Revised relative risks for child underweight and IUGR outcomes (9)
Iron deficiency	Haemoglobin concentrations estimated from prevalence of anaemia	Haemoglobin distributions that halve anaemia prevalence in malarial regions and reduce it by 60% in non-malarial regions, estimated to occur if all iron deficiency were eliminated[b]	Anaemia and its sequelae (including cognitive impairment), maternal mortality	Updated estimates for WHO Member States (11)	Systematic review and meta-analysis of cohort studies (41)
Vitamin A deficiency	Prevalence of vitamin A deficiency, estimated as low serum retinol concentrations (<0.70 µmol/l) among children aged 0–4 years	No vitamin A deficiency	Mortality due to diarrhoeal diseases, measles, prematurity and low birth weight, and neonatal infections (children <5), morbidity due to vitamin A deficiency and its sequelae (all age groups)	Updated estimates of the prevalence of vitamin A deficiency in children <5 for 2004 (9)	From Rice et al. (42) for 6–59 months, new relative risk estimates for 0–5 months (9)

(Continued overleaf)

Table 3.7 Continued

Risk factor	Exposure variable	Theoretical minimum	Outcomes[a]	Exposure estimates	Hazard estimates
Zinc deficiency	Less than the USA recommended dietary allowances for zinc	No zinc deficiency	Diarrhoeal diseases, pneumonia, malaria	Updated estimates of the prevalence of zinc deficiency in children <5 for 2004 (9)	New relative risk estimates from intervention trials (9)
Suboptimal breastfeeding	Prevalence of suboptimal breastfeeding (exclusive, predominant, partial, non-breastfeeding)	100% exclusive breastfeeding from 0–5 months and any breastfeeding from 6–23 months	Diarrhoeal diseases, lower respiratory infections, other causes arising in perinatal period (infectious disease component only)	New estimates of prevalence of suboptimal breastfeeding from recent national survey data (9, 43, 44)	New relative risk estimates from a random effects meta-analysis of 7 studies, including a multicentre study in Ghana, India and Peru (9)
Other nutrition-related risk factors and physical activity					
High blood pressure	Usual level of systolic blood pressure	Mean of 115 mmHg and SD of 6 mmHg	IHD, stroke, hypertensive disease and other cardiovascular diseases	Updated WHO estimates for Member States (39)	Meta-analysis of 61 cohort studies with 1 million North American and European participants (45)
High cholesterol	Usual level of total blood cholesterol	Mean of 3.8 mmol/l and standard deviation of 0.6 mmol/l	IHD, ischaemic stroke	Updated WHO estimates for Member States (39)	Meta-analysis of 61 cohorts with 900 000 participants from Europe and North America (28)
Overweight and obesity (high BMI)	BMI (height (m) divided by weight (kg) squared)	Mean of 21 kg/m² and standard deviation of 1 kg/m²	IHD, ischaemic stroke, hypertensive disease, diabetes, osteoarthritis, colon and uterine cancers, post-menopausal breast cancer	Updated WHO estimates for Member States (39)	APCS meta-analysis for cardiovascular and metabolic outcomes (47) and new meta-analysis of 221 data sets for cancers (46)

Risk factor	Definition	Reference value	Diseases	Data source	Source
High blood glucose	Fasting plasma glucose (FPG) concentration	Mean of 4.9 mmol/l and standard deviation of 0.3 mmol/l	Diabetes mellitus, IHD, cerebrovascular disease	Regional estimates of FPG distribution for people aged 30 years and over (8)	APCS meta-analysis of 13 cohorts with 200 000 participants from the Asia-Pacific region (57)
Low fruit and vegetable consumption	Fruit and vegetable intake per day	600 g (SD 50 g) intake per day for adults	IHD, stroke, colon and rectum cancers, gastric cancer, lung cancer, oesophageal cancer	Systematic review of food consumption surveys and food availability data (49)	Systematic review and meta-analyses of published cohort studies (49, 51–53)
Physical inactivity	Four categories of inactive, low, medium, and high activity levels (50, 55). Activity in discretionary-time, work and transport considered	High activity level: minimum 3 days per week of vigorous intensity activity (minimum 1500 MET-minutes/week), or 7 days per week of any intensity activity (minimum 3000 MET-minutes/week)	IHD, breast cancer, colon cancer, diabetes mellitus	Prevalence estimates for three categories of physical inactivity from Bull et al. (54). Sufficiently active category split into moderate and highly active using data for 28 countries (50, 56)	Systematic review of published cohort studies (50, 54)

Sexual and reproductive health

Risk factor	Definition	Reference value	Diseases	Data source	Source
Unsafe sex	Sex with an infected partner without any measures to prevent infection	No unsafe sex	HIV/AIDS, sexually transmitted infections and cervical cancer	PAF = 1 (STDs excluding HIV/AIDS, cervical cancer); HIV/AIDS proportions from UNAIDS Reference Group estimates (58), updated using information from UNAIDS Monitoring Reports and other sources (59–64)	
Lack of contraception	Prevalence of traditional methods or non-use of contraception	Use of modern contraceptives for all women who want to space or limit future pregnancies	Maternal mortality and morbidity	Data from World contraceptive use 2007 (67)	From CRA 2000 study (66)

(Continued overleaf)

Table 3.7 Continued

Risk factor	Exposure variable	Theoretical minimum	Outcomes[a]	Exposure estimates	Hazard estimates
Tobacco	Current levels of smoking impact ratio (indirect indicator of accumulated smoking risk based on excess lung cancer mortality); oral tobacco use prevalence	No tobacco use	Lung, upper aerodigestive, stomach, liver, pancreas, cervix, bladder, colon, rectum and kidney cancers, myeloid leukaemia, COPD, other respiratory diseases, tuberculosis, all vascular diseases, diabetes	Updated smoking impact ratios calculated from GBD 2004 lung cancer mortality estimates (2); oral tobacco prevalence for South Asia from WHS-India (70)	Relative risks for most causes from the ACS cohort (69, 71, 72), as used by Danaie et al. (50); from meta-analyses for tuberculosis (73) and for mouth and oropharynx cancers from chewing tobacco (74)
Alcohol	Current alcohol consumption volumes and patterns	No alcohol use	IHD, stroke, hypertensive disease, diabetes, liver cancer, mouth and oropharynx cancer, breast cancer, oesophagus cancer, colon and rectum cancers, other cancers, liver cirrhosis, epilepsy, alcohol use disorders, depression, intentional and unintentional injuries	Updated estimates of alcohol consumption for WHO Member States (75, 77)	Relative risks for colon and rectum cancer added (78); other relative risks from Rehm et al. (76)
Illicit drugs	Use of amphetamine, cocaine, heroin or other opioids and intravenous drug use	No illicit drug use	HIV/AIDS, overdose, drug use disorder, suicide, and trauma	Revised based on trends in illicit drug use reported by UNODC (18)	PAFs from Degenhardt et al. (79); HIV/AIDS PAFs updated using information from UNAIDS Monitoring Reports and other sources (59–64)

Environmental risks

Indoor smoke from solid fuels	Use of solid fuel or coal household use taking into account a ventilation factor	No solid fuel or coal use	Lower respiratory infections, lung cancer, COPD	Updated estimates for WHO Member States (83)	Relative risks come from the CRA 2000 study (84)
Unsafe water, sanitation and hygiene	Six categories of exposure: • Ideal situation, corresponding to the absence of transmission of diarrhoeal disease through water, sanitation and hygiene • Regulated water supply and partial sewage treatment • Improved water and basic sanitation • Basic sanitation only • Improved water only • No improved supply or basic sanitation	Absence of transmission of diarrhoeal disease through water and sanitation	Diarrhoeal diseases	Updated estimates for WHO Member States (19)	Relative risks come from the CRA 2000 study (80)
Urban outdoor air pollution	Annual mean fine particulate matter with an aerodynamic diameter greater than 2.5 μm (PM2.5) and 10 μm (PM10)	Mean concentration of 7.5 μg/m³ for PM2.5 and 15 μg/m³ for PM10	Respiratory infections, lung cancers, selected cardiopulmonary diseases	Updated estimates for WHO Member States (81, 82)	Relative risks come from the CRA 2000 study (81)

(Continued overleaf)

Table 3.7 Continued

Risk factor	Exposure variable	Theoretical minimum	Outcomes[a]	Exposure estimates	Hazard estimates
Lead exposure	Mean and standard deviation of blood lead level	Blood lead below 1 µg/dl [c]	Mild mental retardation, raised blood pressure (which increases the risk of IHD), stroke, hypertensive disease and other cardiovascular diseases	Updated WHO estimates for Member States	Relative risks for mild mental retardation and raised blood pressure from the CRA 2000 study (85); relative risks for the effect of blood pressure on cardiovascular outcomes from the prospective cohorts study (45)
Global climate change	Climate scenarios based on actual and counterfactual carbon emissions and concentrations	Average of 1961–1990 climate conditions	Diarrhoea, flood injury, malaria, undernutrition and associated disease outcomes	Climate change that resulted from unmitigated carbon emissions, as projected to 2004 in the 2000 CRA study (86)	Relative risks derived from observed relationships between climate and health, from CRA 2000 study (86)
Occupational risks					
Occupational risk factors for injuries	Current proportions of workers exposed to injury risk factors	Exposure corresponding to lowest rate of work-related fatalities observed: 1 per million per year for 16- to 17-year-olds employed as service workers in the USA	Unintentional injuries	PAFs estimated for CRA 2000 assumed to hold for 2004 (87)	Occupational risk factors for injuries
Occupational carcinogens	Proportions of workers exposed to background, low, and high levels of workplace carcinogens	No work-related exposure above background to chemical or physical agents that cause cancer	Leukaemia, lung cancer, mesothelioma	PAFs estimated for CRA 2000 assumed to hold for 2004 (87); PAFs for mesothelioma are from Driscoll et al. (88)	Occupational carcinogens

Occupational airborne particulates	Proportions of workers with background, low and high levels of exposure	No work-related exposure above background	COPD and asthma, pneumoconiosis, silicosis and asbestosis	PAFs estimated for CRA 2000 assumed to hold for 2004 (87); PAFs for asbestosis, silicosis and pneumoconioses are from Driscoll et al. (89)	Occupational airborne particulates
Occupational ergonomic stressors	High, moderate, and low exposure based on occupational categories	Physical workload at the level of managers and professionals (low)	Lower back pain	PAFs estimated for CRA 2000 assumed to hold for 2004 (87)	Occupational ergonomic stressors
Occupational noise	High and moderate exposure categories (>90 dBA and 85–90 dBA)	Less than 85 dBA on average over 8 working hours	Hearing loss	PAFs estimated for CRA 2000 assumed to hold for 2004 (87)	Occupational noise
Other selected risks					
Unsafe health-care injections	Exposure to at least one contaminated injection	No contaminated injections	Acute infection with HBV, HCV and HIV, cirrhosis and liver cancer	Previous PAFs for HIV (90) adjusted to take into account a recent meta-analysis of the transmission probability for HIV through reuse of a contaminated needle (92), revised estimates for HIV incidence and prevalence (63) and recent data on transmission modes for HIV infection in India (95). Previous PAFs for hepatitis B and C, cirrhosis and liver cancer assumed to apply for 2004.	Unsafe health-care injections

(Continued overleaf)

Table 3.7 Continued

Risk factor	Exposure variable	Theoretical minimum	Outcomes[a]	Exposure estimates	Hazard estimates
Childhood sexual abuse	Prevalence of non-contact abuse, contact abuse and intercourse	No abuse	Depression, panic disorder, alcohol abuse/dependence, drug abuse/ dependence, post-traumatic stress disorder and suicide in adulthood	Prevalences estimated by Andrews et al.for year 2000 assumed to apply for 2004 (25)	Systematic review and meta-analysis of published studies (25)

ACS, American Cancer Society; AIDS, acquired immunodeficiency syndrome; BMI, body mass index; COPD, chronic obstructive pulmonary disease; CRA, comparative risk assessment; dBA, A-weighted decibels (the noise power calculated in dB); GBD, global burden of disease; HIV, human immunodeficiency virus; HBV, hepatitis B virus; HCV, hepatitis C virus; IHD, ischaemic heart disease; IUGR, intrauterine growth restriction; MET, metabolic equivalent; PAF, population attributable fraction; PM, particulate matter; SD, standard deviation; STD, sexually transmitted disease; UNAIDS, Joint United Nations Programme on HIV/AIDS; UNODC, United Nations Office on Drugs and Crime; USA, United States of America; WHO, World Health Organization; WHS, World Health Survey.

[a] Outcomes likely to be causal but not quantified due to lack of sufficient evidence on prevalence and/or hazard size are not listed here.

[b] The theoretical minimum haemoglobin levels vary across regions and age-sex groups (from 11.66 g/dl in children under 5 years in South-East Asian Region (SEAR)-D to > 14.5 g/dl in adult males in developed countries) because the other risks for anaemia (e.g. malaria) vary.

[c] Theoretical minimum for lead is the blood lead level expected at background exposure levels. Health effects were quantified for blood lead levels above 5 μg/dl where epidemiological studies have quantified hazards.

unsafe water, hygiene and sanitation; and 15% to smoke from indoor use of solid fuels. The joint effect of all three of these risk factors is, however, 46%. Similarly, 45% of cardiovascular deaths among those older than 30 years can be attributed to raised blood pressure, 16% to raised cholesterol and 13% to raised blood glucose, yet the estimated combined effect of these three risks is about 48% of cardiovascular diseases.

Risks for child health

In 2004, 10.4 million children under 5 years of age died: 45% in the WHO African Region and 30% in the South-East Asia Region. The leading causes of death among children under 5 years of age are acute respiratory infections and diarrhoeal diseases, which are also the leading overall causes of loss of healthy life years. Child underweight is the leading individual risk for child deaths and loss of healthy life years, causing 21% of deaths and DALYs. Child underweight, together with micronutrient deficiencies and suboptimal breastfeeding, accounted for 35% of child deaths and 32% of loss of healthy life years worldwide. Unsafe water, sanitation and hygiene, together with indoor smoke from solid fuels, cause 23% of child deaths. These environmental risks, together with the nutritional risks and suboptimal breastfeeding, cause 39% of child deaths worldwide.

Risks for cardiovascular disease

The two leading causes of death are cardiovascular – ischaemic heart disease and cerebrovascular disease; cardiovascular diseases account for nearly 30% of deaths worldwide. Eight risk factors – alcohol use, tobacco use, high blood pressure, high body mass index, high cholesterol, high blood glucose, low fruit and vegetable intake, and physical inactivity – account for 61% of loss of healthy life years from cardiovascular diseases and 61% of cardiovascular deaths. The same risk factors together account for over three quarters of deaths from ischaemic and hypertensive heart disease.

Cardiovascular deaths occur at older ages in high-income countries than in low- and middle-income countries. DALYs account for this difference by giving a higher weight to deaths at younger ages. Among adults over 30 years of age, the rate of DALYs attributed to the eight cardiovascular risk factors is more than twice as high in middle-income European countries than in high-income countries or in the Western Pacific Region, where rates are lowest. In all regions, the leading cause of cardiovascular death is high blood pressure, which causes between 37% of cardiovascular deaths in the South-East Asia Region to 54% of cardiovascular deaths in middle-income European countries. The eight cardiovascular risk factors cause the largest proportion of cardiovascular deaths in middle-income European countries (72%) and the smallest proportion in African countries (51%).

Risks for cancer

Cancer rates are increased by many of the risks considered in this report, and some leading cancers could be substantially reduced by lowering exposure to these risks. Worldwide, 71% of lung cancer deaths are caused by tobacco use (lung cancer is the leading cause of cancer death globally). The combined effects of tobacco use, low fruit and vegetable intake, urban air pollution, and indoor smoke from household use of solid fuels cause 76% of lung cancer deaths. All deaths and unhealthy life years attributable to cervical cancer are caused by human papillomavirus infection from unsafe sex. Nine leading environmental and behavioural risks – high body mass index, low fruit and vegetable intake, physical inactivity, tobacco use, alcohol use, unsafe sex, urban and indoor air pollution, and unsafe health-care injections – are responsible for 35% of cancer deaths.

Other cancers are also caused by infections. Worldwide, 63% of stomach cancer deaths are caused by infection with Helicobacter pylori, 73% of liver cancer deaths are caused by infection with viral hepatitis or liver flukes, and as noted above, 100% of cervical cancer deaths are caused by infection with human papillomavirus. The combined effects of seven infectious agents – blood and liver flukes, human papillomavirus, hepatitis B and C, herpesvirus and H. pylori – cause 18% of cancer deaths. Together with the nine environmental and behavioural causes of cancer, these infections explain 45% of cancer deaths worldwide. For specific cancer sites, the proportion is higher: more than three quarters of deaths from mouth and oropharynx cancer, liver cancer, lung cancer and cervical cancer can be explained by infections, and environmental and behavioural exposures.

Conclusions

It is clear that the world faces some large, widespread and certain risks to health. The five leading risk factors identified in this report are responsible for one quarter of all deaths in the world; all 24 risk factors are responsible for almost one half of all deaths. Although some of these major risk factors (e.g. tobacco use or overweight and obesity) are usually associated with high-income countries, in fact, more than three quarters of the total global burden of diseases they cause already occurs in low- and middle-income countries. Health risks are in transition – and health has become globalized – as patterns of consumption change markedly around the world and populations contain a higher proportion of older people, as a result of successes against infectious diseases and decreasing fertility levels.

Developing countries increasingly face a 'double burden' from the risks for communicable diseases and maternal and child outcomes that traditionally affect the poor combined with the risks for non-communicable conditions. The poorest countries still face a high and concentrated burden from poverty, undernutrition, unsafe sex, unsafe water and sanitation, iron deficiency and indoor smoke from solid fuels. At the same time, dietary risk factors for high blood pressure, cholesterol and obesity, coupled with insufficient physical activity, are responsible for an increasing proportion of the total disease burden. Had the risks considered in this report not existed, life expectancy would have been on average almost a decade longer in 2004 for the entire global population, with greater increases in the low-income countries than in the high-income countries.

The results from the report provide powerful input for policy actions when combined with information about interventions, their costs and their efficacy. Although risk exposure estimates are based on less-than-perfect data, they are often conservative because, as health improves, gains can multiply. For example, reducing the burden of disease in the poor may raise income levels, which, in turn, will further help to reduce health inequalities. Many cost-effective interventions are also known, and prevention strategies can be transferred between similar countries. Much of the necessary scientific and economic information, evidence and research is already available for guiding policy decisions that could significantly improve global health.

Box 3.1 Global health risks: progress and challenges (Stevens et al. 2009)

Understanding the effects of health risks is vital to designing and targeting prevention efforts. However, the analysis of risk factors is challenging due to the inherent complexity of finding and interpreting evidence on risks and their causal associations with disease and disability. Risk assessment is limited both by epidemiologic knowledge and by availability of global information on risk factor exposure. To carry out a quantitative risk assessment, evidence must exist first, to show that the exposure to each risk causes disease, second, to quantify the magnitude of harm caused by each exposure, and lastly, to assess the presence of each risk in the population globally.

Some risk factors are easier to assess than others. Exposure to biological risks such as high body mass index (BMI) or vitamin deficiencies can be measured with relatively little error, and can be linked to disease outcomes on an individual basis. In contrast, it is more difficult to precisely measure exposure to dietary, environmental and behavioural risk factors. For these risks, the lack of precise measurements makes it more challenging to link exposures to disease incidence. Because it is more difficult to generate epidemiological evidence about dietary, environmental and behavioural risk factors, they are less likely to be included in a comparative risk assessment. When included, their burden may be estimated with more uncertainty than for risks that are easier to measure. This inevitably produces a set of estimates for risk factors that are not perfectly comparable and must be interpreted carefully.

Risk factors are not all equally easy to measure and similarly, some prove to be more amenable to interventions than others. To ensure consistency across the risk factors, the burden of each risk factor is calculated by comparing the actual situation to a counterfactual one where exposure to the risk factor is at an ideal level. For some risk factors, such as micronutrient deficiencies, effective policies to ensure adequate nutrition in low-cost settings are known. Achieving the ideal exposure level is feasible and affordable. However, for a risk factor such as high body mass index, few effective interventions have been demonstrated. While some isolated populations have a mean BMI in the ideal range, attaining a low population mean BMI is a daunting task for today's societies.

Assessing and interpreting the impact of risks on health is challenging due to the inherent complexity of finding and interpreting evidence on risks and their causal associations with disease and disability at the population level.

Feedback

1 Several differences among the three mortality groups suggest such that demographic changes and a better economic environment are accompanied by a reduction in the relative importance of communicable disease risk factors and an increase in non-communicable disease risk factors. We can see, for example, a gradation in the relative importance of factors such as underweight, unsafe water/sanitation/hygiene, iron deficiency and indoor smoke from solid fuels, these being most important in high mortality developing countries, least important in developed countries, and of intermediate importance in low mortality developing countries. A reverse trend is

observed for factors generally related to non-communicable diseases, including blood pressure, cholesterol, smoking, overweight and low fruit and vegetable intake.

2 The dual burden of nutritional diseases includes the problems caused by malnutrition and micronutrient deficiencies and the chronic, non-communicable diseases of adults. The rapidity of the nutritional transition means that many low- and middle-income countries must now respond to both sets of diseases.

3 The main limitations include:
- lack of data on exposure levels (risk factors) in the population, and limitations of the data available (for example, due to difficulties in measurement and/or lack of risk factor surveillance);
- lack of data on hazard (estimates of relative risks for the exposure-disease relationships examined) and limitations of the data available (for example, due to remaining uncertainty in disease causation for some risk factor-disease relationships, limitations of the studies performed to obtain hazard estimates (for example, case-control or cohort studies), possibility of residual confounding, and so on);
- the need to extrapolate information on exposure levels or hazard from one population (with data available) to another (without data available);
- lack of data stratified to show potential correlations among risk factors;
- uncertainty around the methods used to estimate disease burden.

Summary

This chapter discussed SMPH with an emphasis on the burden of disease. You should now be able to describe the different uses of SMPH, as well as their advantages and limitations. You should also be more familiar with the GBD and Global Health Risks studies, including the methods used and main results.

References

Andreev EM, McKee M and Shkolnikov VM (2003) Health expectancy in the Russian Federation: a new perspective on the health divide in Europe. *Bull WHO* **81**: 778–85.

Lopez AD, Mathers CD, Ezzati M et al. (eds) (2006) *Global Burden of Disease and Risk Factors*. Washington (DC): World Bank.

Mathers CD (2003) Towards valid and comparable measurement of population health. *Bull WHO* **81**: 787–8.

Omran AR (1971) 'The epidemiological transition: a theory of the epidemiology of population change. *The Milbank Memorial Fund Quarterly* **49** (No. 4, Pt. 1): 509–38.

Prüss-Üstün A, Mathers C, Corvalán C and Woodward A (2003) *Introduction and Methods: Assessing the Environmental Burden of Disease at National and Local Levels. Environmental Burden of Disease Series No. 1*. Geneva: World Health Organization.

Stevens G, Mascarenhas M and Mathers C (2009) Global health risks: progress and challenges. *Bulletin of the World Health Organization* **87**(9): 646.

Ustun TB, Chatterji S, Villanueva M, Bendib L, Celik C, Sadana R et al. (2000) *WHO Multicountry Survey Study on Health and Responsiveness 2000–2001. GPE Discussion Paper No. 37*. Geneva: World Health Organization.

World Health Organization (2008) *The Global Burden of Disease: 2004 update*. Geneva: World Health Organization (available at http://www.who.int/healthinfo/global_burden_disease/GBD_report_2004update_full.pdf).

World Health Organization (2009) *Global Health Risks: Mortality and Burden of Disease Attributable to Selected Major Factors*. Geneva: World Health Organization (available at http://www.who.int/healthinfo/global_burden_disease/GlobalHealthRisks_report_full.pdf, last visited February 2011).

📖 Further reading

Mathers CD, Sadana R, Salomon JA, Murray CJ and Lopez AD (2001) Healthy life expectancy in 191 countries, 1999. *The Lancet* **357**: 1685–91.

Morrow RH, Hyder AA, Murray CJ and Lopez AD (1998) Measuring the burden of disease. *The Lancet* **352**: 1859–61.

Murray CJ and Lopez AD (1999) On the comparable quantification of health risks: lessons from the Global Burden of Disease Study. *Epidemiology* **10**: 594–605.

Murray CJL, Salomon JA, Mathers CD and Lopez AD (eds) (2002) *Summary Measures of Population Health: Concepts, Ethics, Measurement and Applications*. Geneva: World Health Organization.

Van der Maas PJ (2003) How summary measures of population health are affecting health agendas. *Bull WHO* **81** (5) (available at http://www.who.int/bulletin/volumes/81/5/en/vandermaas0503.pdf).

4 Inequalities in health

Martin McKee, Fiona Sim and Joceline Pomerleau

Rise up with me against the organisation of misery
Pablo Neruda

(with acknowledgement to Sir Michael Marmot, who uses this quotation to introduce both the report of the WHO Commission on Social Determinants of Health (2008) and the English Strategic Review of Health Inequalities in England (2010))

Overview

In Chapters 2 and 3 you learned about ways of measuring the overall level of health of a population and why these are important for public health planners. In this chapter we will go beyond average measures of health to discuss how health can vary within a population, thus giving rise to health inequalities. You will learn about why these inequalities exist and what can be done about them. Health inequalities are now prominent on the policy agenda. They are recognized as one of the greatest challenges facing the world today: failure to address this problem could have dramatic consequences for global economy, social order and justice, and for civilization as a whole.

Learning objectives

By the end of this chapter you should be able to:

- describe the main developments in the debate about inequalities in health over the past 150 years
- discuss the evidence for and against the explanations proposed for the persistence of health inequalities in the UK in the 1970s
- apply a framework for action on health inequalities to the development of a health strategy

Key terms

Discrimination (based on the definitions of the European Union) *Direct discrimination* occurs where one person is treated less favourably than another is, has been, or would be treated in a comparable situation on grounds of race, ethnic origin or other factor; *indirect discrimination* occurs where an apparently neutral provision, criterion or practice would put persons with a given trait (for example racial or ethnic origin) at a particular disadvantage compared with other persons, unless that provision, criterion or practice is objectively justified by a legitimate aim and the means of achieving that aim are appropriate and necessary.

Health inequalities Differences in health status or in the distribution of health determinants between different population groups (WHO).

Life course epidemiology Study of the long-term effects on later health or disease risk of physical or social exposures during gestation, childhood, adolescence, young adulthood or later adult life (Kuh and Ben-Shlomo 2004).

Regeneration Reviving run-down or deprived areas, for example by providing employment and training schemes, improving housing, developing transport links, offering local health services, landscaping and creating green spaces from derelict areas etc. (Public Health Electronic Library 2005).

Health inequalities and inequities – working definitions

Improving the health of the poor and reducing health inequalities have become the central goals of many international organizations including the World Bank and World Health Organization, and of several national governments within the context of their domestic policies and development assistance programmes. Using a common terminology is thus crucial when discussing this major public health concern.

Health inequalities affect rich and poor nations. Globally, life expectancy is over 80 years in some countries, including Sweden and Japan, and less than 50 years in several African nations. But within countries, similar inequalities prevail: in the UK, for example, life expectancy in the wealthiest parts of London is over 80, while only 55 years in the poorest areas in Glasgow. There is a clear gradient between richest and poorest (see Figure 4.1).

The expression '**health inequalities**' is used to refer to a broad range of differences between different population groups (for example, countries, regions, socioeconomic groups, ethnic groups, genders). It generally reflects population differences in circumstances and behaviours that are in most case socially determined (Leon and collaborators 2001). The expression 'health inequities' represents inequalities that are *unfair* and that, at least in theory, could be remediable. The term 'health care inequities' is often used to describe unjust differential access to health services, a major concern in developing countries and countries in transition (if access to health care was the same for everyone in a region or country, then inequities in access would not exist), but also important in developed countries where some groups may be disadvantaged in access to health care or even, as in the USA, have no coverage. The term 'health disparities' is also used, particularly in the American context, where it usually describes inequalities associated with race. Importantly, the word 'disparities' tends not to convey the same implication of unfairness, echoing the preference for the word 'variations' by the British government in the 1980s. Although the same or similar terms are used in many countries, it is important to note that health inequalities and inequities within countries are not understood in the same way everywhere.

Do Activity 4.1 to see what they mean in your country.

Age

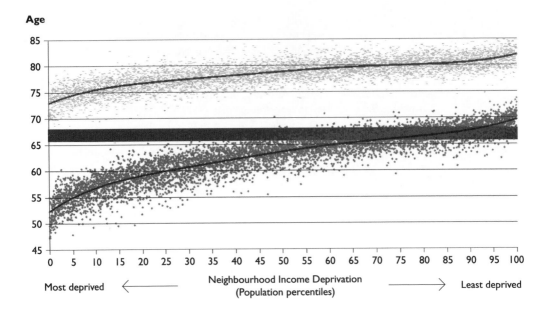

Figure 4.1 The relationship between life expectancy and income deprivation, England

Source: http://www.marmotreview.org/ [ONS data]

Note: DFLE = disability free life expectancy

Activity 4.1

Think about what inequalities in health mean in your country and discuss with some of your colleagues. Write down some examples of these inequalities.

Feedback

In general terms, you might have said, for example, something like:

- Mortality rates are higher in poorer people compared with richer people.
- Poorer people have higher prevalence of mental health problems than more affluent groups in the population.
- Individuals living in a certain region more often suffer from a certain type of cancer.
- People from a certain ethnic background have a higher risk of dying from cardiovascular diseases.
- Poor people suffering from chronic diseases cannot afford regular follow up with a doctor or other qualified health professional.

Your answers will vary according to where you live. Indeed, the way we perceive health inequalities often varies among countries. Some believe that looking at inequalities in health status is what counts. Others prefer focusing on health services as the determinant of health status most readily influenced by health professionals. For example, in some rich countries of Western Europe such as the United Kingdom (UK) or Sweden, health inequalities often focus on socioeconomic gradients in ill health and mortality, while access to health services is relatively universal. However, in some developing countries and countries in transition, the problem is often seen as being related to access to health care, with poorer population sub-groups having a lower probability of obtaining health care when they need it. The constraints that prevent the poor from taking advantage of the available health services thus need to be examined.

Changing concepts of health inequalities – historical background

Research on inequalities in health has a long history, but much of the early work was undertaken in the UK. Indeed, until the latter part of the twentieth century, there was relatively little research, and few explicit policy responses, in many other parts of Europe or elsewhere. There were several reasons for this. The UK was the first country to go through the Industrial Revolution, emerging in large part due to its rich resources of coal and iron ore. It was thus the first country to have to confront the health problems arising in the rapidly expanding, industrializing cities (these conditions have been described graphically by Frederick Engels in his classic book on the *Condition of the Working Class in England*). At that time those in authority felt under pressure to develop systems of social solidarity to prevent the worst consequences of the growing inequality between rich and poor.

By 1860 William Farr was using English mortality data to document differences in mortality between localities. He argued that we needed to understand the differences in the environments in which different classes worked. However, a major step in our understanding of inequalities came in 1911 when the British government introduced into the national Census questions on occupation (rather than simply what industry someone worked in). In 1913, T.H.C. Stevenson, a medical statistician in the General Register Office, used this classification by occupation to generate a set of tables of mortality according to what was described as 'social grades', and later referred to as 'social classes'.

Until then, social class had been thought of simply in terms of upper, middle and working classes. However, Stevenson produced an eight-fold classification, with intermediate classes between the upper and middle and between the middle and working classes and by adding three industrial groups for those working in mining, textiles and agriculture.

In 1921 this system was revised. The industrial classes re-allocated to the other classes to create the new five class scheme in use since then in the UK. The scheme is as follows:

I   Professional occupations
II   Managerial and technical occupations
III   Skilled occupations:
(N)   Non-manual
(M)   Manual
IV   Partly skilled occupations
V   Unskilled occupations

In a paper given to the Royal Statistical Society in 1928, Stevenson argued that 'culture' was more important than material factors in explaining the lower mortality of the 'wealthier classes'. 'Culture', in which Stevenson included knowledge of health and hygiene, was more closely linked to occupation than to income or wealth. He conceded that the allocation of occupations to classes was largely a matter of judgment but he argued that the system was validated by the emergence of a uniform increase in mortality moving down the scale, although there is also some evidence that the allocation process was designed to show this.

For much of the twentieth century, the UK was unique in publishing mortality data by social class, although other measures were used elsewhere. For example, mortality data were disaggregated by race in the USA, showing a large gap in life expectancy (Levine and collaborators 2001).

By the early 1970s there was a widespread sense of optimism in much of Europe. Economies were booming and welfare states were in place. It was widely assumed that a combination of economic growth and social protection would ensure that health inequalities would soon be a thing of the past (this was, of course, before the global economic shock caused by the 1974 oil crisis). Consequently it came as a surprise to many people when a report on patterns of mortality in the UK showed that the gap was as large as ever. The 1970–72 Decennial Supplement of Occupational Mortality took advantage of the fact that, at the time of a census, it was known with considerable precision both how many people in each social class had died (that was always known) but also how many had been alive. By putting the two together it was possible to specify with some accuracy the scale of any inequality. The report showed that men in social class V (unskilled) were 2.5 times as likely to die before age 65 than those in social class I (managerial and professional) and that children in social class V families were twice as likely to die as those in social class I.

Partly stimulated by these findings, a large research effort began in other countries to determine the scale and nature of health inequalities. To the surprise of many, it soon became apparent that inequalities could be found almost anywhere one looked. For example: a study in Australia found that children with no parent in paid work were 25 per cent more likely than those with one working parent to have serious chronic illness; a study in Norway found that the proportion of unskilled men reporting a chronic illness was 1.4 times that of professionals; in the USA the age-adjusted mortality of men with lowest level of education was 2.5 times that of those with the highest education; in France men in low status jobs had 5 times the death rate of those in high status jobs. The precise relationship varied among countries but the general pattern was clear.

In the face of this evidence the then UK Labour government commissioned a report into the causes of inequalities in health. The Black Report, named after its chair, Sir Douglas Black, was completed just after the election that brought Margaret Thatcher's Conservative government to power in 1979. It was immensely controversial. The new government was determined to minimize its impact so it cancelled the planned press conference and made available only a few poorly reproduced photocopies. However, although the government of the day made no use of the report in formulating health or social policy, their desire to suppress the report failed; an unofficial press conference attracted major interest. The text was subsequently published commercially, rapidly becoming a bestseller. The government, meanwhile, proceeded to develop policy acknowledging 'variations' in health, implying 'natural' occurrences not amenable to change and not an emotive term, but *not* health inequalities.

The Black Report confirmed that health inequalities were not narrowing in the UK. It proposed four possible mechanisms to explain the increasing gap: artefact, selection, behavioural, and materialist. These are now considered in turn:

1 Artefact

This is based on the possibility that biases could arise in the Decennial Supplement as the numerator derived from death certificates and the denominator derived from census. It is possible that an individual may not be described in the same way in the two sources. However this would tend to reduce the scale of inequalities as more deaths would be recorded in the higher classes as people posthumously promoted their departed relatives.

Another possibility was that inequality appeared to be widening simply because social class V was shrinking, with fewer people who were completely unskilled. As a result, the average level of health in social class V moved further from that in social class I (Figure 4.2).

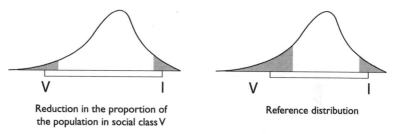

Reduction in the proportion of the population in social class V

Reference distribution

Figure 4.2 The impact of a reduction in the size of social class V

Other possible factors included the changing meaning of social class over time, as old jobs disappear and new ones emerge. For these reasons it was argued that we really could not be sure what the data were showing.

2 Social selection

This was based on the idea that healthy individuals tend to be promoted whereas unhealthy ones lose their jobs. In other words, it is not that low social class makes you unhealthy but rather that poor health causes you to move down the social scale. Evidence in favour of this mechanism included the finding that tall women (by implication who were healthier) marry into higher social classes than their fathers. But it was also known that health inequalities were as great in the retired (and who could not move down the scale as their classification was based on their last employment) as in those of working age.

3 Behaviour

This theory held that the poorest people have the worst health because they indulge in health damaging behaviour. Evidence in favour of this is that smoking is more common in lower socioeconomic groups. However, there was also considerable evidence that behavioural factors and the traditional risk factors that go with them can only explain some of the variation in health. Two other points were also noted: (a) behaviour is determined, in part, by social position, for example when smoking is used as a coping strategy in adversity; and (b) patterns of behaviour by social class, again using the example of smoking, have changed considerably over time and are influenced by government policies.

4 Material circumstances

This saw poverty as the principle cause, with many studies linking levels of deprivation at area level with poor health. To many it was an obvious assumption that poverty would lead to poor health.

At the time the Black Report was published it was not possible to determine with certainty which of these theories was correct. However several research projects in the UK were underway that would soon provide important new insights. One of the most important of these was the Office of Population, Censuses and Surveys (OPCS – now the Office for National Statistics, ONS) Longitudinal Survey. Undertaken in England and Wales, it involved identifying a 1 per cent sample of the 1971 Census and following them up until death. It had several advantages over previous studies. In particular it avoided posthumous promotion and it was able to detect any selection from downward mobility. It confirmed the existence of large inequalities in health, with little evidence that selection was taking place and it identified the importance of factors that had previously not been considered as important, and which led to gradations within the existing social class system, such as housing tenure or car ownership.

Another landmark study also involved following people over many years (a cohort study). This was the Whitehall Study of British civil servants which began in 1967. Even though it looked solely at males who were in employment in the British civil service – hardly a complete cross-section of the population – it still found marked inequalities in health and mortality according to employment grade. Unlike the OPCS study it collected detailed information on risk factors, such as weight, cholesterol, smoking and blood pressure. It showed that, even when all of these were taken into account, they could only explain about one third of the variation observed. The Whitehall II Prospective Study, which started in 1985, is continuing this line of research among London based male and female office staff aged 35 to 55 years working in 20 civil service (government) departments.

Later in the 1980s, several more studies emerged, looking at other measures of health. For example, the Health and Lifestyle Survey, which was a survey of self assessed and objective measures of health in 9,000 subjects in 1985–86. Its results showed that a wide range of health measures varied with social class (for example, self-perceived health, body mass index and lung function).

This UK-based research, together with a growing body of evidence emerging from other countries, showed convincingly by the end of the 1980s that many aspects of health are determined by social class. The explanations based on artefact and social selection had been dismissed and the emerging consensus, which remains, is that health inequalities can be explained largely by a combination of material and behavioural factors. Of course, life is never quite so simple ...

Activity 4.2

Assuming that health inequalities would come from differences in material circumstances (fourth theory above), describe a few possible ways in which poverty could lead to poor health.

Feedback

There are numerous ways in which poverty could lead to poor health. The following description sums it up well.

...damp housing leading to increased amounts of respiratory infection; household overcrowding facilitating the spread of infection; inadequate diet associated with low incomes ... failure to perceive the seriousness of childhood illnesses by poorly educated and informed parents; stresses leading to child abuse; a generally poor environment increasing the risks of child accidents; together with the everyday strain of coping with a demanding young family in inadequate circumstances in areas suffering from multiple deprivation.

(Robinson and Pinch 1987)

Emerging potential mechanisms to explain health inequalities

There are two other themes that are increasingly recognized as important. One is the evidence that it is not just one's circumstances now that determine one's health but instead the accumulated experience throughout life (and in some cases in-utero). This idea is sometimes referred to as the Barker hypothesis, after David Barker, whose research found that poor intrauterine growth (identified from surviving birth records from the 1930s) was associated with disease in adulthood, especially cardiovascular disease and stroke. This has led to a mass of research in what has become known as **life course epidemiology**. There is now compelling evidence to link conditions in early childhood and before birth with a wide range of common (and less common) diseases. The mechanisms vary. For example, cardiovascular disease and cancers may be due to a phenomenon known as programming, in which certain physiological responses are determined in early life, or by exposure to specific agents, such as helicobacter pylori infection which leads to later stomach cancer. The policy implication is that, to tackle inequalities, interventions should primarily focus on the circumstances of children and those with young families.

A second theme is the importance of psychosocial factors. Research has shown that people working in conditions described as 'non-learning' or monotonous have higher mortality from cardiovascular disease after adjustment for social class, or that increased mortality is associated with poor social integration. This highlights the need to look beyond the more obvious material factors to include broader measures of wellbeing. In the past decade, the associations between mental health and health inequalities have been extensively studied: these associations are complex (Friedli 2009). It is now well recognized that poverty is causally linked with increased risk of poor mental health in many diverse societies; it is also likely that long-term and severe forms of mental illness may impact on a person's socioeconomic status. For more detailed account of mental health inequalities in the UK context see the London Health Observatory's coverage of this topic (London Health Observatory 2005).

During the 1980s and most of the 1990s health inequalities were off the political agenda in the UK. When the (New) Labour party returned to power in 1997, their first Secretary of State for Health, Frank Dobson commissioned a report, essentially updating the Black report. The result, the Acheson Report (1998) on health inequalities (not to be confused with the earlier Acheson report on the public health function, 1988) noted that the number of people living below the poverty line had increased considerably in the UK during the 1980s and that the gains in health among the highest social class had not been shared by those in the lowest class. The Acheson Report summarized the evidence on the causes of and responses to inequalities available at the time and made 123 recommendations for action (only a few of which were directed at the health service). This attracted some criticism for being somewhat of a shopping list, since the recommendations were neither prioritized nor costed. Nevertheless, it provided a useful update of the evidence on health inequalities. A major theme, drawing on the work on life course epidemiology, was the need to focus attention on children ('the early years') and families.

Since then government policy to tackle health inequalities focused on intersectoral action, and the resultant Plan for Action (2003) was supported by no less than twelve government departments including Health. Despite the efforts of central government and numerous policy initiatives implemented locally, health inequalities – or 'the Gap' as it came to be known – narrowed only slightly by 2010. Prior to this, WHO had invited Sir Michael Marmot of University College London, to chair a global Commission on the Social Determinants of Health, which reported in 2008 (*Closing the Gap in a Generation*, Marmot 2008) and interest in the subject had climbed every political agenda. In what some feared was history repeating itself, the outgoing Labour government in the UK had commissioned Sir Michael to review progress and make further recommendations. This led to publication of the report, *Fair Society, Healthy Lives* in 2010 (Marmot 2010), after the election that brought a Conservative/Liberal Democrat Coalition government to power. However, this time, the report was published and the new government has stated that it endorses its findings.

The main recommendations of *Fair Society, Healthy Lives* require interventions across the life course, while retaining emphasis on those that will influence the early years of life:

- give every child the best start in life
- enable all children, young people and adults to maximize their capabilities and have control over their lives
- create fair employment and good work for all
- ensure a healthy standard of living for all
- create and develop healthy and sustainable places and communities
- strengthen the role and impact of ill-health prevention.

Potential actions to tackle health inequalities

So what can be done to reduce health inequalities? Goran Dahlgren and Margaret Whitehead developed a framework for action that included four broad areas: strengthening individuals; strengthening communities; improving access to essential facilities and services; encouraging macroeconomic and cultural change. We will look at each of these in turn.

Strengthening individuals involves giving people the ability to make health choices. It recognized that giving people 'Knowledge' does not necessarily lead to changes in either their 'Attitudes' or 'Practices' (the 'KAP' model). It includes, for example, advice on smoking cessation, healthy nutrition and the benefits of exercise. However it understands that this will be less effective with disadvantaged individuals, although it is not ineffective. It also understands that the poor face major barriers to changing their behaviours. For example, in the early 1990s it was shown that families with children in the UK living on social security benefits did not have enough money to meet the basic necessities for life. As a consequence there is a growing focus on empowerment of individuals: this was a major focus of the 2004 English White Paper, 'Choosing health: making healthier choices easier', and government's enthusiasm for Social Marketing as a tool for achieving behaviour change. The UK government since 2010 has largely retained this focus on the individual in its 2010 English Public Health White Paper, 'Healthy lives, healthy people – our strategy for public health in England', although it also favours what is described as the 'Big Society', which, in theory at least, may lead to a more community-wide inclusive approach to health and wellbeing. However, critics have argued that this is a cover for the withdrawal of the role of the state in health promotion. A risk remains that the poorest will continue to be marginalized unless special efforts are made to ensure everyone's engagement. This links with the second strategy.

Strengthening communities can take two forms. One is **community development**, in which local groups identify what are problems to them and develop local alliances to address them. The second is **community regeneration**. This involves integrated action to improve social conditions, with an emphasis on economic regeneration. This is especially challenging as it is often a top-down initiative and faces problems gaining local ownership. There is, however, a growing body of research on what works and what does not. Thus, success is associated with: strong citizen groups; integrated programmes; priority given to employment and alleviating poverty; a sense of partnership; a long-term commitment; and adequate, protected resources. Failure is most likely where there is mainly physical refurbishment, a short timescale, and no locally managed infrastructure in place.

Improving access to services. This recognizes that the poor face many barriers to services (not only health services but also all types of social services), such as the time involved, the cost of getting there, distance (big supermarkets see little point in investing in poor areas), and knowledge of what is available (increasingly important with the growing use of the Internet and the creation of a digital divide). It invokes a concept originally proposed by a Welsh general practitioner, Julian Tudor Hart, who argued that 'the availability of good medical care tends to vary inversely with the need for it in the population served', in other words, those who need health care most are least likely to have access to it ('the **inverse care law**').

The neo-liberal agenda, with privatization of services and commercial consolidation in some countries, has often exacerbated this situation. In many countries, health care and social reforms may make access more difficult. For example, the growth of supermarkets has led to closures of small shops and in the UK rural bus services collapsed following privatization. Consequently, in some parts of the UK, such as the run-down suburbs of some large cities, it is almost impossible to obtain fresh fruit and vegetables at affordable prices (although the situation is considerably worse in American cities, where the term 'food deserts' has been coined). Health care reforms have often led to more centralized specialist services, creating access difficulties for those people who have no means of transport.

There are, however, ways to overcome these problems, including development of local cooperatives, making available finance for small enterprises, and outreach activities by health services.

Encouraging macroeconomic and social change. This addresses the big political issues, specifically to what extent should we redistribute resources within society? The argument can be made on two grounds. One is simply fairness: it is unfair to concentrate ever more resources in the hands of the already rich. However a second argument is attracting more attention from some political commentators. It stipulates that countries with large income inequalities tend to experience lower rates of economic growth, higher rates of crime, and greater social disorder. There is growing evidence that this can be accounted for by the tendency of such countries to under invest in the less well off in their population, and not just in housing and health but also in the skills that are ever more important to compete in a knowledge based economy.

One of the most controversial issues in recent years in the area of health inequalities has been whether societies that have less equal income distributions have worse health. This was originally proposed by Richard Wilkinson and has been developed further in his book *The Spirit Level* (2009) written with Kate Pickett. This research shows that death rates among a group of industrialized countries, from which there were data on income distribution, were higher in those with more unequal income distributions. Research in the USA, at the level of individual states (Kaplan and collaborators 1996), seemed to support this view. You can see in Figure 4.3 the relation (statistically significant) between the proportion of total household income received by the less well off 50 per cent of the population in each state in 1990 and mortalities adjusted for age.

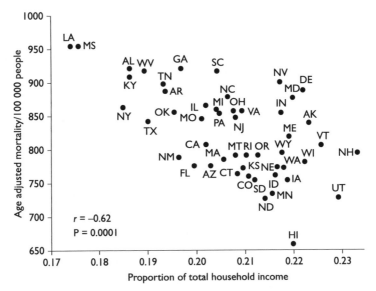

Figure 4.3 Inequality in income in the United States, 1990

Source: Kaplan and collaborators (1996)

This research has been highly controversial, not least because the idea that inequality may be more important than absolute income challenged the neo-liberal belief in the 'trickle down theory'. This theory suggested that as the wealthy became even richer, larger amounts of their wealth would trickle down to the poor and so benefit everyone. As everyone was gaining it did not matter whether the gap between top and bottom was widening.

Subsequent work, however, cast doubt on the generalizability of this relationship. In particular, it was shown that with a larger number of countries the relationship was no longer present, as was also the case when income per individual rather than income per family (with no adjustment for family size) was used. A subsequent study by the same researchers (Ross and collaborators 2000), showed that the association they had reported for states in the USA was not seen among Canadian provinces.

Nonetheless, there is now considerable evidence that income inequality in a country is an important determinant of many aspects of overall health. One of the mechanisms proposed is that knowledge of one's relative position in society leads to psychosocial stress, and subsequently to illness.

The following extract from a paper by Lynch and colleagues (2001) addresses this relationship. You will see that the authors refer to the Gini coefficient.

The Gini coefficient is a measure of income inequality. Consider a society in which income was distributed perfectly equally. If you plotted a graph of the cumulative percentage of individuals (or households, depending on what you were interested in) against the cumulative percentage of income, you would get a straight line (AB in Figure 4.4). But in practice, this never happens. Typically the poorest receive quite a bit less than 10 per cent of the overall income (illustrated by the dots – representing deciles – and the curved line). The Gini coefficient is simply a mathematical representation of this situation, calculated as the area ABC (shaded) divided by the area ABD. The smaller it is, the more equal is the distribution of income. Lynch and colleagues express the Gini coefficient as a percentage; more usually it is expressed as a proportion, typically taking a value between 0.2 and 0.4.

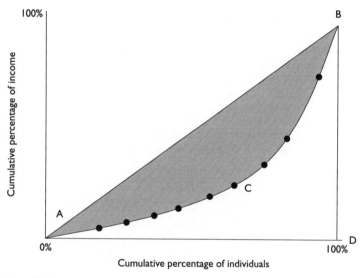

Figure 4.4 The Gini coefficient

Activity 4.3

As you read the next extract (Lynch et al. 2001) below, try to answer the following questions:

1 What are the main challenges faced in describing patterns of income inequality in a country?
2 What do the authors mean by the term 'social capital'?
3 The authors found a strong correlation between the Gini coefficient and life expectancy when they compared all 22 countries. Why was this?

4 What explained the association between income inequality and child mortality?

5 The authors describe the USA as the exception, not the rule. Why?

6 What does this paper add to the debate on the relationship between income inequality and health?

Income inequality, the psychosocial environment and health: comparisons of wealthy nations

Important questions remain about the underlying empirical evidence to support claims that countries with more income inequality and poorer psychosocial environment have worse population health. Previous research has been based on small numbers of countries and limited health indicators, such as life expectancy – a synthetic, overall measure of population health which can mask differences in the age and cause of death structure between countries. Across Europe, between country differences in the cause of death structure have been shown to be important in interpreting differences in the extent of within country health inequalities.

We aimed to assess associations between income inequality and low birthweight, life expectancy, self-rated health, and age-specific and cause-specific mortality among countries providing data in wave III of the Luxembourg Income Study (LIS). The LIS is widely regarded as the premier study of income distribution in the world. We have also examined how aspects of the psychosocial environment were associated with between-country variations in health.

Methods
Country selection
Wave III (1989–92) of the LIS provides the most recent, complete income inequality data available and includes 23 countries – Taiwan, Czech republic, Hungary, Israel, Poland, Russia, Slovak republic, Australia, Belgium, Canada, Denmark, Finland, France, Germany, Italy, Luxembourg, Netherlands, Norway, Spain, Sweden, Switzerland, UK, and USA. Taiwan was excluded because health data were not available. We first examined income inequality and life expectancy among the remaining 22 countries. However, all subsequent analyses were limited to 16 countries after excluding Russia, Poland, Hungary, Slovak and Czech republics, and Israel. We limited the sample because the period under study witnessed the break-up of the Soviet Union, collapse of other eastern bloc governments, and the continuing struggles in Israel. Such social instability may directly affect both income inequality and measures of the psychosocial environment thus making comparisons with countries having more stable political, economic, and social institutions difficult to interpret.

Assessment of income inequality
We used the Gini coefficient, based on equivalised household disposable income, as our measure of income inequality. This is a standard measure providing an overall estimate of inequality that ranges from 0 to 1 – higher values mean greater inequality.

Assessment of the psychosocial environment

We used data from the 1990–91 wave of the World Values Survey (WVS) to generate measures of the quality of the psychosocial environment. The WVS was conducted through face-to-face interviews of nationally representative samples in 43 countries and collected data on political, cultural, economic, and civic beliefs, and other aspects of life. All measures were weighted to generate valid national estimates. 'Distrust' was measured by the question 'generally speaking, would you say that most people can be trusted or that you can't be too careful in dealing with people.' 'Belonging to organisations' and 'volunteering' was the mean number of organisations to which respondents reported belonging and doing unpaid work. Both these questions were asked in regard to a variety of organisations – social welfare, religious, education/cultural, political, local community, third world development/human rights, conservation/environment, professional, youth, recreation, women's groups, peace, animal rights, health-related, or other groups. Mean perceptions of 'control' were assessed from a question on how much 'freedom of choice and control you feel you have over the way your life turns out'. 'Belonging to a trade union' was the per cent of respondents reporting trade union membership. We had a priori distinguished 'belonging to trade unions' from belonging to other types of organisations because of the specific role trade unions play in affecting socioeconomic policies and in mediating social class relations. We also included an additional social indicator from the UN Human Development Report – 'females in government' – which represents the per cent of elected seats in national government held by women.

Assessment of health outcome

Life expectancy at birth (1991–93) was taken from the WHO's statistical information system. Mortality rates were calculated from age-specific and sex-specific numbers of deaths and population counts from the WHO mortality database. All-cause death rates were standardised in 5-year age groups using the new European Standard populations for men and women. We calculated rates for all ages combined and age groups <1, 1–14, 15–44, 45–64, and 65 years plus. Standardised mortality rates were also computed for the following causes of death: coronary heart disease, stroke, lung cancer, breast cancer, prostate cancer, diabetes, infectious, chronic obstructive pulmonary disease, cirrhosis, unintended injury, and homicide. We compared mortality rates for 1989–92 for all countries except Germany, where only 1990–92 data were available. Rates of low birthweight (<2500 g) were obtained from WHO's statistical information system and were available for 1991–93 for all study countries except Canada and the USA (for which 1989–90 rates were used). Low birthweight data were not available for the Netherlands. Self-rated poor health was taken from the WVS, and represents the per cent of the population reporting their health to be 'fair, poor, or very poor'. All outcomes were calculated from pooled rates for the years described above except for self-rated health which was based on point prevalence for the 1990–91 group of the WVS survey.

Statistical analyses

We calculated Pearson correlation coefficients for associations between income inequality, measures of social capital, and health outcomes. All analyses were

weighted by population size and adjusted for gross domestic product, using the
Penn World Tables purchasing power parity.

Results

We first examined data on income inequality and life expectancy for 22 countries in
the wave III LIS database, in figure 4.5, which shows that income inequality was
strongly and negatively associated with life expectancy (p=0·0001). However, this
association was largely induced by the data point for Russia, where the level of
income inequality vastly exceeded all other countries. For the reasons explained
above all subsequent analysis excluded Russia, Poland, Hungary, Czech and Slovak
republics, and Israel.

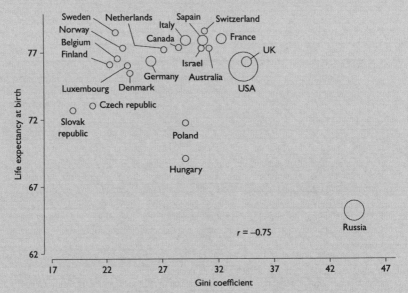

Figure 4.5 Income inequality (gini coefficient) and life expectancy for all
22 countries reporting to the Luxembourg Income Study, for the period 1989–91

Source: Lynch and collaborators (2001)

Table 4.1 shows sex-specific associations of income inequality with mortality by age
and cause, and with life expectancy, for 16 countries. Higher income inequality was
strongly associated with greater mortality among infants, and more moderately
associated with mortality among those aged 1–14 years in both sexes. Associations
between income inequality and mortality declined with age at death, and then
reversed, so that among those aged 65 years or older, higher income inequality was
moderately, but not conventionally significantly, associated with lower all-cause
mortality. Income inequality was not related to life expectancy differences. In analyses not shown, exclusion of the USA substantially diminished the associations
between income inequality and child mortality (eg, female infant mortality from
r=0·69 to r=0·26).

Table 4.1 Correlation weighted by population size between income inequality (gini coefficient) with mortality and life expectancy OECD among 16 countries (1989–92), adjusted for gross domestic product per capita

	Women	p value	Men	p value
Mortality by age				
<1 year	0·69	0·004	0·74	0·002
1–14 years	0·53	0·04	0·60	0·02
15–44 years	0·46	0·09	0·45	0·09
45–64 years	0·35	0·20	0·09	0·75
>65 years	−0·41	0·12	−0·47	0·08
All ages	−0·28	0·32	−0·26	0·34
Mortality by cause				
Coronary heart disease	0·03	0·93	−0·04	0·88
Stroke	−0·46	0·09	−0·56	0·03
Lung cancer	0·65	0·01	0·21	0·44
Breast cancer	0·04	0·89	..	..
Prostate cancer	..	..	−0·16	0·57
Diabetes	−0·21	0·45	−0·05	0·85
Infectious	0·50	0·06	0·47	0·08
Chronic obstructive pulmonary Disease	0·63	0·01	0·12	0·68
Cirrhosis	−0·31	0·26	−0·32	0·25
Unintentional				
<1 years	0·48	0·07	0·46	0·08
1–14 years	0·35	0·20	0·49	0·06
15–44 years	0·44	0·10	0·34	0·22
45–64 years	0·23	0·41	0·07	0·79
>65 years	−0·35	0·20	−0·20	0·47
Suicide	−0·49	0·07	−0·28	0·31
Homicide	0·66	0·01	0·65	0·01
Life expectancy	0·04	0·89	−0·11	0·70

Source: Lynch and collaborators (2001)

Income inequality was inconsistently associated with specific causes of death. Among women, higher inequality was at least moderately associated with higher rates of homicide, lung cancer, chronic pulmonary obstructive disease, infectious disease, and unintentional deaths under age 1 year. However, it was also moderately associated with lower stroke and suicide rates among women. For men, higher inequality was associated with high rates of homicide, infectious disease, and unintentional death from ages 0–14 years, but it was also associated with lower stroke mortality. Income inequality was not associated with CHD, breast or prostate cancer, cirrhosis or diabetes. Exclusion of the USA removed associations between income inequality and deaths from unintentional injury, infectious disease, and homicide (data not shown).

Low birthweight and poor self-rated health were available only for both sexes combined. Higher income inequality was strongly associated with a greater proportion of low birthweight infants ($r=0\cdot79$, $p=0\cdot001$). This association was reduced with exclusion of the USA. Income inequality was only moderately associated with poorer self-rated health ($r=0\cdot46$, $p=0\cdot12$).

Table 4.2 shows that belonging to organisations, distrust, and control were unrelated to mortality at any age. However, countries that had greater trade union membership and political representation by women had better child mortality profiles. For instance, lower male infant mortality was associated with greater trade union membership and female political representation. Similar but weaker patterns emerged for mortality between ages 1–14 years. No social indicators were strongly related to mortality at higher ages, except volunteering, which was related to lower mortality among elderly people.

Measures of the quality of the psychosocial environment showed generally weak and somewhat inconsistent associations with cause-specific mortality. Greater distrust was associated with lower CHD mortality among both women and men. Since distrust and control were strongly negatively correlated, higher levels of perceived control were also significantly correlated with higher CHD mortality in both men and women. Distrust was also moderately associated with greater cirrhosis and unintentional injury deaths under 1 and above 65 years of age. Belonging to organizations was associated with lower cirrhosis among men and women. The amount of volunteering was negatively associated with stroke and cirrhosis mortality. Associations with measures of social capital were unchanged by excluding the USA. Greater trade union membership and having more women in government were both moderately associated with lower unintentional injury death, especially among the young. None of the psychosocial indicators were associated with female or male life expectancy. Only trade union membership and per cent women in government were associated with reduced rates of low birthweight. Poor self-rated health was only associated with volunteering.

Discussion

Our findings seem consistent with a previous study that compared the USA and Canada. Although the extent of inequality was strongly related to health differences between US metropolitan areas, there was no association between income inequality and mortality across such areas in Canada. Evidence comparing states and cities within the USA has been used extensively to support the income inequality psychosocial environment theory of population health. It seems likely that the USA is the

Table 4.2 Correlations between mortality, life expectancy, low birthweight, self-rated health, and distrust, organisation membership, volunteering, control, trade union membership, and the % of women elected to national government among OECD countries (1989–92), adjusted for gross domestic product per capita and weighted by population size

	Distrust (n=14)	p value	Belonging to organisations (n=13)	p value	Volunteering (n=12)	p value	Control (n=14)	p value	Belonging to trade union (n=14)	p value	% women in government (n=16)	p value
Women												
Mortality by age												
<1 years	0·07	0·82	−0·21	0·51	0·25	0·47	0·14	0·64	−0·56	0·04	−0·63	0·01
1–14 years	0·12	0·70	0·13	0·70	0·23	0·49	0·32	0·29	−0·52	0·07	−0·41	0·13
15–44 years	0·36	0·22	−0·10	0·76	0·05	0·89	0·10	0·75	−0·38	0·20	−0·37	0·18
45–64 years	−0·33	0·28	0·24	0·45	−0·31	0·36	0·40	0·18	0·15	0·62	−0·19	0·50
>65 years	−0·33	0·28	0·19	0·56	−0·59	0·06	0·28	0·35	0·40	0·17	0·43	0·11
All ages	−0·33	0·27	0·20	0·53	−0·59	0·06	0·33	0·27	0·36	0·23	0·33	0·24
Mortality by cause												
CHD	−0·61	0·03	0·30	0·35	−0·14	0·67	0·63	0·02	0·46	0·11	0·16	0·56
Stroke	−0·29	0·33	0·02	0·95	−0·55	0·08	0·23	0·45	0·31	0·29	0·44	0·10
Lung cancer	−0·44	0·13	0·17	0·59	0·53	0·10	0·54	0·06	−0·06	0·84	−0·46	0·08
Breast cancer	−0·21	0·49	0·37	0·23	−0·22	0·51	−0·10	0·75	0·20	0·50	−0·12	0·68
Diabetes	−0·08	0·78	−0·04	0·91	−0·13	0·69	−0·02	0·95	−0·26	0·39	0·19	0·51
Infectious	0·26	0·39	0·01	0·96	0·33	0·32	0·11	0·71	−0·39	0·19	−0·38	0·16
Chronic obstructive pulmonary disease	−0·32	0·29	0·18	0·57	0·13	0·70	0·42	0·15	−0·16	0·61	−0·51	0·05
Cirrhosis	0·50	0·08	−0·58	0·05	−0·66	0·03	−0·37	0·22	−0·28	0·35	0·16	0·57
Unintentional												
<1 years	0·63	0·02	−0·33	0·29	0·10	0·76	−0·15	0·64	−0·59	0·03	−0·46	0·08
1–14 years	0·21	0·49	0·02	0·94	0·30	0·38	0·23	0·44	−0·40	0·18	−0·30	0·27

(Continued overleaf)

Table 4.2 Continued

	Distrust (n=14)	p value	Belonging to organisations (n=13)	p value	Volunteering (n=12)	p value	Control (n=14)	p value	Belonging to trade union (n=14)	p value	% women in government (n=16)	p value
15–44 years	0·34	0·25	−0·28	0·37	0·37	0·27	0·18	0·55	−0·54	0·06	−0·42	0·12
45–64 years	0·42	0·16	−0·31	0·34	0·42	0·20	−0·09	0·77	−0·28	0·35	0·24	0·38
>65 years	0·53	0·06	−0·33	0·29	−0·25	0·46	−0·78	0·002	0·07	0·82	0·18	0·52
Suicide	0·34	0·26	−0·04	0·89	−0·38	0·25	−0·45	0·12	0·45	0·13	0·39	0·15
Homicide	−0·03	0·93	−0·01	0·98	0·40	0·22	0·37	0·22	−0·42	0·16	−0·45	0·09
Life expectancy	0·45	0·12	−0·33	0·29	0·41	0·20	−0·44	0·13	−0·31	0·30	−0·14	0·62
Low birthweight (both sexes combined)	0·07	0·84	0·13	0·70	0·22	0·55	0·22	0·49	−0·57	0·05	−0·71	0·005
Self-rated poor health (both sexes combined)	0·47	0·11	−0·36	0·25	−0·80	0·003	−0·29	0·33	−0·17	0·58	0·29	0·34
Men												
Mortality by age												
<1 years	0·20	0·51	−0·23	0·47	0·19	0·58	−0·02	0·95	−0·58	0·04	−0·73	0·002
1–14 years	0·13	0·67	0·01	0·98	0·23	0·50	0·32	0·28	−0·57	0·04	−0·48	0·07
15–44 years	0·39	0·18	−0·31	0·33	0·23	0·50	0·13	0·67	−0·52	0·07	−0·34	0·21
45–64 years	0·41	0·16	−0·21	0·51	0·39	0·24	−0·04	0·88	−0·15	0·63	−0·05	0·87
>65 years	−0·32	0·28	0·34	0·29	−0·51	0·11	0·11	0·73	0·48	0·10	0·43	0·11
All ages	−0·06	0·84	0·17	0·59	−0·53	0·09	0·13	0·67	0·25	0·42	0·27	0·33
Mortality by cause												
CHD	−0·63	0·02	0·36	0·25	−0·11	0·74	0·55	0·05	0·53	0·06	0·23	0·41
Stroke	−0·15	0·62	−0·08	0·81	−0·60	0·05	0·04	0·90	0·31	0·30	0·50	0·06
Lung cancer	−0·07	0·83	0·33	0·30	0·27	0·43	−0·19	0·52	−0·34	0·26	−0·39	0·15

Prostate cancer	−0·16	0·60	0·48	0·12	0·07	0·84	−0·003	0·99	0·52	0·07	0·22	0·43
Diabetes	−0·23	0·44	−0·01	0·97	−0·02	0·95	0·12	0·70	−0·25	0·41	0·09	0·74
Infectious	0·30	0·32	−0·06	0·85	0·24	0·48	0·13	0·68	−0·42	0·16	−0·33	0·12
Chronic obstructive pulmonary disease	−0·40	0·18	0·41	0·18	−0·11	0·74	0·34	0·25	−0·02	0·94	−0·16	0·58
Cirrhosis	0·56	0·05	−0·58	0·05	−0·71	0·01	−0·31	0·31	−0·30	0·31	0·19	0·49
Unintentional												
<1 years	0·67	0·01	−0·33	0·30	0·13	0·70	−0·22	0·48	−0·64	0·02	−0·47	0·08
1–14 years	0·12	0·71	−0·04	0·90	0·32	0·33	0·38	0·20	−0·52	0·07	−0·40	0·14
15–44 years	0·33	0·26	−0·36	0·26	0·33	0·31	0·21	0·49	−0·55	0·05	−0·30	0·27
45–64 years	0·28	0·35	−0·33	0·29	0·46	0·16	0·06	0·84	−0·22	0·47	−0·002	0·99
>65 years	0·47	0·10	−0·32	0·31	0·11	0·74	−0·60	0·03	−0·02	0·95	0·11	0·70
Suicide	0·35	0·25	−0·13	0·68	−0·08	0·81	−0·25	0·40	0·29	0·33	0·23	0·41
Homicide	0·04	0·89	−0·07	0·84	0·40	0·23	0·28	0·36	−0·46	0·11	−0·45	0·09
Life expectancy	−0·14	0·65	−0·07	0·82	0·28	0·40	−0·21	0·49	0·13	0·68	0·06	0·82

All available data have been used but sample sizes differ because some questions in the WVS were not asked in some countries.

Source: Lynch and collaborators (2001)

exception, not the rule, and it is possible that evidence drawn from studies within the USA has less direct applicability to other wealthy nations. Higher income inequality within the USA is overwhelmingly associated with more unequal distribution of many powerful determinants of health. This may not be the case in other wealthy countries where there has been more widespread and more evenly distributed social investments in public health relevant goods and services. As we have argued elsewhere, there is no necessary association between income inequality and population health – it may depend on the distribution of other health-relevant resources and exposures that exist within a country. For example, low CHD in southern Europe may be related to high prevalence and low social inequality in healthy diets, while the relatively low life expectancy of Danish women is likely related to the historical patterns of relatively high prevalence and low social inequality in smoking. Understanding how different countries generate particular patterns and trends in population health is likely to be historically and culturally contextualized. It may not be income inequality or the quality of the psychosocial environment that drives population health in these stable healthy nations. Rather, what may be most important are the current and historical links between income inequality and the distribution of health relevant resources and exposures, and how these links have played out over the life course of different birth cohorts. Levels of health within a country are the product of complex interactions of history, culture, politics, economics, and the status of women and ethnic minorities. These complex interactions might not be adequately described by current levels of income inequality or aggregate indicators of the psychosocial environment.

Feedback

1 Current indicators of income inequalities may be of limited value. Some researchers have raised doubt about their accuracy for international comparison (for example, difficult to assess household income, income is a sensitive topic, different tools may have been used in different countries, difficulty with sampling, measurement bias, and so on). They may also be too simplistic, the authors suggesting that they do not take account of other important factors on health such as history, culture, politics, economics, women's status and ethnic minorities.

2 Social capital is a multidimensional concept used to describe the total mix of relationships individuals have. It is a network of social relations characterized by norms of trust and reciprocity.

3 The association was largely due to the data from Russia as the level of income inequality largely exceeded that of the other countries. The number of data points being small, one such country can have an important effect on the correlation coefficient.

4 The association observed was mainly due to data from the USA, a country that has a very high income inequality and poor child health.

5 Studies that compared states or cities in the USA have often shown strong relationships between inequality levels and health differences. However, this does not seem to be the case when we compare other wealthy countries where there have been more widespread and more evenly distributed social investments in public health relevant goods and services.

6 This study challenges the theory suggesting that differences in psychosocial environments are keys to explaining health differences among countries. It suggests that the

understanding of differences in health patterns needs to be historically and culturally contextualized. The interactions between history, culture, politics, economics, status of women and ethnic minorities need to be considered.

This chapter has concentrated thus far on social inequalities in health, although there are many others, often very complex, in particular in respect to access to services. For example, older people are often less intensely investigated and treated than younger people, even though they are equally able to benefit. Another factor is ethnicity. Gender inequity also exists as exemplified in the South Asian context where gender **discrimination** at each stage of the female life cycle contributes to health disparity, sex selective abortions, neglect of girl children, reproductive mortality, and poor access to health care for girls and women (Fikree and Pasha 2004).

Activity 4.4

Read the following extract from a paper by Raj Bhopal (1997) on ethnicity and health, and answer the following questions:

1 Bhopal mentions the concept of 'black box epidemiology'. What do you understand by this concept?
2 What are the potential pitfalls of research on ethnicity and health, and how can they be avoided?

Is research into ethnicity and health racist, unsound, or important science? Research into ethnicity and health

Expectations of researchers
Scientists want to discover the causes and processes of disease, while health policy makers and planners want to meet the needs of ethnic minority groups. Historical analysis reveals motives such as a wish to reverse the health and social disadvantages of ethnic minority groups, curiosity about racial and ethnic variation, and an interest in ranking races and ethnic groups.

The message from most publications on ethnicity and health is that this opportunity must not be missed. Marmot and colleagues' report *Immigrant Mortality in England and Wales* opens with the statement: 'Studies of mortality of immigrants are useful for pointing to particular disease problems of immigrants, investigating aetiology and validating international differences in disease'.

Black box epidemiology
Does such research discover aetiology? Thousands of associations between racial and ethnic groups and disease have been published with the promise that they will help in elucidating aetiology. The data are usually published in the style of aetiological epidemiology to show relative frequency of disease by means of standardised mortality ratios or similar measures. Few variations have been explained in a way that gives new insight into aetiology.

Most ethnicity and health research is 'black box' epidemiology. Skrabanek argued that science must open and understand the black box. He cited a review of 35 case-control studies of coffee drinking and bladder cancer which failed to provide important information and likened such epidemiology to repeatedly punching a soft pillow.

We need to move from the repetitious demonstration of disease variations that have already been shown in research into ethnicity and health or in work on international variations or in social and sex variations and move to new territory. Studies of ethnicity and health should be able to provide models and contexts for advancing aetiological knowledge if questions for research are clearly articulated and pursued with sound methods.

Is such research unsound epidemiology?

Much research into ethnicity and health is unsound. The key variables of ethnicity and race are vaguely defined, and the underlying concepts are poorly understood and hard to measure. There is inconsistent use of terminology: for example, Asian, white, Caucasian, and Hispanic are common terms in research but have inconsistent and non-specific meanings. There are difficulties in collecting comparable data across cultural groups: for example, do questions on stress or alcohol consumption have equivalence across cultures? There are problems in recruiting representative and comparable population samples.

Data need to be adjusted for known confounding variables and interpreted with the recognition that adjustment is probably incomplete. Rigour is needed for sound epidemiology in ethnicity and health, but the literature is littered with elementary errors (see Table 4.3).

Table 4.3 Basic errors in epidemiological studies of ethnicity

---

- *Inventing ethnic groups* – A study labelled a group as Urdus on the basis of the language spoken, thus inventing an ethnic group

- *Not comparing like with like* – Inner city populations are different from whole population samples, but studies of ethnicity and health continue to focus on them for convenience

- *Lumping groups together* – A paper on smoking and drinking habits in British residents born in the Indian subcontinent did not describe sex and regional variations, creating the impression that smoking and drinking were unimportant in the 'Asian' population. As has been shown, smoking and drinking are important problems in some subgroups.

- *Not adjusting for confounding factors* – Inferences can change radically once interacting and confounding factors are accounted for

---

Harm from such research

Perceiving ethnic minorities as unhealthy – The perception that the health of ethnic minority groups is poor can augment the belief that immigrants and ethnic minorities are a burden.

The focus on a few 'ethnic' problems (such as high birth rates, 'Asian rickets,' the haemoglobinopathies, and congenital defects said to be linked to consanguinity) has been at the expense of major problems. Health education material for ethnic minority groups in the 1980s tackled birth control, lice, child care, and spitting, but there was nothing on heart disease and little on smoking and alcohol.

The comparative approach – Most research into ethnicity and health (including mine) is based on the comparative paradigm and presents data using the 'white' population as the standard. Inevitably, attention is focused on diseases that are commoner in ethnic minority groups than in the white population, thereby displacing problems like cancer and respiratory disease that are very common but less so than in the white population from their rightful place as high priorities for ethnic minority groups.

Ignoring quality of services – The misperception that the needs of ethnic minorities are so different from those of the majority that separate strategies are necessary (but which may not materialise) provides a rationale for national strategy to exclude consideration of ethnic minority groups. The promise of aetiological understanding has meant a focus on variation in diseases, as opposed to the quality of services. There is a huge gap in the research record on the quality of care received by ethnic minority groups.

Fuelling racial prejudice – Finally, racial prejudice is fuelled by research portraying ethnic minorities as inferior to the majority. Infectious diseases, population growth, and culture are common foci for publicity.

Conclusion

Knowledge of the interplay of cultural, genetic, and environmental factors is valuable, and research into race and ethnicity is one way to achieve it. Contemporary researchers also justify such research as necessary to help meet the needs of ethnic minority groups and point out that lack of data can hinder health policy. Inequalities in the health status of ethnic minority groups demand attention. For these reasons, scientists' interest in the relation between race, ethnicity, and health will increase.

Participation by ethnic minorities in research, policy making, and the development of services might be one safeguard against repeating the mistakes of the past.

Senior and I made nine recommendations to help make ethnicity a sound epidemiological variable (see Table 4.4). To these I would add (or re-emphasise) the following:

- Researchers, policy makers, and professionals in the subjects of race, ethnicity, and health should understand the ignoble history of race science and be aware of the perils of its return
- In the absence of consensus on the nature of ethnicity and race, researchers must state their understanding, describe the characteristics of both the study and comparison populations, and provide and justify the ethnic coding
- Editors must play a greater role in developing and implementing a policy on the conduct and reporting of research on race, ethnicity, and health
- There should be wide recognition that, like data on social class, information on race and ethnicity has a key role in raising awareness of inequalities and stimulating policy and action.

Table 4.4 Summary of recommendations to improve the value of ethnicity as an epidemiological variable

- Ethnicity should be perceived as different from race and not as a synonym for it
- Ethnicity's complex and fluid nature should be appreciated
- The limitations of methods of classifying ethnic groups should be recognised, and reports should state explicitly how such classifications were made
- Investigators should recognise the potential influence of their personal values, including ethnocentricity
- Socioeconomic differences should be considered as an explanation of differences in health between ethnic groups
- Research on methods for ethnic classification should be given higher priority
- Ethnicity's fluid and dynamic nature means that results should not be generalised except with great caution
- Results should be applied to the planning of health services
- Observations of variations in disease should be followed by detailed examination of the relative importance of environmental, lifestyle, cultural, and genetic influences

Source: Senior and Bhopal (1994)

Feedback

1 This means that, although we see an association between a given risk factor (here ethnicity) and an outcome, we cannot explain it, we do not understand the mechanism behind it. In the current example, we see health differences among ethnic groups but we do not know what factors might explain them.

2 The author describes various potential pitfalls:
   - ethnicity is hard to define (for example, there are inconsistent and non-specific meanings used, ethnic groups invented, groups sometimes lumped together, and so on);
   - its underlying concepts are poorly understood;
   - it is hard to measure with accuracy or validity;
   - there are inconsistent and non-specific meanings used;
   - there are problems in recruiting representative and comparable population samples;
   - adjustment for confounding factors and interactions is not always done;
   - differences are rarely studied in details in an attempt to explain them (going beyond the 'black box');
   - research on ethnicity and health can be 'harmful' (for example, if ethnic groups are perceived as unhealthy, if the conclusions focus on a few 'ethnic' problems, if they minimize the importance of some problems, if the importance of the quality of care is forgotten, if it fuels racial prejudice).

Suggestions on how these can be avoided include:
- researchers should understand how research into race and health was misused in the past;
- ethnicity should be perceived as different from race and not as a synonym for it;
- the complex and fluid nature of ethnicity should be appreciated;
- the limitations of the methods of classifying ethnic groups should be recognized;
- researchers should provide a better description of the characteristics of their study and comparison populations and an explicit description of the ethnic coding used in their research;
- research on methods for ethnic classification should be given higher priority;
- researchers should recognize the potential influence of their personal values, including ethnocentricity;
- analyses should take account of potential confounders including socioeconomic status;
- results should not be generalized except with great caution;
- results should be applied to the planning of health services;
- ethnic minorities should be involved in research, policy making, and the development of services;
- a partnership between scientists from ethnic minority and ethnic majority groups should be developed;
- a wider and constructive debate on mounting criticisms should exist;
- the presentation and interpretation of research into ethnicity and health should change – from aetiological research to being a tool for assessing needs and inequality and for stimulating and guiding policy action (observations of variations in disease should be followed by detailed examination of the relative importance of environmental, lifestyle, cultural, and genetic influences);
- editors should have a greater role in developing and implementing a policy on the conduct and reporting of research on race, ethnicity and health.

Activity 4.5

Now think about your own country, or one in which you have worked, and identify any groups within the population of this country that are disadvantaged in relation to access to health care. Consider the reasons for this and the nature of any policy response. In particular, think of whether there is any direct or indirect discrimination (see list of key terms) that should be overcome. A potential source of help for this task is the website of the London Health Observatory, in particular its Health Inequalities Interventions Toolkit.

Feedback

The answer will obviously depend on the country you are considering. However you may wish to think of groups that are defined in terms of:

- their social, demographic, or functional characteristics: elderly people, women, the poor, prisoners, disabled people, rural inhabitants, inner city inhabitants;
- minority populations: Australian aborigines, New Zealand Maoris, Native Americans, First Nation Canadians, African-Americans, Roma in central Europe, San (Bushmen) in Namibia and Botswana, or other linguistic and ethnic minorities in many countries worldwide;
- new migrants: refugees and asylum seekers in industrialized countries.

The reasons why discrimination exists are many and often reflect country-specific features. However you should consider concepts of citizenship (who is eligible), the size and political voice of the group concerned, attitudes to multi-culturalism, legal rights, etc.

Tackling health inequalities

Interventions to tackle health inequalities can be introduced at local, national or even international policy level – for example, the WHO initiative to convene a global Commission on the Social Determinants of Health, chaired by Sir Michael Marmot, which reported in 2008, recommended actions to be taken by governments worldwide, with three overarching recommendations:

1 improve daily living conditions;
2 tackle the inequitable distribution of power, money and resources;
3 measure and understand the problem and assess the impact of action.

At a more local level, it is also possible to prioritize addressing health inequalities. In London, for example, the Greater London Authority (GLA) has focused particularly on effective interventions in childhood, following the recommendations of the Marmot Review (Marmot 2008) and its own Health Inequalities Strategy (2010), the publication of which is a requirement under the GLA Act of 2007. The economic arguments for public health interventions are often those most likely to gain the attention of policy makers. This is well illustrated in the report, *Early Years Interventions to Address Health Inequalities in London – The Economic Case* (Greater London Authority 2011).

Summary

In this chapter you were introduced to the concept of health inequalities, including the reasons behind them and the potential actions to tackle them. The chapter discussed the main developments in the debate about inequalities in health, and examined the evidence for and against the explanations proposed for the persistence of health inequalities in the UK in the 1970s. It also described how strengthening individuals and communities, improving access to services and encouraging macroeconomic and social changes could be used as actions for the development of an evidence-based health strategy tackling health inequalities.

References

Acheson Report (1998) *Independent Inquiry into Inequalities in Health*, chaired by Sir Donald Acheson (available at http://www.dh.gov.uk/en/Publicationsandstatistics/Publications/PublicationsPolicyAndGuidance/DH_4097582).

Bhopal R (1997) Is research into ethnicity and health racist, unsound, or important science? *Br Med J* 314: 1751–6.

Department of Health (England) (2010). *Healthy lives, healthy people – our strategy for public health in England* (available at http://www.dh.gov.uk/prod_consum_dh/groups/dh_digitalassets/@dh/@en/@ps/documents/digitalasset/dh_122347.pdf).

Fikree FF and Pasha O (2004) Role of gender in health disparities: the South Asian context. *Br Med J* **328**: 823–6.

Friedli L (2009) *Mental Health, Resilience and Inequalities*. London. Mental Health Foundation & WHO.

Greater London Authority (2010) *Greater London Authority Health Inequalities Strategy* (available at www.london.gov.uk/priorities/health/tackling-inequality).

Greater London Authority (2011) Early years interventions to address health inequalities in London – the economic case. (available at www.london.gov.uk/who-runs-london/mayor/publication/early-years-interventions-economic-case)

Kaplan GA, Pamuk ER, Lunch JW, Cohen RD and Balfour JL (1996) Inequality in income and mortality in the United States: analysis of mortality and potential pathways. *Br Med J* **312**: 999–1003.

Kuh D and Ben-Shlomo Y (eds) (2004) *A Life Course Approach to Chronic Disease Epidemiology: Tracing the Origins of Ill-health from Early to Adult Life*, 2nd edn. Oxford: Oxford University Press.

Leon DA, Walt G and Gilson L (2001) International perspectives on health inequalities and policy. *Br Med J* **322**: 591–4.

Levine RS, Foster JE, Fullilove RE, Fullilove MT, Briggs NC, Hull PC, Husaini BA and Hennekens CH (2001) Black-white inequalities in mortality and life expectancy, 1933–1999: implications for healthy people 2010. *Public Health Rep* **116**: 474–83.

London Health Observatory (2005) *Health in London – Population groups – Ethnic minorities*. London, London Health Observatory (available at http://www.lho.org.uk/HIL/Population_Groups/Ethnicminorities.htm).

Lynch J, Smith GD, Hillemeier M, Shaw M, Raghunathan T and Kaplan G (2001) Income inequality, the psychosocial environment, and health: comparisons of wealthy nations. *The Lancet* **358**: 194–200.

Marmot M (2010) *Fair Society, Healthy Lives*. Strategic Review of Health Inequalities in England Post-2010 (available at http://www.marmotreview.org/AssetLibrary/pdfs/Reports/FairSocietyHealthyLives.pdf).

Marmot M (2008) *Report of the WHO Commission on Social Determinants of Health: Closing the Gap in a Generation*. Geneva: WHO.

Public Health Electronic Library (2005) *Glossary*. London: Health Development Agency and National Institute for Health and Clinical Excellence (available at http://www.phel. gov.uk/glossary/glossary.asp).

Robinson D and Pinch S (1987) A geographical analysis of the relationship between early childhood death and socio-economic environment in an English city. *Soc Sci Med* **25**: 9–18.

Ross NA, Wolfson MC, Dunn JR, Berthelot JM, Kaplan GA and Lynch JW (2000) Relation between income inequality and mortality in Canada and in the United States: cross sectional assessment using census data and vital statistics. *Br Med J* **320**: 898–902.

Senior P and Bhopal RS (1994) Ethnicity as a variable in epidemiological research. *BR Med J* **309**: 327–9.

Tudor-Hart J (1971) The inverse care law. *The Lancet*, 27 February.

Further reading

Bhopal RS (2007) *Ethnicity, Race and Health in Multicultural Societies: Foundations for Better Epidemiology, Public Health and Health Care*. Oxford: Oxford University Press.

Bulletin of the World Health Organization (2000) Special issue on inequalities in health. *Bull World Health Org* **78**: 1–152. This series of papers explore inequalities in health with an international perspective.

Centre for evidence in ethnicity, health and diversity, University of Warwick (available at http://www2.warwick.ac.uk/fac/med/research/csri/ethnicityhealth/).

Evans T, Whitehead M, Diderichsen F, Bhuiya A and Wirth M (eds) (2001) *Challenging Inequities in Health: From Ethics to Action*. Oxford: Oxford University Press. This is an excellent collection on health inequalities globally.

Healy J and McKee M (2004) *Accessing Health Care: Responding to Diversity*. Oxford: Oxford University Press. This book explores issues involved in providing health care to a wide range of diverse populations in many different countries.

Kinyanda E, Woodburn P, Tugumisirize J et al. (2009) Poverty, life events and the risk for depression in Uganda. *Soc Psychiatry Epidemiol* (e publication).

London Health Observatory Health Inequalities Intervention Toolkit: (available at http://www.lho.org.uk/ LHO_Topics/Analytic_Tools/HealthInequalitiesInterventionToolkit.aspx).

Marmot Review Website, UCL: (available at www.marmotreview.org/).

Sainsbury Centre for Mental Health (2009) Mental health inequalities: measuring what counts. Report of Seminar 2009 (available at http://www.centreformentalhealth.org.uk/pdfs/mental_health_ inequalities_seminar_report.pdf).

Taylor L, Taske N, Swann C, Walker S (2007) Public health interventions to promote positive mental health and prevent mental health disorders among adults. NICE (available at http://www.nice.org.uk/nice-Media/pdf/mental%20health%20EB%20FINAL%2018.01.07.pdf).

WHO (2010) Definition of health inequalities (available at http://www.who.int/hia/about/glos/en/index1. html).

Wilkinson R and Pickett K (2009) *The Spirit Level: Why Equality is Better for Everyone*. London: Allen Lane. The second (paperback edition, Penguin), published in 2010, includes an additional chapter responding in detail to the criticisms, many ideological, that were made against the first edition. http://www.who. int/bulletin/archives/78(1)3.pdf [31/12/10] Bulletin of the WHO, Health inequalities and the health of the poor, extract from special themed issue, Inequalities in Health, 2000.

The impact of health care on population health 5

Ellen Nolte, Martin McKee, Fiona Sim and Joceline Pomerleau

Overview

By now you will recognize that a very broad range of activities in all sectors can affect the health of a population. This chapter will specifically discuss the role of the health care sector in promoting population health.

Learning objectives

By the end of this chapter you should be able to:

- discuss the changing views on the contribution of health care to population health, citing evidence from published sources
- discuss ways of assessing the contribution of health care to health, including the concept of **avoidable mortality** and the use of specific indicators
- describe ways in which health provision can be used to promote health

Key terms

Avoidable mortality   Premature deaths that should not occur in the presence of timely and effective health care.

Health system   A health system includes all the activities whose primary purpose is to promote, restore or maintain health (World Health Organization 2000).

Health system goals   Improving the health of the population they serve, responding to people's expectations, providing financial protection against the cost of ill health (World Health Organization 2000).

Changing views on the role of health care

Prior to the twentieth century, it would have seemed ludicrous to most people that health services could contribute to better health at a population level. Whether one survived or died was seen largely as a matter of divine will. This began to change in Europe when, for example, Florence Nightingale (1820–1910) showed that it was possible to reduce substantially the mortality among soldiers injured in the Crimean War by applying strict sanitary routines in a hospital in Turkey. Ignaz Semmelweis (1818–1865) a Hungarian physician, also showed that something could be done when he instituted hand (and later equipment) washing with chlorinated water and reduced the death rate among mothers following childbirth.

Until then, with no anaesthesia, an inadequate understanding of infection, and only a very few pharmacologically active drugs, going in to hospital was, quite correctly, seen as a process that made death rather more likely. By the beginning of the twentieth century, however, things had changed in the more advanced nations. Anaesthesia was relatively safe, aseptic techniques were in use, as were new drugs to fight infection, such as sulphonamides.

Throughout the twentieth century, scientific knowledge grew and with it, advances in health care. The Second World War provided a major impetus for innovation in health care just as in the technologies of warfare, such as aviation. It also led to a vast expansion in the number of people with surgical training, some of whom went on to become responsible for innovation in surgical techniques. By the 1960s many commentators, viewing the shining new hospitals and health centres that were springing up in industrialized countries, were caught up in unprecedented optimism about the achievements attributable to health care, even predicting the eradication of infections and cancer.

In the mid-1960s, however, some contrary voices began to be heard. Thomas McKeown, Professor of Social Medicine in Birmingham, looked at the large decline in mortality that had occurred over the previous 100 years in England and argued that it had been due largely to broader social change rather than to access to health care. He showed that the largest declines in mortality had taken place before the introduction of effective medical treatments. McKeown postulated, for example, that in England and Wales declining mortality from tuberculosis was largely a function of improved nutrition during the nineteenth and early twentieth centuries, by using mortality data plotted against the introduction of specific interventions (Figure 5.1), to which he credited little impact on the reduction of mortality.

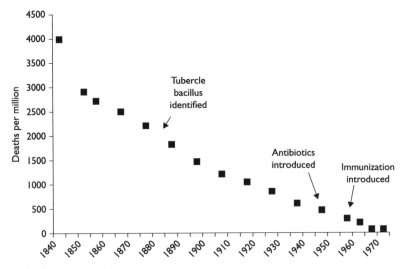

Figure 5.1 Decline in mortality from tuberculosis in England and Wales over time
Source: Derived from McKeown (1979)

Soon afterwards, another dissenting voice was heard. This was Ivan Illich, who in his book *Medical Nemesis* (Illich 1976) argued that medicine was not only useless, but was actually harmful. He argued that patients suffered from side effects of drugs, hospital acquired infection, and the effects of poorly performed surgery. He saw the newly developed technology that allowed for a scatter gun approach to testing as leading to a situation in which apparent abnormalities (which may simply be the one in 20 tests that lie outside the 95 per cent confidence intervals conventionally used to signify the bounds of normality) led to increasingly invasive investigations and treatment, each in turn carrying an unnecessary risk. He described the harm done to patients as *clinical iatrogenesis*, but he also identified a resulting dependency on medicine, and with that a diminution of autonomy for patients, which he described as *social iatrogenesis*. The term iatrogenesis is derived from the Greek, meaning physician (*iatros*) created (*genesis*).

The concept of social iatrogenesis resonated with an emerging movement among mental health specialists that challenged the widespread practice of institutionalizing people with psychiatric illness and the growing use of powerful drugs, which were seen by some as a means of social control of deviancy. Leading writers on this topic included the radical psychiatrist RD Laing and the libertarian commentator Thomas Szasz.

The views of McKeown and Illich have been highly controversial and several commentators have revisited McKeown's arguments. For example, Simon Sretzer argued that McKeown was wrong in some important aspects and, while individual health care may not have been very important during the period in question, social and public health interventions, such as improved housing to reduce overcrowding, clean water supplies, and implementation of regulations on quality of food played a much more important role than that acknowledged by McKeown. Johan Mackenbach examined changing mortality in the Netherlands between 1875–79 and 1970, and agreed with McKeown that antibiotics were only introduced *after* mortality from infectious diseases had already fallen substantially. However he showed how their use was associated with acceleration in the rate of decline. Thus, assuming a general introduction of antibiotics in the Netherlands around 1946, he estimated that between 1.6 and 4.8 per cent of the total decline in infectious disease mortality between 1875–79 and 1970 could be attributed to medical care. He also analysed the impact of improvements in surgery, anaesthesia and antenatal and perinatal care since the 1930s. Taking account of all of these factors he estimated that between 5 and 18.5 per cent of the total decline in all-cause mortality in the Netherlands between 1875–79 and 1970 could be attributed to health care.

Several physicians challenged Illich from a biomedical perspective. While they conceded that in the past many treatments were useless or harmful (examples included the application of hot cups to the skin, the use of strong purgatives, or even rolling a cannonball on the abdomen), they asserted that medicine had moved on from those times and that the treatments made available by the enormous growth in medical knowledge that had taken place in the 1960s and 1970s were much more likely to have been evaluated and found to be effective.

A rather less complacent view was taken by Archie Cochrane, who argued, in a landmark 1972 publication, *Effectiveness and Efficiency: Random Reflections on Health Services*, that far too much contemporary health care remained unevaluated. He argued for much greater use of the randomized controlled trial, in which subjects are allocated, at random, to different treatments (or placebo) and the outcomes measured. In recognition of his pioneering work, the Cochrane Collaboration, an international collaboration dedicated to the systematic review of evidence of effectiveness in health care, was named after him.

Activity 5.1

Many of the commentators mentioned above were writing in the 1970s. Do you believe that their views still apply? Explain why.

Feedback

Clearly the world has moved on and many new treatments are now available. For example, in the field of cancer there are many new chemotherapeutic agents, and some forms of cancer, such as much childhood leukaemia and some forms of testicular cancer are effectively curable. The management of ischaemic heart disease has changed beyond recognition, with the introduction of thrombolysis, angioplasty and other increasingly less invasive techniques, and effective methods of secondary prevention in those who have already suffered a heart attack. Thus, Robert Beaglehole estimated that 42 per cent of the decline in deaths from cardiovascular disease in New Zealand between 1974 and 1981 could be attributed to advances in medical care and Luc Bonneaux and his colleagues showed that the long-term decline in mortality from coronary heart disease in the Netherlands between 1969 and 1993 accelerated significantly after 1987 coinciding with the wider availability of interventions such as coronary care units and thrombolysis. Similarly deaths from major trauma have declined, reflecting improved methods of resuscitation.

However, at the same time as advances in medical care, we have seen that many of the criticisms voiced by Illich, Cochrane and others have been accepted (even if only reluctantly) and systems have been put in place in many countries to ensure that clinical iatrogenesis is reduced (such as surveillance of adverse effects of drugs and quality assurance programmes) and that interventions are based on evidence (for example, through technology assessment agencies).

Yet, we cannot assume that these changes have taken place everywhere. In many countries there are still health care workers who have been relatively untouched by the growth of evidence-based health care and whose practices are embedded in the past. There is a particular problem in some parts of the world, such as the countries of the former Soviet Union, where, primarily because of the long period of scientific isolation before 1990, many obsolete and ineffective interventions, such as those involving light and magnetic therapy, are still in use today (McKee 2007).

But does it work in practice?

If we think that modern, evidence-based health care holds the potential to improve population health, can we test this hypothesis? Although some attempts have been made to judge the achievements of health care by looking at the overall levels of mortality, this is somewhat simplistic. A more sophisticated approach was led by Rutstein and collaborators (1976), for example.

The important study conducted by David Rutstein and colleagues, proposed the concept of *unnecessary untimely deaths*. These were deaths from certain conditions that should be avoidable, on the basis of current medical knowledge, by timely intervention and that could therefore serve as an indicator for the quality of medical care. Medical care was defined in its broadest sense as prevention, cure and care:

the application of all relevant medical knowledge [...],the services of all medical and allied health personnel, institutions and laboratories, the resources of governmental, voluntary, and social agencies, and the co-operative responsibility of the individual himself.

(Rutstein and collaborators 1976)

Using this broad definition, they proposed a list covering over 90 conditions including childhood infections and diabetes. Rutstein and his team acknowledged that the chain of responsibility to prevent the occurrence of a case of death from any of the conditions they selected may be complex, and that the physician cannot be solely responsible for failures that result in a death. However, they argued that the physician nevertheless has a crucial role as being the 'one competent to provide the leadership and the professional guidance' to inform (community) action to prevent such events. Information on these events was therefore seen as providing an index of the quality of care delivered by health care providers, agencies and institutions or by health care sectors. Following this line of reasoning, their list includes not only conditions where the role of medical care appears to be obvious, as for example in the case of appendicitis, but also conditions where the contribution of medical care in prevention of unnecessary untimely death is usually believed to be relatively small, such as lung cancer.

Charlton and colleagues subsequently adopted this approach and applied it at the community level. Accepting that we all must die some time (Benjamin Franklin famously said that 'only two things are certain, death and taxes') they imposed an upper age limit on 'avoidability' at age 65. They also reduced the very lengthy list of conditions created by Rutstein to 14 disease groups, chosen to reflect different aspects of health care including primary care, general practice referrals to hospitals and hospital care. Their work formed the basis for the European Community (EC) Concerted Action Project on Health Services and 'Avoidable Deaths' that resulted in the publication of the EC Atlas of 'Avoidable Death' in 1988. This document was further updated in 1993 and 1997. This work broadened the definition of health care to include collective health services such as screening and public health programmes, for example immunization. The conditions considered 'avoidable' were chosen on the basis of having 'identifiable effective interventions and health care providers'. Now named 'avoidable death indicators', these deaths were intended to 'provide warning signals of potential shortcomings in health care delivery'.

Since then the concept has been refined and extended, in particular by increasing the range of diseases included as new treatments become available and by increasing the upper age limit, as life expectancy increases generally.

There have since been a large number of studies from different countries. They show that, in almost all industrialized countries, deaths amenable to medical care have declined at a faster rate than those that are not so amenable. For example, Johan Mackenbach argues that, in the Netherlands between 1950 and 1984, improvements in preventing deaths from amenable causes contributed almost three years to male life expectancy and almost four years to female life expectancy at birth.

The concept has also been used to compare countries, as in a study that found that about a quarter of the difference in mortality between east and west Europe in the 1980s could be accounted for by deaths from causes that would have been avoidable through consistent application of health care provision. A 2008 paper showed how, at a time when most industrialized countries were seeing large declines in avoidable mortality, the United States was making very little progress (Nolte and McKee 2008).

More recent work on avoidable mortality has increasingly focused on distinguishing more clearly between causes that are amenable to medical intervention, through secondary prevention and treatment ('treatable' conditions) and those amenable to interventions that are usually outside the direct control of the health services, through healthy public policies ('preventable' conditions). This approach was used in a study in Valencia in Spain. It showed how deaths from causes amenable to medical care fell between 1970 and 1990 but those amenable to national health policies (such as traffic injuries and lung cancer) rose.

While the concept of avoidable mortality provides a broad picture of how things are changing, it says little about what might be causing any change. For this it is necessary to look in more detail at specific conditions. In general, there are two types of indicator of health care performance. One involves looking at things that clearly should not happen and such events are recognized in health care as serious untoward incidents and normally lead to a full enquiry into the causes and how to prevent recurrence. Examples include cases of vaccine preventable disease, deaths after routine surgery, or deaths at young ages from conditions where death should not occur if care is adequate. The second group includes diseases that are not always cured and for which both incidence and mortality can be measured: the best example here is cancer, and in many countries much valuable information, including trends, is accessed from cancer registry data.

Imaginative use of available indicators makes it possible to look at different levels of the health care system (although always recognizing that health systems are complex, with each level continually interacting with others). For example, rates of measles infection (which should be prevented by immunization) indicate the quality of public health and primary care services. However, caution is required in interpreting such data. Increases in numbers of measles cases in parts of England since the early 2000s have been associated with the reduction in uptake of childhood immunizations, particularly MMR, following the publication of a paper in the *Lancet*, subsequently withdrawn, which falsely indicated links between the MMR vaccine and autism. This demonstrates how the understanding and acceptability of health promoting interventions within a community is a major determinant of their uptake (Salathé and Bonhoeffer 2008). The existence, in some countries, of diabetes registers, makes it possible to compare survival rates and to draw conclusions about the quality of primary (mainly) and secondary care and, specifically, the co-ordination between them (Figure 5.2). Mortality from diabetes has been found to be a very sensitive measure of health systems performance (Nolte et al. 2006).

The use of more specific indicators also makes it possible to identify when whole health systems are facing problems. For example, in the 1990s, deaths among young people with Type 1 diabetes increased up to eight times in some countries of the former Soviet Union as supplies of insulin became erratic and existing health services faced growing financial pressures. More recently we have seen instances of serious resistance to antibiotics with major consequences for individuals and groups of patients, as a result of widespread excess prescribing over decades of these valuable and easily accessible drugs.

As this section has shown, there is now compelling evidence that health care can play an important role in improving population health. To do so, however, it has to be related to the health needs of the population and to be based on evidence of effectiveness.

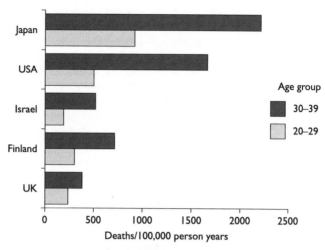

Figure 5.2 Age-specific all-cause death rates in cohorts of young people with diabetes
Source: derived from DERI (1995) and Laing and collaborators (1999)

How can health services be used to promote health?

This section goes beyond the immediate consequences of diagnosis and treatment to ask whether health care facilities offer opportunities to promote health more generally.

Ways in which health care can promote health

One way to reach this objective is by designing facilities in ways that promote health, both physical and mental. In a classic study of patients undergoing cholecystectomy in a Pennsylvania hospital, those given rooms with windows looking out onto trees and lawns had shorter postoperative hospital stays and required less pain relief than matched controls in similar rooms with windows facing a brick wall (Ulrich 1984). Results of focus groups indicate concerns not only about the view from beds, especially among bedridden patients, but also the quality of washing facilities, privacy, and the ability to control noise levels. Other aspects of the environment are also important, with a German study identifying colour preferences for rooms, furnishings and bed linen, in that case beige, white, green and pink (of course, given the importance of cultural norms, we cannot assume that the same colours would be selected elsewhere – what colours do you think would be preferred in your country?). Hospital building design is nowadays more likely to take account of the relationship between environment and health, including the use of colour, open space and works of art. One manifestation of the benefits of a therapeutic design is the international movement promoting the Planetree model (see http://www.planetree.org/).

It is also important that health services meet the needs of those who cannot make their voices heard, the people who, historically have often been invisible to policy-makers, such as those who are homeless legal and illegal migrants, people with disabilities, those with mental health problems and many chronic diseases. For example, in a British study, most hospital lifts were inaccessible to those with limited mobility or with visual or hearing impairments. Surprisingly, health care facilities, which were often built many decades ago, are often inaccessible to people in wheelchairs, but the introduction of legislation, for example in the UK – the Disability Discrimination Act, 2005, superseded by the Equality Act, 2010 – has latterly helped to improve access for disabled people.

Another way for health services to promote health is to send consistent messages. For example, if we accept that the decline in deaths from heart disease reflects improvements in clinical care, and also in people's diet, then it seems strange that we spend vast amounts to unblock someone's coronary arteries using angioplasty but then fail to discourage them from blocking them up again with fried food, a lack of fresh fruit and vegetables, and by being physically inactive. Recent research in the UK has suggested that one in three hospital in-patients are at risk of malnutrition, which is not always dealt with during their hospital stay. Duration of hospital stay is shorter if nutritional status is addressed, so it is both effective for patients and in the interests of the institution and wider society to ensure patients are well fed. A person's nutritional status is dependent on several factors, including access to adequate appropriate meals; poor nutrition among elderly people, for example may implicate a failure of social care provision through 'meals on wheels'. So, in addition to interventions by hospitals alone, a whole systems approach is necessary for health care to play its part most effectively in improving health.

Further, given that tobacco consumption is among the leading causes of premature death in industrialized countries and causes harm to not only those who are smoking but also those around them, it seems strange that we often fail to discourage smoking after an episode of ill health that has necessitated hospitalization. In many countries smoking has been banned on hospital premises within the past few years only in response to legislation. Where action was taken voluntarily to ban smoking prior to a legal ban, the experiences of hospitals demonstrated that it required commitment by managers and health professionals to achieve (McKee and colleagues 2003).

Health care professionals are especially well placed to bring about change. They are still (for the most part) respected sources of advice. Their influence can be deployed at either the institutional or the individual patient level. At an organizational level, institutions that engage senior health professionals in leadership positions have been shown to have better outcomes. At the individual patient 'behaviour change' level, a systematic review of smoking cessation strategies found that one in 35 smokers given brief advice to give up by a physician will do so, and if nicotine replacement therapy is added, this increases to one in 17. Similarly, brief interventions by physicians are effective in reducing alcohol consumption by problem drinkers. The evidence for the exemplar or role model effect of the health professional should not be dismissed, but there is evidence to suggest that brief interventions by a health professional that lack sincerity are less likely to be sustained. So, arguably, all health care professionals should act as exemplars of healthy behaviour, but the reality is that health professionals are human, too.

A recent initiative in England has been the introduction of the NHS Health Check programme for risk assessment, prevention and early detection of cardiovascular disease, diabetes and kidney disease among adults aged 40–74 years. Local Primary Care Trusts have begun to implement the checks very differently, with some targeting areas of greatest deprivation – and usually of greatest need – and others taking a more opportunistic approach. It is likely that uptake will vary with the approach used. The results of evaluation are awaited with interest. So far, for those attending, effective communication of risk and signposting people to appropriate services for further management seem to be important.

It is also important to recall the saying often attributed to Hippocrates 'Primum non nocere' – or 'first do no harm'. The struggle against infection has always been finely balanced, with humans remaining only slightly ahead over the past century as micro-organisms mutate in response to our actions. Antibiotic resistant infection is a growing problem in industrialized countries but rates vary enormously within Europe and across the world. In Europe, rates are low in Scandinavia and high in Southern Europe. Antibiotic resistant infection is clearly linked to prescribing policies and poses a major threat to the way we provide health care in the future. Regarding hospital acquired infection, many hospitals still have inadequate or inaccessible hand-washing facilities and physicians often fail to wash their hands between patients even where there is a clear risk of cross-infection. The introduction of mandatory 'bare below the elbow' policies for medical and nursing staff and the use of alcohol-based hand wipes are among recent attempts to reduce hospital infection in the UK and many other countries. (See more in Chapter 7.)

Finally, it is important to remember that patients are not the only people who use health care facilities. Public health professionals should also be concerned about the health needs of staff and they may also be interested in the health of others visiting their institution. For example, the prominent presence of fast-food outlets within hospitals in many developed countries is difficult to reconcile with a health promoting environment. Outside hospital, community-based health care provision provides scope for health promotion and disease prevention. The long-established health visiting service is an obvious example, but working across agencies to ensure that effective health promoting messages are delivered by workers in education, social care and leisure facilities, for example, offer opportunities for people working across all sectors to contribute to improvement in population health (Sim et al. 2007). See Chapters 4 and 6 for more about the contributions of other sectors to improving public health.

Regarding health care staff, it is estimated that, within the European Union (EU) work-related injuries in the health care sector are 34 per cent higher than the average across all sectors. Increased flexibility of work and insecurity of employment in the health sector have been associated with excessive fatigue, high rates of burnout, reduced employee morale, absenteeism and high turnover. Beyond the immediate impact on individuals working in health care this may also have implications for the quality of care they deliver.

Read the following extract by Yusuf (2002) in which he discusses ways of reducing the burden of cardiovascular diseases.

Two decades of progress in preventing vascular disease

In the mid-1950s, myocardial infarction and strokes were not considered to be preventable. This view persisted until the early 1980s. Over the past two decades, reliable data have emerged indicating that smoking cessation, β-blockers, antiplatelet agents, inhibitors of angiotensin-converting enzyme (ACE), and lipid-lowering agents (today's HPS results), each reduce the risk of vascular events to a moderate but important degree. Today's issue of *The Lancet* has two reports from the MRC/BHF Heart Protection Study (HPS), a large and well-designed 2×2 factorial randomised trial that reliably evaluates the effects of cholesterol-lowering with simvastatin and a cocktail of antioxidant vitamins in preventing vascular events.

The results of cholesterol-lowering with simvastatin are a culmination of experimental and epidemiological studies as well as randomised trials over the past 30–40 years. Early trials of cholesterol-lowering were not convincing because the available interventions (drugs or diet) lowered cholesterol to only a modest degree, the interventions were not well-tolerated, or the studies lacked adequate statistical power. With the discovery of statins, large reductions in cholesterol concentrations were easily and safely achievable, and this finding led to a series of trials that demonstrated benefits in selected populations. The MRC/BHF-HPS extends the knowledge to much broader populations. A 1 mmol difference in LDL led to a 25 per cent reduction in relative risk of vascular events (coronary heart disease and strokes) overall. This reduction is probably an underestimate of the true benefits that 40 mg simvastatin would confer, because a substantial proportion of patients in the placebo group also received a statin as the results of other trials became available during the HPS. Therefore, the real benefits are likely to be somewhat larger, perhaps around a one-third reduction in relative risk.

Clear benefits were also seen in several subgroups of patients who were poorly represented in previous trials. These subgroups include those over 75 years of age, women, those with concentrations of LDL below 2·5 mmol/L, individuals with diabetes and no vascular events, and those with known cerebrovascular or peripheral arterial disease. The reduction in ischaemic stroke, without an excess of haemorrhagic stroke is noteworthy, and confirms the findings from previous trials. The reductions in vascular events were observed in addition to other effective therapies, such as aspirin, β-blockers, and ACE inhibitors.

The implications of these findings are profound. Cholesterol-lowering with a statin is of value in much broader populations than currently recognised, including those with 'low' and 'normal' lipid values. Thus, practically all patients with vascular disease today in western countries will benefit from statins. Perhaps clinicians will choose to initiate and continue treatment with statins in high-risk individuals without routine lipid measurements. The extremely low rates of myopathy and increases in liver enzymes confirm the safety of simvastatin used at 40 mg a day. The lack of liver toxicity suggests that in most patients, muscle or liver enzymes need not be measured routinely. Minimising measurements of lipids and muscle or liver enzymes will simplify the clinical use of statins, and reduce the costs associated with their use. The current results from the HPS study on efficacy and safety were obtained with simvastatin at 40 mg a day. Higher doses of simvastatin may not be as safe, and the recent withdrawal of cerivastatin on safety grounds [in 2001] emphasises the importance of using specific drugs at doses proven to be both effective and safe.

The HPS trial, with three other major trials, also shows the lack of efficacy of antioxidant vitamins in preventing vascular complications. Indeed the small increases in LDL and triglycerides with vitamins in HPS call for caution, as it could well be that prolonged use of these antioxidant vitamins (at least in western populations without nutritional deficiencies) is not only ineffective but may also potentially lead to some increase in vascular disease. Therefore the routine use of such vitamins in large doses should be discouraged.

The lack of benefit of antioxidant vitamins in several large randomised trials contradicts the claims from observational studies that suggested protection against cardiovascular disease and cancers. Several other contradictions between the randomised trial results and the observational data are highlighted by the HPS results. For example, observational studies have described no consistent relation between lipid concentrations and ischaemic strokes, and some have even suggested an increase in haemorrhagic strokes at low concentrations of lipid. Yet an important reduction in ischaemic strokes, with no excess in haemorrhagic strokes, is seen with lipid-lowering in the HPS trial. Furthermore, observational studies have suggested lower rates of fractures with statins and vitamins, higher rates of obstructive airways disease at low cholesterol concentrations, lower rates of cataracts, and lower rates of dementia with both interventions – yet none of these observations have been confirmed by randomised trials, including HPS. These apparent contradictions are likely due to confounding from other factors that may be associated with use of vitamins or statins, which cannot be adequately adjusted for in observational studies. These findings emphasise the need to generally view claims of treatment benefit from observational studies with considerable scepticism, unless confirmed by large well-designed randomised trials.

The past 25 years have seen the establishment of aspirin, β-blockers, ACE-inhibitors, and lipid-lowering therapies to lower the risk of future vascular events, by about a quarter each, in high-risk patients. The benefits of each intervention appear to be largely independent, so that when used together in appropriate patients it is reasonable to expect that about two-thirds to three-quarters of future vascular events could be prevented. Add to this the potential benefits of quitting in smokers (which lowers the risk of myocardial infarction by a half), and blood-pressure lowering (a 10 mm Hg reduction in systolic blood pressure could reduce the risk of vascular events by a quarter) in hypertensive patients, and it may be possible to lower the risk of future events by more than four-fifths in high-risk individuals. Therefore, the potential gains from the combination of currently known preventive strategies are large. Given that over 80 per cent of cardiovascular disease occurs in developing countries, a priority is to make these interventions affordable, accessible, and convenient (perhaps even a combination pill). Ensuring that patients worldwide receive these treatments will lead to substantial clinical and public health benefits.

It is worth noting that simvastatin, one of five statins currently in use, has been made available in the UK for over-the-counter sales in pharmacies since July 2004. NICE guidance (NICE 2006), which promotes the use of statins for both primary and secondary prevention, is based on evidence of consistently low incidence of adverse effects.

The next extract by Robert Beaglehole (2001) also discusses ways of reducing the burden of cardiovascular diseases but from a different approach.

Activity 5.2

As you read the extract below by Robert Beaglehole (2001) make notes comparing and contrasting his policy implications with those of Yusuf (in the extract above).

 Global cardiovascular disease prevention: time to get serious
This year there will be an estimated 56 million deaths globally. The two leading causes, coronary heart disease and stroke, will be responsible for 7·0 million and 5·5 million deaths, respectively. For demographic reasons, most of these deaths occur in the poorer regions of the world. The pattern will probably be unchanged in 2020.

Causes of cardiovascular disease

The proximal causes of the cardiovascular disease epidemics are well known. The major risk factors – inappropriate diet and physical inactivity (as expressed through unfavourable lipid concentrations, high body mass index, and raised blood pressure), together with tobacco use – explain at least 75 per cent of new cases of cardiovascular disease. In the absence of these risk factors, cardiovascular disease is a rare cause of death. The optimum levels of cardiovascular disease risk factors are known; unfortunately, only about 5 per cent of the adult population of developed countries are at low risk with optimum risk factor levels.

There is now a strong case for diverting scientists, the bodies that fund them, and the journals that publish their work, away from aetiological research and towards the more challenging task of identifying the best ways of enabling people and populations to lower their risk of cardiovascular disease.

Prevention priorities

The important policy question now, especially for less-developed countries, is the appropriate balance between primary and secondary prevention and between the population and high-risk approach to primary prevention. The only strategy with the potential to greatly increase the proportion of the population at low-risk status is the population-wide approach to primary prevention. All other strategies will, at best, only restrain the epidemics; they will not prevent them. The challenge is to implement the population approach to primary prevention, that is, to shift the population risk factor distributions to the left. Since the aim should be reduction of population risk, and since 95 per cent of the population is not at the optimum risk level, most resources should be directed towards this aim. This challenge will require strong government leadership including fiscal, taxation, and other cross-sectoral policies appropriate for less-developed countries. The real challenge is to redirect resources to population-wide measures, away from strategies directed towards individuals.

Evidence is available in support of the policies needed for the task of shifting risk factor distributions. Data from the Asia Pacific Cohort Studies Collaboration, for example, indicate that a 2 per cent reduction of mean blood pressure (about 3 mm Hg in blood diastolic pressure), achieved by a shift of the blood pressure distribution to the left, has the potential to prevent 1·2 million deaths from stroke (about 15 per cent of all deaths from stroke) and 0·6 million from coronary heart disease (6 per cent of all deaths from coronary heart disease) every year by 2020 in the Asia Pacific region alone. Reductions in mean population blood-pressure values of this magnitude have been achieved in the USA, and could readily be achieved in many populations by reducing the salt content of manufactured food. Favourable shifts in the population distributions of abnormal blood lipid concentrations could be achieved by the maintenance of healthy diets in the face of urbanisation, and the promotion of the traditional Mediterranean diet. The promotion of physical activity is a public health priority, especially in the context of nutritional abundance, and to counter the pandemic of obesity; serious attention should be given to the environmental determinants of obesity and physical inactivity.

Control of the tobacco industry remains an absolute health priority for all countries. The two main aims in tobacco control are to support the expressed desire of most adult smokers in many countries to give up smoking, and to reduce the uptake of smoking by young people. Achievement of the adult cessation goal will have a major positive effect on the burden of the tobacco pandemics in a relatively short time; strong government action – ie, the provision of subsidised cessation therapies – is needed. Smoking cessation by health workers and in patients with clinical cardiovascular disease are two obvious immediate priorities. The long-term aim is for smoke-free societies; the health effect of successful population-based youth programmes will not, however, be evident for decades. The relations between risk factors and disease events are continuous, and most events occur in people in the middle range of the risk factor distribution who are not normally judged high risk. The effort expended on measuring risk factors in individuals is, therefore, questionable. Since most of the population is at risk in developed countries, and because this strategy is particularly inappropriate for less-developed countries, promotion of the measurement of risk factors, such as blood pressure and cholesterol concentrations, should be stopped, except for surveillance purposes. Perhaps high-risk status can be assessed simply with information on age, family history, past history of disease, and smoking status. On the basis of these questions, health professionals might be able to identify people who would warrant tobacco cessation help and cheap blood pressure and cholesterol lowering medication, even in the absence of knowledge of their biomedical risk factor levels. There is, after all, increasing evidence of benefits at all levels of risk factors in high risk individuals. These issues are of special relevance to less-developed countries, where resources used for individual risk assessment could be used for the primary aim of reducing population risk or for treatment. In these countries, only cheap and effective secondary preventive interventions should be used – that is, aspirin after myocardial infarction.

Advancement of global cardiovascular disease prevention needs strong international leadership and a willingness to work with communicable disease control initiatives in rebuilding public health infrastructures. WHO is again assuming this role, but support is also needed from non-governmental organisations.

Feedback

Beaglehole argues that the major and well known risk factors for cardiovascular disease (inappropriate diet, physical inactivity and smoking) explain up to 75 per cent of new cases of cardiovascular disease. For this reason research should divert its efforts away from aetiological studies into new risk factors towards identifying ways that are suitable to reduce levels of risk factors in populations (that is, the public health approach). In view of the high burden of cardiovascular disease worldwide and the knowledge about factors causing this burden already accumulated he strongly argues that available resources and policy strategies should be directed towards the population approach to primary prevention ('Measures seeking to prevent the initial occurrence of a disease by personal and communal efforts'), that is, increasing the proportion of the population at low risk, rather than promoting further the individualistic approach, that is, identifying and treating individuals at high risk.

Yusuf reviews the progress that has been made in preventing (cardio)vascular disease over the last 20 years, focusing on the benefits gained from treating high-risk individuals through secondary prevention efforts ('Measures seeking to arrest or retard disease through early detection and appropriate treatment or to reduce the occurrence of and the establishment of chronicity'). Recognizing that about 80 per cent of the global burden of cardiovascular disease occurs in developing countries he argues that the priority should be to make secondary prevention interventions affordable, accessible and convenient to ensure that patients worldwide will benefit from treatment.

The arguments given by Beaglehole and Yusuf emphasize different approaches that are ultimately both aimed at reducing the global burden of cardiovascular disease. There is no right or wrong answer; both approaches are valid, moreover, they complement each other in achieving this aim. The perspective adopted by each writer very much reflects the work they are involved in as will the perspective you may have adopted in reading the two papers. Again, both visions have advantages and disadvantages; a comprehensive and effective strategy to combat the global burden of cardiovascular disease will adopt an approach balancing both views.

Infant mortality

Infant mortality has traditionally been used as a key measure of population health in international comparisons. It is commonly regarded as a sensitive indicator of living conditions and of the coverage and quality of health care in a given country. In England, for example, infant mortality was chosen as one key indicator within the National Health Services (NHS) Performance Framework that is also viewed as supporting the UK's national health inequalities target to narrow the gap in infant mortality rates between children of fathers in manual social groups and the population as a whole. However, aggregate measures such as infant mortality provide only limited information about the determinants of health in early life. They may conceal different trends in neonatal and postneonatal mortality, since *postneonatal* mortality is strongly related to socioeconomic factors while *neonatal* mortality may more closely reflect the quality of medical care. The impact on neonatal mortality has been studied to monitor changes in European countries during periods of major transition, where access to health care, drugs and equipment changed markedly in a relatively short period of time in the 1990s. Koupilová and colleagues compared neonatal mortality in Sweden with the Czech Republic and demonstrated the impact of transition (Koupilová et al. 1998).

So it is generally considered that infant mortality can be a useful indicator of the quality of medical care but:

- it should be looked at in association with other measures, such as avoidable mortality; and
- in considering infant mortality one should take account of differences in underlying factors that increase the risk of a death in infancy. This, as several groups noted, can most easily be done by adjusting for differences in birth weight. Low birth weight is associated with adverse socioeconomic factors.

Causality

The question of whether one thing causes another is at the heart of epidemiology. In an ideal world, we would take a group of people, divide them into two groups at random, so that each group was identical, in every way, to the other, and expose one to the factor in question while keeping the other group unexposed. This is essentially what we do when we test the effectiveness of drugs – the randomized (because which individual receives the intervention is decided randomly) controlled (because there is a control group to compare with) trial. In risk factor epidemiology this is not so easy. Think about the practicalities and ethical issues involved in, say, looking for the effects of smoking or diet. As a consequence, we often have to look for associations between potential risk factors and diseases, for example, the observation in the 1950s that people who smoke seemed to be especially likely to get lung cancer. However, just because two things are associated, it does not mean that they are related causally, in other words, that one causes the other. They may simply occur in the same people – lots of risk factors cluster (think about the things people who live in deprived areas are exposed to).

Epidemiologists have, inevitably, given this issue some thought. In 1965 Sir Austin Bradford Hill developed a series of nine criteria of causality. When applying them it is still necessary to use judgement: not all might apply in a given set of circumstances and as Bradford Hill said, these are not hard and fast rules. However, if only a few of the criteria apply, you should think carefully about whether a causal relationship really exists.

The criteria are:

Strength of association: A strong association is more likely to be causal (although a weak association can be too).

Consistency: Where an association is seen consistently in different circumstances it is more likely to be causal. Again, inconsistency does not exclude causality as something may be causal only in certain circumstances, such as people with particular genetic make-up.

Specificity: The cause should lead to a single, rather than multiple outcomes. This criterion has since been criticized and is generally seen as not very helpful as it is clear that some factors, such as tobacco, cause many diseases.

Temporality: Exposure to the cause should occur before the outcome.

Biological gradient: There should be a dose-response curve – the greater the exposure, the greater the risk of disease. There are, of course, exceptions.

Biological plausibility: It should make sense in the light of what is known about bio-logical mechanisms. Of course, epidemiological research may stimulate research in basic science that may revise what is known about biological mechanisms.

Coherence: It should be consistent with common sense. Given that tobacco is inhaled and not painted on the skin or eaten, it makes sense that it causes lung cancer and not skin or colon cancer.

Experimental evidence: This is rarely available for humans but animal studies may help.

Analogy: For example, if one drug can cause birth defects then it is plausible that another one might.

Clearly these criteria are not perfect, and they have been criticized by some. For example, Ken Rothman favours the view that scientists should simply report the evidence and leave it to others to make judgements, suggesting that scepticism is preferable in science. However, for those in public health who feel that we have an obligation to make a judgement, these criteria may help. See *Introduction to Epidemiology* in this book series for much more on epidemiology.

Activity 5.3

Look at Figure 5.3 which shows trends in infant, neonatal, and postneonatal mortality in East and West Germany between 1972 and 1997. Analyse these trends and prepare

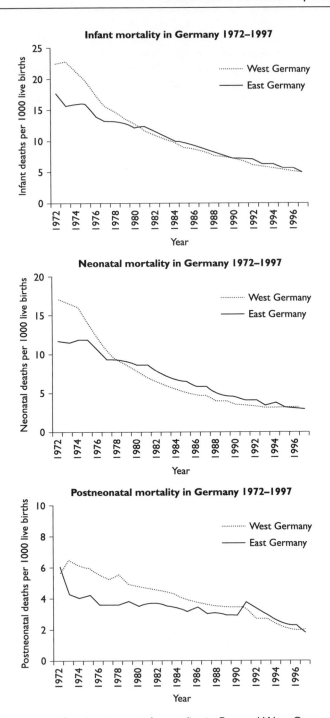

Figure 5.3 Trends in infant, neonatal and postneonatal mortality in East and West Germany between 1972 and 1997

Source: Nolte et al. (2000)

a briefing note (of no more than 800 words) for the German health minister that answers the following questions:

1 What do the figures tell us about health care in east and west Germany?
2 What do they tell us about other factors that may have influenced trends?
3 Make a recommendation on whether infant mortality is an appropriate indicator for quality of health care, justifying your point of view.

Feedback

1 Both parts of Germany experienced considerable declines in the infant mortality rate (IMR) between 1972 and 1997. Until 1980, infant mortality was higher in west Germany than in east Germany; since then, IMR was very similar in both parts.

The decline in infant mortality was due to a decline in both neonatal and postneonatal mortality in both parts of Germany although the pattern differed between the two countries. Thus, neonatal mortality (NMR), although initially (until 1978) higher fell much more steeply in the west, resulting in higher NMR in the east from 1978 onwards until 1995, when rates became similar to those in the west. Until 1990, postneonatal mortality (PNMR) was consistently higher in west Germany than in the east, where rates had fallen steeply already in the early 1970s. In 1990, east Germany experienced a small increase in PNMR, which soon fell again to become similar to PNMR in the west by 1997.

2 Based on the observed declining trends in infant mortality one may conclude that both countries experienced improvements in living standards and health care, both impacting on infant health. However, since NMR was lower in the west throughout the 1980s one may speculate that access to and/or quality of peri/neonatal care may have been better in west Germany in the 1980s than in the east since NMR is usually more closely related to health care. To support this statement one would need to look at additional data, for example birthweight-specific neonatal mortality. In contrast, looking at PNMR one may conclude that access to and/or quality of postnatal care may have been superior in the east throughout much of the 1970s and 1980s. One may wish to look at the causes of death to explore this assertion further, for example, looking at the frequency of sudden infant death (SID) or data on utilization of postnatal care.

Finally, in looking at IMR across different countries one needs to be aware of possible limitations of data comparability regarding completeness of registration of live births and deaths. For example, until 1990 east Germany used a definition of a live birth which was more restrictive (the definition requires the presence of a heart beat *and* breathing) than that used in the west (the definition requires the presence of a heart beat *or* breathing *or* pulsating umbilical cord). As a consequence, infant mortality in east Germany was slightly underestimated as some of the deaths occurring immediately after birth would have been considered stillbirths and so excluded, unlike in west Germany.

3 Following from the above: infant mortality can be a good indicator of the quality of medical care but
  - it should be looked at in association with other measures, such as avoidable mortality.
  - you should ideally take account of differences in underlying factors that increase the risk of a death in infancy. This, as several groups noted, can most easily be done by adjusting for differences in birth weight. Low birth weight is associated with adverse socioeconomic factors.

Source of data on health care systems in Europe

The Health Systems in Transition Profiles (HiTs) provide comparative and analytical views into health care systems in Europe. These reports are produced by the European Observatory on Health Systems and Policies, in which LSHTM is a partner, along with the London School of Economics, a number of European governments, the European Commission, the European Investment Bank and the World Bank. In addition to the HiTs, the Observatory produces overviews of a wide range of issues relating to health systems in high- and middle-income countries.

Activity 5.4

The HiTs can be obtained freely from the European Observatory website. They are about 80 to 120 pages long so you will probably want to read them online rather than printing them out.

Go to the Observatory website (http://www.euro.who.int/en/home/projects/ observatory, European Observatory on Health Systems and Policies). Select 'Health Systems Profiles'.

Select the 2009 HiT for Slovenia. Browse through the document and find the following information (take advantage of this exercise to see the type of information provided in the HiTs – they all use the same format):

1 life expectancy in Slovenia in 2006; life expectancy in Austria in 2006
2 number of acute hospital beds per 1000 population in 2007 in Slovenia

Feedback

1 Life expectancy 78.4 years in Slovenia; 80.2 years in Austria
2 3.77 acute care beds per 1000 population

Summary

You should now be familiar with the main views and issues related to the role of health care in promoting and ensuring the health of a population. This chapter examined the changing views on the contribution of health care to population health. It discussed different approaches used to assess the contribution of health care to health and described how health services can be used to promote health.

References

Beaglehole R (2001) Global cardiovascular disease prevention: time to get serious. *The Lancet* **358**: 661–3.
Cochrane AL (1972) *Effectiveness and Efficiency: Random Reflections on Health Services.* London: Nuffield Provincial Hospitals Trust.
DERI (Diabetes Epidemiology Research International) Study (1995) International analysis of insulin-dependent diabetes mellitus mortality: a preventable mortality perspective. *Am J Epidemiol* **142**: 612–18.

European Observatory on Health Systems and Policies (2005) *Home page*. Brussels: European Observatory on Health Systems and Policies (available at http://www.euro.who.int/observatory).

Illich I (1976) *Medical Nemesis: The Expropriation of Health*. New York: Pantheon Books.

Koupilová I, McKee M and Holčík J (1998) Neonatal mortality in the Czech Republic during the transition. *Health Policy* **46**: 43–52.

Laing SP, Swerdlow AJ, Slater SD et al. (1999) The British Diabetic Association Cohort Study, I: all-cause mortality in patients with insulin-treated diabetes mellitus. *Diabet Med* **16**: 459–65.

McKee M (2007) Cochrane on Communism: the influence of ideology on the search for evidence. *International Journal of Epidemiology* **36**: 269–73.

McKee M, Gilmore A and Novotny T (2003) Smoke-free hospitals. *Br Med J* **326**: 941–2.

McKeown T (1979) *The Role of Medicine: Dream, Mirage or Nemesis?* Oxford: Blackwell.

NICE (2006) *NICE Guidance, Technology Assessment 94: Statins for the prevention of cardiovascular events*. London: NICE.

Nolte E, Bain C and McKee M (2006) Diabetes as a tracer condition in international benchmarking of health systems. *Diabetes Care* **29**: 1007–11.

Nolte E, Brand A, Koupilová I and McKee M (2000) Neonatal and postneonatal mortality in Germany since unification. *J Epidemiol Community Health* **54**: 84–90.

Nolte E and McKee CM (2008) Measuring the health of nations: updating an earlier analysis. *Health Affairs* **27**(1): 58–71

Rutstein DD, Berenberg W, Chalmers TC et al. (1976) Measuring the quality of medical care. *N Engl J Med* **294**: 582–8.

Salathé M and Bonhoeffer S (2008) The effect of opinion clustering on disease outbreaks doi: 10.1098/?rsif.2008.0271 *J. R. Soc. Interface* **5**(29): 1505–8.

Sim F, Lock K and McKee M (2007) Maximising the contribution of the public health workforce: the English experience. WHO Bulletin, Dec 2007 doi: 10.2471/BLT.07.044289.

Ulrich RS (1984) View through a window may influence recovery from surgery. *Science* **224**, 420–1.

World Health Organization (2000) *The World Health Report 2000. Health System Improving Performance*. Geneva: World Health Organization.

Yusuf S (2002) Two decades of progress in preventing vascular disease. *The Lancet* **360**: 2–3.

📖 Further reading

Bailey L, Vardulaki K, Langham J and Chandramohan D (2005) *Introduction to Epidemiology*. Maidenhead: Open University Press.

Evaluation of NHS Health Check in Tower Hamlets: http://www.uel.ac.uk/ihhd/projects/EvaluationoftheTowerHamletsPilotVascularCheckProgramme.htm

Frampton SB, Gilpin L and Charmel PA (eds) (2003) *Putting Patients First: Designing and Practicing Patient-centered Care*. San Francisco, CA: Jossey-Bass. For those who would like to read about the international movement entitled the Planetree model.

Mackenbach JP (1996) The contribution of medical care to mortality decline: McKeown revisited. *J Clin Epidemiol* **49**: 1207–13.

NHS Health Check:

a) Public information: http://www.nhs.uk/Planners/NHSHealthCheck/Pages/Thetests.aspx
b) Information for NHS staff: http://www.dh.gov.uk/en/Publicationsandstatistics/Publications/DH_097490

Nutrition screening survey in the UK and Republic of Ireland in 2010, BAPEN, 2011: http://www.bapen.org.uk/pdfs/nsw/nsw10/nsw10-report.pdf

6 Assessing the impact on population health of policies in other sectors

Karen Lock, Fiona Sim, Martin McKee and Joceline Pomerleau

Overview

In Chapter 5 you learned about how health care can contribute to making a population healthier. In this chapter, you will examine how to determine the effects that activities and policies in non-health sectors, such as transport, agriculture and the environment, have on the health of the public. This chapter will introduce health impact assessment (HIA), its principles, uses, advantages, limitations, and how it is performed.

Learning objectives

By the end of this chapter you should be able to:

- describe the broad determinants of health and recognize the range of policy sectors that influence population health
- explain how public health can have a role in addressing these wider determinants of health in policy-making
- describe the key elements of a HIA process
- outline the application of HIA to policies from the non-health sector, illustrated by examples of HIA worldwide
- comment on the strengths and limitations of current HIA methods in helping policy-makers decide on priorities and activities
- have a basic understanding of how HIA can be applied in a real policy-making situation

Key terms

Health inequalities Differences in health experience and health status between countries, regions and socioeconomic groups.

Health Impact Assessment (HIA) A means of assessing the health impacts of policies, plans and projects in diverse economic sectors using quantitative, qualitative and participatory techniques.

What is health impact assessment?

The most widely quoted definition of health impact assessment (HIA) was developed at a consensus conference of the World Health Organization (WHO): 'HIA is a combination of procedures, methods, and tools by which a policy, programme, or project may be judged as to its potential effects on the health of population and the distribution of those effects within the population' (World Health Organization European Centre for Health Policy and World Health Organization Regional Office for Europe 1999).

All definitions highlight that HIA is concerned with the health of populations and attempts to predict the future consequences of health decisions that have not yet been implemented.

The purpose of HIA

HIA is a flexible and adaptable approach helping those developing and delivering policies. It is intended to influence decision-makers so that policies, projects and programmes in all areas lead to improved public health, or do no harm to population health (Lock 2000).

In 2006, during the Finnish Presidency, the European Union introduced the 'Health in every policy' initiative, under which the health impact of proposed policies in any sector were expected to be assessed (Stahl et al. 2006). The English Department of Health has included Health Impact Assessment (HIA) as part of the mandatory 'Impact Assessment' required by Government for all relevant policies for developing better, evidenced-based policy by careful consideration of the impact on the health of the population (DH 2011). While this is a positive statement and there is abundant advice about how HIA can be conducted, there is no requirement to conduct it rigorously, but just that it should be done.

Recently, the concept of integrated impact assessment has become more prominent, whereby health impact assessment is integrated into Sustainability Assessment and Strategic Environmental Assessment. Obviously, this is a more complex process than HIA alone, but the additional effort may be valuable, particularly in circumstances when one of the elements of impact assessment is mandatory and the others are not, as in local government in England (London Health Commission 2011).

HIA can influence decisions in four ways:

1 by raising awareness among decision-makers of the relationship between health and other factors such as the physical, social and economic environment, so that they consider health effects in their planning;
2 by helping decision-makers identify and assess the potential impact of a specific proposal on population health and wellbeing, and on the distribution of those effects within the population (that is, issues of equity by considering health inequalities or the impact on specific vulnerable groups);
3 HIA can also identify practical ways to improve and optimize the outcome of proposals, by producing a set of evidence-based recommendations which feed into the decision-making process;
4 by helping stakeholders affected by policies to participate and contribute to decision-making.

Whatever approaches or methods are used, it is important to maintain a clear focus on the ultimate purpose of HIA. This is to inform and influence subsequent decision-making. HIA is not merely a research tool, it is a political tool to aid decision-making.

HIA within the context of a broad health model

The HIA approach is grounded in the broad determinants of human health. These include personal, social, cultural, economic, environmental and other factors that influence the health status of individuals and populations. You will have covered some of these earlier in the book, for example in Chapters 3 and 4.

Activity 6.1

Think about the determinants of human health. Then, list some examples of determinants for each of the following categories:

- Pre-conceptual/in utero: _____
- Behavioural/lifestyle: _____
- Psycho-social environment: _____
- Physical environment: _____
- Socioeconomic status: _____
- Provision of and access to public services: _____
- Public policy: _____
- Global policy issues: _____

Feedback

You will find below a few examples of health determinants. The list is of course not exhaustive (it could almost be endless) and you may have provided other good examples. This exercise simply reminds us that health is determined by a complex combination of factors affecting all aspects of our lives, many of which will interact. This is important to consider in many aspects of public health practice and especially in HIA, where we would inadequately be able to look at the health effects of wider policy if we limited our analysis to impacts on death and incidence of medically defined disease.

- Pre-conceptual/in utero: maternal health, health of foetus during pregnancy
- Behavioural/lifestyle: diet, smoking, physical activity, risk taking behaviour (for example, unsafe sex, illicit drugs)
- Psycho-social environment: community networks, culture, religion, social inclusion
- Physical environment: air, water, housing, noise, waste
- Socioeconomic status: employment, education, training, household income
- Provision of and access to public services: transport, shops, leisure, health and social services
- Public policy: economic, welfare, crime, agriculture, health policies
- Global policy issues: international trade, European Union policy, multi-national industries (for example for tobacco, food, oil)

This broad model of health helps to show that virtually every area of human activity influences health, and therefore that most public or political decisions have the potential to impact on health both positively and negatively. This obviously means that the greatest scope for improving the public's health often lies outside the control of the health services, through interventions in economic, housing, agriculture, transport, education and other 'non-health' areas.

In most countries the interface between the health and non-health sectors is still fairly limited, for example, to links between health care and social care, and public health and environmental health. Health is not routinely on the agenda of other ministries or agencies. However, the financial burden of negative health impacts of their policies usually falls on the health sector.

Policies and programmes, and the way they are implemented, represent important influences on people's health and well-being. HIA is one concept that has emerged to identify those activities and policies likely to have major impacts on the health of a population. It is increasingly proposed as a way of bringing together stakeholders from diverse backgrounds (including those from the public, private and voluntary sectors as well as the community) to identify and address how the development and implementation of a policy or programme will affect the wider determinants of health.

Many health determinants are interrelated and there are several cross cutting issues that affect health (for example poverty). The systematic nature of HIA is designed to allow health impacts to be considered by way of a number of categories. The categories cover a series of intermediate factors that are determinants of health, through which changes due to a policy or project can impact on people's health. The precise categories used and their component parts may vary according to the nature of the proposed policy, programme or other development thus providing sufficient flexibility in the application of the health impact assessment concept in different circumstances. The categories of health determinants used in Activity 6.1 illustrate one example of such a classification.

Activity 6.2

Explain, using an example of your choice, how certain policies unrelated to health can have a negative impact on the health sector.

Feedback

Numerous policies set by government departments other than health ministries can have indirect negative effects on the health of populations.

For example, the British and US Ministries of Trade have promoted the activities of multi-national tobacco companies overseas in the past. Yet, it is Ministries of Health that have to treat people with smoking-related disease (approximately 20 per cent of the burden of disease in the USA).

Another example is the European Union Common Agricultural Policy (CAP) which determines which crops are grown, and the prices they are sold at throughout the European Union (EU). Certain CAP regimes maintain the livelihoods of farmers by subsidizing production of 'unhealthy crops' such as tobacco and high fat dairy products. Often this production is more than what is consumed by people in Europe creating surpluses, for example of butter fat, which is sold cheaply to food companies to produce high-fat processed food. The US Department of Agriculture does the same with high fructose corn syrup, explaining the sweet sauces in much American fast food. The CAP also determines the prices of crops imported from other (usually developing) nations, thus affecting livelihoods and the socioeconomic status of people worldwide.

Historical background of HIA

The basic concepts of HIA are not new and they will be familiar to those working in public health. HIA builds on and brings together many existing methods and disciplines including policy appraisal, risk assessment, stakeholder analysis, evidence-based health care, and environmental impact assessment.

HIA has its roots in two main developments:

1 the promotion of healthy public policy; and
2 environmental impact assessment.

Healthy public policy was a key component of the Ottawa charter for health promotion. The concept included policies designed specifically to promote health (for example, banning cigarette advertising) and policies not dealing directly with health but acknowledged to have a health impact (for example, transport, education, economic).

The WHO Health for All programme (adopted in 1977 and launched at the Alma Ata Conference in 1978) and the WHO's Healthy Cities programme (launched in 1988) stimulated interest in the important part local authorities and communities can play in improving health, including urban regeneration strategies. More recently this has been updated as the WHO global health policy 'Health for All for the 21st Century' which includes a recommendation to undertake HIA.

Sustainable development plans by national and local authorities have further added to wider policy initiatives, which have implications for improving population health. These initiatives have been strengthened by increased public awareness of social and environmental effects on health, exemplified by the 2008 report of the WHO's Commission on Social Determinants of Health. The open debate of these issues at international, national, and local levels has dramatically increased between the mainly environmental focus of the UN Earth summit in Rio de Janeiro (in 1992), and the World Summit on Sustainable Development in Johannesburg (in 2002) whose agenda had a much greater focus on poverty and human health issues (United Nations 2003).

The principles of HIA are similar to social impact assessment and environmental impact assessment (EIA). Initially it developed as a natural extension of these methods. Many countries, including the countries of the EU and the USA, have long had a legal requirement to carry out EIA. Article 129 of the Maastricht treaty (signed in 1992) and its subsequent revisions in the Treaties of Amsterdam, Nice and Lisbon, require the EU to check that policy proposals do not have an adverse impact on health or create conditions that undermine health promotion.

It has been argued that procedures for HIA could be most easily introduced with the inclusion of health in existing processes for EIA. While health effects are currently supposed to be dealt with within the EIA legislation, they are actually poorly assessed or not at all. There are some initiatives that are attempting to strengthen the health elements in other impact assessments. One approach is so-called 'integrated impact assessment tools'. Another approach is to strengthen the health component of Environmental Assessment. For example, in a European legal protocol on Strategic Environmental Assessment (World Health Organization Regional Office for Europe

2001). Mostly HIA has developed as an independent tool for promoting public health in policies and programmes.

What has HIA been used for?

HIA has been used in many countries in the world and for various types of policies and programmes in a wide range of policy sectors. We will examine this in Activity 6.3.

Activity 6.3

What are the main policy sectors or projects that HIA has been applied to? To explore this you are invited to search for and read examples of completed HIAs of programmes, projects or policies at both local and national levels. You can select examples by searching the following websites for subjects or countries that interest you. It may be best to start with the WHO website or HIA gateway website (see those listed below). While exploring these websites, you will see that HIA can be used for different purposes. Prepare a list of the main applications of HIA.

1 HIA Gateway (http://www.apho.org.uk/default.aspx?QN=P_HIA) Association of Public Health Observatories. This site is the easiest place to start. It was launched in December 2000 and moved to the Association of Public Health Observatories in 2004. It has numerous links and HIA resources, including an introductory guide, many examples of HIA toolkits and case studies, information about HIA training opportunities, as well as links to reviews of evidence. It is useful for anyone interested in Integrated Impact Assessment, Mental Well-being Impact Assessment and health-related Strategic Environmental Assessment as well as 'standard' HIA. It began as a national site, but has evolved to become an international resource. Note, however, that the future of the HIA Gateway is uncertain at the time of writing, due to proposed changes to the structure and delivery of Public Health in England.
2 World Health Organization HIA website (http://www.who.int/hia/en/) (World Health Organization 2005). This website was set up in 2003 and has worldwide examples and links.
3 Liverpool University. International Health Impact Assessment Consortium, established 2000 (http://www.liv.ac.uk/ihia/) Provides research, consultancy, training and capacity building in HIA.
4 National Institute for Public Health and the Environment. Environmental Impact Assessment (http://www.rivm.nl/en/).
5 London Health Commission – Health Impact Assessment (http://www.london.gov.uk/lhc/hia/) Although the focus is London, the site offers examples applicable elsewhere and helpful explanatory documents for non-specialists.

Feedback

Your summary of the main applications of HIA may include:

1 *Urban and transport planning* Urban regeneration schemes and policies, for example in London and Wales. Transport strategies, for example in Scotland, Merseyside, London.

2 *Political lobbying* There was for example the input of a rapid HIA to the Public Inquiry into the Manchester Airport Second Runway expansion.

3 *National Policy Appraisal* Examples can be found in The Netherlands, Canada and Thailand.

4 *Environmental HIA (often called EHIA)* Examples can be found in New Zealand, Australia, Central and Eastern Europe (through National Environmental Health Action Plans). This usually covers issues such as waste disposal, air quality and transport, water pollution.

5 *Developing country policies and programmes* This has mainly been used to appraise donor aid projects (for example, World Bank, Asian Development Bank, UN Food and Agriculture Organisation). Examples include agricultural and water policies and the World Commission on Dams. The method was based on a more medical model of health, considering health impacts in five main disease categories: communicable disease, non-communicable disease, nutrition, injury and mental disorder. The likelihood of specific health risks related to the project was considered and risk reduction strategies proposed. More recently the approach taken in developing countries has adopted a broader view of the determinants of health.

6 The WHO website alone refers (in alphabetical order) to 15 different sectors of HIA activity, from agriculture, culture, energy, to mining, tourism, waste and water.

This list and the one you prepared confirm that HIA covers a wide range of policy sectors.

Methods of HIA

It should be clear that HIA is a multidisciplinary, intersectoral process within which a range of evidence about the health effects of a proposal is considered in a structured framework. It takes into account the opinions and expectations of those who may be affected by a proposed policy. Evidence for the potential health impacts of a proposal are analysed and recommendations for improving health are fed into the decision-making process.

HIA has been undertaken in a range of different ways. The choice of the approach depends on the timeframe and resources available. There are many different toolkits and methods proposed (many of which can be accessed via the weblinks given above). This can appear confusing for a newcomer. However, in many ways this is not as important as it seems, as all methods have similarities. It also serves to highlight the inherent flexibility of HIA, and the ability to adapt the process to the requirements of the particular circumstances.

Core stages of the HIA process

There is a general consensus about the core stages of HIA which are summarized in Figure 6.1. These stages are briefly described below. Further details can be found in various methodological guides available (see the list of optional readings and additional resources given at the end of the session). It should be noted that not every HIA necessarily has to follow this framework rigidly. HIA is a flexible approach which can be adapted to specific circumstances.

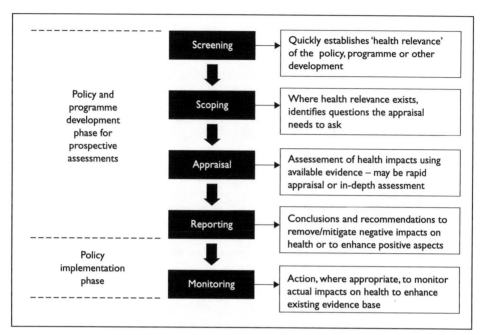

Figure 6.1 A schematic representation of an HIA process

Screening Systematic screening of policies and programme proposals provides a quick preliminary assessment of the relevance to health of the proposals. It is an important first stage of the health impact assessment and can be done with or without the assistance of screening tools and checklists. It enables any significant issues relating to health to be identified and a decision to be made on whether or not there is a need for more detailed assessment to take place.

Scoping If there is felt to be a need for further consideration of the health impacts or potential impacts, the scoping stage identifies the questions that need to be addressed in the assessment process, and the scope of the HIA for example, the geographical area, the population and the timescales to be covered.

Appraisal The appraisal stage itself also has in-built flexibility. It can take the form of a rapid appraisal, which might be done over the course of a few days, or an in-depth appraisal, which may require a period of weeks or several months. The appraisal may include quantitative and/or qualitative assessments that cover both risks and hazards to health, and opportunities to help people to improve their health by adjusting elements of the proposals or by integrating new elements within it.

Reporting recommendations to decision-makers The conclusions of the appraisal and assessment are reported to those responsible for the decision-making and should meet political timeframes. The report should make any recommendations necessary to remove or to mitigate any negative impacts on the health of a population or on specific groups within a population. Similarly, the report should identify ways on which the proposal could be enhanced in order to positively encourage and support people to improve their health and wellbeing.

Using evidence to make recommendations

A key consideration in HIA is identifying and assessing potential evidence. Evidence for actual or potential impacts can come from many sources including epidemiological evidence, local routine data sources from health and other sectors, and qualitative sources of data collection (some of which may be gathered specifically for the HIA). Due to the broad nature of the determinants of health, the evidence base available to support the HIA process may be of poor quality, detailed but still inconclusive, incomplete or difficult to locate. Unfortunately epidemiology and related health sciences, which could contribute to HIA, are currently limited in their ability to explore outcomes other than death or disease incidence, and are unable to quantify causal pathways and the multiple interactions between risk factors. This emphasis on health determinants means that HIAs will confront considerable uncertainty in making definitive conclusions about potential health impacts. For many policies, especially those implemented at a national level where even the immediate effects are often unclear, the causal pathways are very complex, with the current evidence base patchy and often irrelevant to concrete policy options. For this reason, HIA practitioners have to acknowledge the constraints of only being able to make recommendations based on the 'best available' evidence given the time and other resource limitations.

There is much debate about what is the 'best available' evidence. Many scientists argue that quantified estimates are more influential but it should be remembered that not everything that can be quantified is important, that things should not be quantified if not done robustly, and that not everything that is important can be quantified. So in HIA it is accepted that evidence from a variety of sources is necessary.

However, this creates its own problems. Prioritizing and making recommendations using evidence from different sources and methodologies is fraught with difficulty. HIA also has to be aware that the evidence can be mixed, contradictory or limited, and so an important part of the process is involving key stakeholders to ensure that any recommendations are based on a clear understanding of their different perspectives, and are reached by consensus.

Other methodological difficulties

Several issues are unresolved in the methodology of HIA. Although there is increasing agreement about the wide variety of factors that influence health, the comparative importance of these varies across professional and public views. In order for HIA to be a valid tool, a shared definition of health is needed. This affects the ability to measure health impacts in various settings. At present, different models measure health impacts in different ways. Most use some checklist procedure, which uses the perceived determinants of health as markers for changes in health risks for example, using employment levels as a marker for the status of community health. The difficulty with this is that causal pathways are so complex that it is not often possible to say if an outcome will definitely be good or bad for the health of a population. Will a development such as replacing a derelict industrial site with new offices increase local employment? And if it does will this improve health? Such health indicators can potentially measure progress towards possible health improvement but this is not necessarily equivalent to a measure of health impact.

One of the major criticisms of HIA is that the methods of collecting and analysing evidence are not sufficiently rigorous to withstand scrutiny and challenge. The current evidence base for many health determinants is inadequate for accurately informing a process of assessment. In completed studies the principal sources of evidence have come from literature reviews and qualitative methods. A range of data sources including economic, epidemiological, quantitative, and qualitative information should be routinely taken into account. However, often the most useful information is not being routinely collected. Seldom is there going to be the time or money available for collection of primary data. Although it may be preferable for decision-makers to have a quantitative measure of health impact, the limitations of qualitative estimates may have to be accepted as the best evidence available. This may limit the strength of the recommendations an assessment can make both in terms of the certainty and size of an impact.

HIA aims to influence the decision-making process in an open, structured way. To do this it has to acknowledge that assessing and ranking evidence is not a wholly objective process and involves a series of value judgments. There are no evaluated methods for prioritizing evidence from different sources, and political imperatives are likely to affect the outcome. The balance between objective evidence and subjective opinion should be explicitly recognized in reports of assessments. In evidence-based medicine there is a weighted hierarchy of epidemiological evidence, with randomized controlled trials at the top. Obviously this is not useful in assessments where evidence comes from a range of quantitative and qualitative sources. There is a need for developing a new framework for gathering, interpreting, and prioritizing evidence from different origins for evidence-based policy-making.

The findings of a HIA are often limited by financial and time costs. There is a need for a balance between rigorous methods that require specialist skills and high levels of resources and those that can be used more easily and cheaply. The two approaches are not mutually exclusive and can be combined in a continuum of options for assessment, which includes preliminary project screening, rapid appraisal, and in-depth assessment. The choice of method to use may relate to whatever will have most weight in influencing the decision-making process in a timely way. Ultimately there will have to be a trade-off between costs and quality to make the impact assessment a realizable goal.

Note that HIA need not be a discrete activity at a given time, but sometimes needs to continue over a long period, evolving over time alongside the project whose health impact it is studying. One such example is the HIA associated with the major and very complex plan to redevelop the Kings Cross area of central London over a twenty-year period to 2020. The HIA, which commenced in 2002, was led by Camden Primary Care Trust (PCT), and involved the London Boroughs of Camden and Islington, with stakeholders from all sectors. Its overarching objective was to minimize the risk of increasing health inequalities and social exclusion that might result from regeneration, which would bring with it redevelopment and **gentrification** of the local area (Ison 2003; Collins and Taylor 2007).

Another interesting example of HIA is the rapid assessment conducted in 2004, prior to the outcome of London's bid to host the 2012 Olympics (Buroni 2004). This HIA explored the health impact of having versus not having the Olympics in London. It sought 'to examine the nature and extent of health impacts over the period 2006–2012 and beyond' on the local community. Many potential health impacts (positive and negative) were identified, and the HIA stakeholder workshop concluded that 'participants considered that risk to health from construction activities, employment impacts and gentrification as being significant. However, the most significant influence on health raised was a potential lack of community involvement.' Further work will attempt to ascertain the actual health legacy of the Olympics, not only for the local people, but for the country as a whole.

Benefits of using HIA

Activity 6.4

Despite the current limitations of the methods, process evaluation has shown that HIA leads to many benefits for 'healthy decision-making'. Suggest what these benefits might be.

Feedback

The benefits of deploying HIA include:

• providing a mechanism for health to inform decision-making;
• improving intersectoral working;
• creating a structured approach for demonstrating the broad health agenda to other agencies/policy sectors;
• raising community awareness of health;
• encouraging and enabling public participation in decision-making;
• increasing the transparency of some aspects of decision-making.

The way forward

HIA is a developing process worldwide, at local, regional and national levels. It can be usefully used by public health departments, policy-makers, community groups, non-governmental organizations and individuals working in a range of settings to push public health issues up the political agenda. Its flexibility often means that it can be easy to integrate into existing processes. However, it is important to plan before introducing it. Important things to consider include:

1 identifying and using existing public health expertise and resources;
2 raising awareness about HIA, and the broad determinants of health across health and non-health sectors;
3 looking for opportunities to use HIA to promote intersectoral approaches to health improvement, for example public or political concern;
4 deciding on your approach: rapid or in-depth, projects or policies;
5 managing the expectations of the HIA process and its outcomes: remember there is no single, perfect method; HIA is not a decision-making tool, it helps inform decision-making; there are insufficient resources to do an in-depth HIA of every project/policy.

Activity 6.5

Designing and conducting a HIA of a new agricultural policy

In this activity you will design a rapid HIA of a new agricultural policy. This exercise is deliberately not set in any specific country in order to allow you to think about the issues in the place where you live. These types of policies have been introduced in both

Europe and developing countries. Although some issues will vary depending on the context (that is, the level of economic development, geography and climate) there are also core issues that will be the same (such as access to food, employment, environmental factors).

By working through the three questions described below you will outline the key public health issues that the HIA needs to cover, the main people that it should involve and the types of information that should ideally be collected to present a report and recommendations on the health issues to the Ministry of Agriculture (see scenario below). You will be able to do this using your own knowledge and experience as well as the materials provided. You are not expected to use any other resources.

Practical points to consider before you start

Experience of previous HIAs has shown the value of rapid appraisal sessions. Evaluation of these activities has also identified some potential problems or barriers that it is important to dispel before you start:

- You may feel that you need to become an expert in the process of HIA or agriculture, and that you lack the experience or knowledge necessary. **THIS IS NOT TRUE!** Like any piece of work the focus remains on answering the task you are set, and you should concentrate on the practical things that you are being asked to do. An HIA will appraise policies not just on the basis of the evidence, but also in the light of your views and your knowledge gained through a variety of experience and information. However, if you want to see another example of an HIA looking at agriculture and food, you can check the papers from Gabrijelcic and collaborators (2004) and Lock and collaborators (2003) (both available on the Internet). You can read them before or after the activity as they are not required to do it.
- Some of you may feel that you need more information about specific aspects of the Policy before you can reach a view. If you are not careful, this may result in getting stuck on one point of detail. Try to avoid this. If you feel you are unable to decide on one aspect then note this down, and move forward to the next issue.
- You only need to use the materials provided to you, and it is not expected that you read any more references.

You should set aside approximately one and a half hours to do this activity.

Think broadly about the effects of agriculture, and have fun!

Organization of the work

The exercise includes 3 components:

1 Policy appraisal: apply a 'determinants of health' framework to the policy proposals, to identify the range of public health issues the HIA should consider and which ones you believe may potentially have positive and negative effects on population health.
2 Conduct a stakeholder analysis to identify the key people affected by the policy who should be involved in the HIA.
3 Outline a rapid appraisal of the policy and decide what information you would want to collect to make an analysis of the likely health impacts. You will use this information to propose three recommendations to promote public health.

Scenario

You work in the Public Health Department of the Ministry of Health. You have been asked to conduct a rapid HIA of the possible health effects of a new national policy proposed by the Ministry of Agriculture. This policy aims to increase agricultural productivity and farmers' income. Its objectives are as follows:

1 to increase growth of cash crops for sale or export: including fruits and vegetables, tobacco and non-food crops.
2 to increase productivity through two mechanisms: a) intensification of land use by enforced purchase and amalgamation of the current pattern of small holdings and family farms, and b) technical education and support to increase the use of improved technology (including fertilizers, pesticides, mechanization and irrigation techniques).

Questions to answer

1 What health determinants should be considered when planning an HIA of this policy? Consider the policy proposal and identify what health determinants may be affected. You should remember that health impacts can be both positive and negative, so you need to include both 'risks to health' and issues positively affecting wellbeing. You can develop a table such as Table 6.1. Some examples are given in it to help you start, but these are not exhaustive.

Table 6.1 Health determinants to consider for the new agricultural policy

Category of health determinants	Area of health impact	Type of impact (indicate whether positive or negative)
Pre-conceptual/in utero	Maternal nutrition	
Behavioural/lifestyle	Diet	
Psycho-social environment	Cultural impact	
Physical environment	Land use Water	
Socioeconomic status	Employment	For example, merging of small family farms may remove the source of nutrition from subsistence farmers and families (negative) Commercial farms may become source of employment and income (positive)
Provision of and access to public services		
Public policy		
Global policy issues	Global trade agreements, e.g. Common Agricultural Policy	

2 Who are the stakeholders that the HIA should involve? Most HIAs aim to involve stakeholders that may be affected by or that can influence the policy or project, to allow their opinions to input into decisions. Stakeholder analysis can be used to ensure that stakeholders who normally have low impact or influence 'can be heard' as part of the decision-making process (assuming that the HIA and community involvement are conducted well, which is another problem!). A stakeholder analysis is one technique you can use to identify and assess the importance of key people, groups of people, or institutions that may influence the success of your activity or project (Gil and colleagues 2010). It should be used early in the HIA or other types of project planning. Stakeholder analysis can also be used to develop the most effective support possible for any project and reduce any obstacles to successful implementation.

To conduct a stakeholder analysis you can follow the following steps:

- Develop a **Stakeholder Analysis Table** such as Table 6.2
- Identify all the people, groups, and institutions that will affect or be affected by the policy and list them in the column under 'Stakeholder' (column 1).

Table 6.2 Stakeholder analysis for the new agricultural policy

Stakeholder	Interest(s) in the project	Assessment of Influence
Ministry of Agriculture	Policy proponent, increased production, increased revenue, improved agricultural practices	A

- Once you have a list of all potential stakeholders, review the list and identify the specific interests these stakeholders have in the policy. Consider issues like: the policies benefit(s) to the stakeholder; the changes that the policy might require the stakeholder to make; and the policy activities that might cause difficulty or conflict for the stakeholder. Record these under the column 'Stakeholder Interest(s) in the Project' (column 2).
- Now review each stakeholder listed in column one. Ask the question: how important are the stakeholder's interests to the success of the proposed policy? Consider:
  a) The role the key stakeholder must play for the project to be successful, and the likelihood that the stakeholder will play this role
  b) The likelihood and impact of a stakeholder's negative response to health implications

Assign 'A' for extremely important, 'B' for fairly important, and 'C' for not very important. Record these letters in the column entitled 'Assessment of Influence' (column 3).

3 Conduct a rapid HIA of the proposed policy. This requires you to look in more detail at some aspects of the proposed policy. Choose three issues that you identified in Table 6.1. You also need to outline what information and evidence you would

want to collect to make an analysis of the likely health impacts. Use a table such as Table 6.3 to assist you.

Table 6.3 Information and evidence to be collected for the HIA

Policy-related issue	Potential effects of policy	Health determinants which may be affected	Evidence required and sources of information to assess potential health impacts	Relevant stakeholders

Then outline three clear recommendations that result from this rapid appraisal. You need to identify ways in which the proposed policies could potentially be strengthened to support and promote public health. You should consider ways to both maximize potential positive impacts on health, and to minimize potential negative impacts on health. This should also consider the relevant stakeholders.

Feedback

There is no 'correct' response to this type of rapid HIA exercise. HIA aims to include stakeholder opinion as one part of the information which directs the appraisal of evidence, hence there could be a number of different answers depending on the people involved and their perspective.

You should propose the evidence required to support your statements. Obviously what you will be able to do will be limited by the time and evidence available. It is difficult to replicate these issues in a paper based exercise. However, it is crucial not to be speculative (that is, prioritize the issues you want if the evidence does not justify it), nor just repeat political rhetoric.

In an HIA you must interpret the policy or project details to identify issues which have potential or known health effects. You then need to back up this 'hypothesis' of a health impact by citing evidence to support your conclusions.

You will increasingly learn that policy-makers often say they make 'evidence-based policy' although they use evidence very selectively. In contrast, anyone challenging policy or plans (such as in an HIA) needs to cite as much detailed evidence as possible to ensure their conclusions are robust. The responses to the questions you had to answer are meant as a guide, you may have come up with others.

1 What health determinants should be considered when planning an HIA of this policy?

When considering the proposed policy you need to understand how agricultural can affect the health of different people in different ways. It is important to think broadly about the range of issues, not just nutrition. These include:

a) Access to and availability of food:

- food production – change in types of food produced
- food marketing and distribution, changes in patterns of marketing and distribution (that is, from local to regional, national or international)
- access to different foods by specific population groups, on the basis of their age, socioeconomic status, living in urban/rural areas

b) Methods of agricultural production including:
- use of pesticides and agrochemicals
- intensive agriculture techniques and intensive land use for limited types of crops

c) Working and living conditions of those involved in the food chain and their families including:
- owners of small farms, family gardens or subsistence farmers
- agricultural workers in large farms
- food processing workers
- distributors and retailers – owners and workers running market stalls, small shops and large outlets, such as supermarkets

d) Socioeconomic factors and employment:
- rural poverty – including subsistence farmers or small family farmers who supplement their income in other ways
- high rates of unemployment and low rates of pay in agricultural communities
- the effect of the supermarket retail sector on what the producer is paid for products
- the effect of global trade policies on the price of agricultural products on world markets

e) Travelling patterns and need for travel by different means/modes of transport
- increasing transport of food stuffs long distances to 'market'

f) Tourism and niche markets including:
- agri-tourism
- production of local products 'on farm' for specialized markets (for example, expensive handmade cheese)

You might have come up with a table similar to Table 6.4.

Table 6.4 Health determinants to consider for the new agricultural policy

Category of health determinants	Area of health impact	Type of impact (indicate whether positive or negative)
Pre-conceptual/in utero	Maternal nutrition	Could be positive or negative health impact. If the policy focuses on cash crops, could reduce availability of subsistence food locally, however if small farmers benefited from increased productivity and income this may offset the reduction in home food production
Behavioural/ lifestyle	Diet	The most direct effect between agriculture and health is nutrition. If the fruits and vegetable are available locally could improve diet and health (positive). However, this could also reduce local availability of food (negative, see below).
	Accidents and injury	Increased mechanization or use of pesticides without adequate training (negative impact on rates accidents and poisonings)

(Continued overleaf)

Table 6.4 Continued

Category of health determinants	Area of health impact	Type of impact (indicate whether positive or negative)
Psycho-social environment	Cultural impact	This will depend on whether the crops grown are part of the normal local diet. Often farming of cash crops for export causes change in food grown from local fruits and vegetables to those required by the market (that is, negative impact on food availability)
Physical environment	Water	1. Increased use of pesticides may cause pollution of water supplies (negative). If severe this may cause issues such as:
		2. Food safety: Need to ensure what crops are grown with what water, for example, potential microbial contamination of salads if the water used for irrigation is untreated wastewater (negative). Also heavy metal accumulation in soil or plant uptake (negative).
		3. Irrigation may increase production (positive) but only if this does not deplete home water sources (negative).
	Land use	Will the policy force farmers to sell or merge small farms into large intensively farmed units (for example as the Common Agricultural Policy (CAP) favours). Intensification can lead to increased soil pollution if use of agrochemicals is poorly managed (negative). But intensification can increase production (which could increase food supply, positive).
	Transport pollution	Increasing exports will involve increased transport of foods long distances. There may be some local increases in air pollution around processing and warehouse sites (negative).
Socioeconomic status	Employment	For example: Merging of small family farms may remove source of nutrition from subsistence farmers and families and increase unemployment (negative). Commercial farms may become a source of employment and income (positive). Agricultural processing industries may have positive effects (employment) but also potential negative effects if poor occupational health (dust induced lung diseases etc).
Provision of and access to public services	Occupational and primary care health services, agricultural education services	Occupational health services and agricultural technical education services (positive impact by reduction of accidental injuries and poisonings from new technology and agrochemical use).
Global policy issues	Global trade agreements for example Common Agricultural Policy (CAP)	The CAP effects the price that products can be imported into the European Union, often causing developing countries to accept lower prices for their products. So commercial production may not benefit local farmers (negative).

2 Who are the stakeholders that the HIA should involve?

Table 6.5 provides you with an example of a stakeholder analysis for the new agricultural policy.

Table 6.5 Stakeholder analysis for the new agricultural policy

Stakeholder	Interest(s) in the project	Assessment of influence
Ministry of agriculture	Increased production, intensification of farming	A
Farmers (commercial)	Increased production, increased profits	A
Farmers (family or subsistence)	Increased income or fulfilling family nutritional needs	B
Retailers – local markets	Will it affect local food supply?	B
Food processors	Increased opportunities for processing products for export or sale, increased profits	A
Retailers – supermarkets	Increased dependable supply of fruits and vegetables for their national or global market	A
Consumers	Will it affect the type and quantity or produce available for local consumers?	C
Rural population	Will it increase or decrease unemployment?	C
Ministry of Health	Probably have little interest except food safety issues	C
Rural primary care	Will there be greater risks to the population, will this result in more demand for local health services?	C
Rural education and training services	Is there resources for holding adequate education for those remaining in the more technical agricultural production?	C
Regional development agencies	How will this feed into regional development plans?	B

3 Conduct a rapid HIA of the proposed policy.

Table 6.6 provides you with some examples of HIA for the proposed policy.
For more information, you may be interested to read the paper from Lock and collaborators (2003).
Examples of recommendations that could have resulted from the above policy issues include:

a) Agrochemical use on farms must be accompanied by official training in safe handling, and occupational health inspections to ensure the correct safety equipment is worn, and that agrochemicals are stored safely (that is, correctly labelled).

b) Any compulsory merging of small farm units should not totally remove the ability
   of a rural family to continue home-growing of food. Subsistence farmers should
   be assisted in finding other sources of employment or income by rural education
   and extension schemes.

Table 6.6 Information and evidence to be collected for the HIA

Policy-related issue	Potential effects of policy	Health determinants which may be affected	Evidence required and sources of information to assess potential health impacts	Relevant stakeholders
Increased use of pesticides and agrochemicals.	1. Increased productivity could be positive (increased income, increased food grown) but it depends on who will benefit.	Behavioural/ lifestyle – food consumption, accidents and injury.	1. Amount of crops grown before and after similar schemes elsewhere. Long term sustainability of increased production, for example, from literature reviews.	1. Commercial farmers, farm workers, Ministry of agriculture.
	2. Negative health impacts resulting from accidental poisoning, or environmental contamination due to overuse of agrochemicals, for example, water quality.	Physical environment – water quality	2. Surveillance data for current rates of accidental poisonings amongst farm workers. Literature review of the rates of accidental injury with increasing pesticide use, and ways of minimizing hazards.	2. Farm workers, agricultural technical education workers, occupational health.
Change in land use could cause loss of small family farms.	May reduce access to essential food source or income for many families.	Cultural, socioeconomic.	Survey of how much food eaten is home grown. Also household budget surveys of how much a low income family spends on food, and where the food supply comes from.	Farm workers and their families, consumers.
Intensification of agricultural production.	A source of local employment (although due to efficiency of intensive methods likely to be less farm workers than current land use). Increased mechanization and transport of products – could increase accidents and pollution.	Socioeconomic, physical environment – transport related.	Current rates of road traffic accidents.	Commercial farmers, family farmers, retailers, Ministry of agriculture.

c) The effects on the local rural populations of increased traffic to transport the produce to market should be minimized. This should aim to reduce road traffic accidents and air pollution.

Summary

This chapter introduced you to HIA. It first described the range of policy sectors that influence the main determinants of health, and how public health can have a role in addressing these wider determinants of health in policy-making. It then examined the key elements of a HIA process and described different applications of HIA to policies from the non-health sector. The strengths and limitations of the current HIA methods in helping policy-makers decide on priorities and activities were described. Finally, the last activity provided you with a practical example of how HIA can be applied in a real policy-making situation. You can find more on this theme in this book, particularly in Chapters 10, 11 and 12.

References

Buroni A (2004) Rapid Health Impact Assessment of the Proposed London Olympic Games and Their Legacy. The London Health Commission and the London Development Agency (available at http://www.apho.org.uk/resource/item.aspx?RID=61057).

Collins K and Taylor L (2007) A large-scale urban development HIA: focusing on vulnerable groups in London, England, in M Wismar, J Blau, K Ernst and J Figueras *The effectiveness of health impact assessment: scope and limitations of supporting decision-making in Europe 2007*. Copenhagen: WHO on behalf of European Observatory on health systems and policies, pp. 81–93. (The whole book can be accessed at: http://www.euro.who.int/__data/assets/pdf_file/0003/98283/E90794.pdf)

Department of Health (2011) *Health Impact Assessment* (available at http://www.dh.gov.uk/en/Publicationsandstatistics/Legislation/Healthassessment/DH_647).

Gabrijelcic M, Zakotnik J and Lock K (2004) Health impact assessment: implementing the CAP in Slovenia after Accession. *Eurohealth* 10: 17–21 (available at http://www.euro.who.int/Document/Obs/Eurohealth10_1.pdf).

Gil A, Polikina O, Koroleva N et al. (2010) Alcohol policy in a Russian region: a stakeholder analysis. *Eur J Publ Health* 20(5): 588–94.

Ison E (2003) The Response of Camden PCT King's Cross HIA Project to LBC and LBI on the Argent St George Planning Applications for King's Cross Central (available at http://www.kxrlg.org.uk/news/PCTonASG1.pdf).

Lock KJ (2000) Health Impact Assessment. *Br Med J* 320: 1395–8.

Lock K, Gabrijelcic-Blenkus M, Martuzzi M et al. (2003) Health impact assessment of agriculture and food policies: lessons learnt from the Republic of Slovenia. *Bull WHO* 81: 391–8 (available at http://www.scielosp.org/pdf/bwho/v81n6/v81n6a05.pdf).

London Health Commission (2011) *Integrated Impact Assessment* (available at http://www.london.gov.uk/lhc/hia/iia.jsp).

Stahl T, Wismar M, Ollila E, Lahtinen E and Leppo K (eds) (2006) Health in all Policies. EU, 2006: eu2006.fi (available at http://ec.europa.eu/health/archive/ph_information/documents/health_in_all_policies.pdf).

United Nations (2003) *Johannesburg Summit 2002. World Summit on Sustainable Development in Johannesburg*. New York: United Nations.

World Health Organization Regional Office for Europe (2001) *Health Impact Assessment as Part of Strategic Environmental Assessment*. Copenhagen: World Health Organization Regional Office for Europe.

World Health Organization European Centre for Health Policy and World Health Organization Regional Office for Europe (1999) *Gothenburg Consensus Paper. Health Impact Assessment. Main Concepts and Suggested Approach.* Brussels: European Centre for Health Policy.

📖 Further reading

Barton H, Grant M and Guise R (2010) *Shaping Neighbourhoods: For Local Health and Global Sustainability,* 2nd edn. London: Routledge.

Birley MH (1995) *The Health Impact Assessment of Development Projects.* London: HMSO. Although slightly dated, this book is the original approach developed for developing countries. It contains useful examples.

Birley MH (2011) *Health Impact Assessment: Principles and Practice.* London: Earthscan.

Bulletin of the World Health Organization (2003) Volume 81, Number 6, 387–472. This is a special edition of the journal devoted to articles about HIA from around the world.

Kemm J, Parry J and Palmer S (2004) *Health Impact Assessment.* Oxford: Oxford University Press. This book gives an in-depth perspective on HIA theory, techniques and applications. It has multiple examples from all around the world.

SECTION 2

Major determinants of health

The changing nature of infectious disease | 7

Richard Coker, Fiona Sim, Joceline Pomerleau and Martin McKee

The history of medicine:
- 2000 B.C.—Here, eat this root.
- 1000 A.D.—That root is heathen. Here, say this prayer.
- 1850 A.D.—That prayer is superstition. Here, drink this potion.
- 1920 A.D.—That potion is snake oil. Here, swallow this pill.
- 1945 A.D.—That pill is ineffective. Here, take this penicillin.
- 1955 A.D.—Oops ... bugs mutated. Here, take this tetracycline.
- 1960–1999 A.D.—39 more 'oops.' ... Here, take this more powerful antibiotic.
- 2000 A.D.—The bugs have won! Here, eat this root.

Anonymous, as cited by the World Health Organization (WHO 2000a)

Overview

In the twenty-first century infectious diseases remain a major global public health problem. Public health measures that can both detect and respond to known and unknown risks, linked to the development and monitoring of prevention and control programmes, are crucial to better health worldwide. In this chapter you will learn about how measures to reduce infectious diseases have changed over time. You will also be introduced to the changing patterns of infectious diseases and to the factors underlying these changes, and how these in turn have influenced the way we have tried to contain infectious diseases.

Learning objectives

After completing this chapter you should be able to:

- describe some of the measures used to contain infectious diseases historically
- describe the nature of how infectious diseases are changing
- describe factors behind the changing profile of infectious diseases
- comment on the shifting relationship between the state and individuals in controlling infectious diseases

Key terms

> **Germ theory**   The theory that all contagious diseases are caused by micro-organisms.

The evolution of human disease and our understanding of it

Infectious diseases have always afflicted humanity. Understanding the history of the interrelationship between the agents responsible and their host provides insights into current trends in infectious diseases, some understanding of how environmental and social changes impact upon disease and how contemporary responses to public health threats are frequently reflect those of the past.

The human race originated in the tropical climate of Africa and was affected by the same parasites as other primates in these areas. As these early hunters migrated into more temperate zones, then the infectious agents they were exposed to changed.

As hunting gave way to agriculture, populations grew and stabilized. The development of agriculture, and with it a situation in which domestic animals lived in close proximity to humans, created the opportunity for many **zoonotic infections** (such as measles, which may have arisen from distemper in dogs or rindepest in cows) to spread to humans. The increase in population size and density provided the ideal conditions for further person-to-person spread of infectious micro-organisms. Humans, food and water became established reservoirs for many infectious agents (Diamond 1997).

As civilizations developed further and trade routes became established the movements of people and goods carried new pathogens to susceptible populations. Explorers and armies performed similar functions. By the Middle Ages epidemics of infectious diseases such as plague, smallpox and typhus devastated communities, reduced armies to waste, and generated fear among populations and their leaders.

Of course, a good understanding of disease and its causes is necessary to develop appropriate responses. But before the role of micro-organisms in the causation of disease was understood, responses to epidemics of disease often focused on individuals or groups of individuals perceived as the originators of disease. History is replete with examples of people being subjected to severe measures to protect the wider population. The perceived association of minority populations and disease, in a climate of irrational fear, has been a common feature of responses to infectious diseases for many centuries. For example, the Jewish population in Europe was especially vulnerable as their observance of strict laws on food preparation often spared them infections that affected the remainder of the population. In response to the threat of plague, for instance, 900 Jews were burned alive at Strasbourg in 1349, even before the plague arrived.

Control of infectious diseases became possible through the work of Robert Koch and Louis Pasteur and the isolation and identification of etiologic agents. The epidemiology and clinical picture of infectious diseases could then be described, measures to support control introduced, and the impact of these measures determined. Understanding of the 'germ theory', first plausibly articulated in the 1870s, improved. As a result, the focus of measures to contain disease became narrower. This focus sometimes highlighted the inherent tension between the individual and public health, as noted in Chapter 1. Examples include the following:

- in England the Contagious Diseases Acts of the 1860s were aimed at countering sexually transmitted infections in the armed forces through the compulsory medical inspection of 'streetwalkers' in garrison towns and ports; note that in the culture of that time, only the women sex workers were inspected and not the male soldiers

- the forcible removal of children with suspected polio to specially outfitted pavilions in New York in 1916;
- the detention for life of Mary Mallon ('Typhoid Mary') on North Brother Island (in the East River in New York City) in 1915 (she died in 1938);
- the incarceration of 30,000 prostitutes during World War I in the United States.

Activity 7.1

Think about other legal measures that might be used to influence the control of infectious diseases. List some examples.

Feedback

There are numerous other legal measures that have been used or that are currently being used to control infectious diseases. These include for example:

- the power to tax and spend (for example government spending on treatment of the human immunodeficiency virus (HIV));
- the power to alter how information is received (through health promotion activities – an example might be restrictions on the use of explicit language in campaigns to control sexually transmitted diseases);
- direct regulation of individuals (removal of freedom to decline treatment for tuberculosis, for example);
- indirect regulation through litigation (or **tort**) (for example, suing hospitals that fail to promote infection control to reduce wound infection rates from methicillin-resistant *Staphylococcus Aureus* (MRSA));
- deregulation (for example, removal of legal obstacles for brothels).

For other examples, see also Gostin (2001) and Chapter 9 in this book.

Activity 7.2

The advent of effective anti-microbial agents along with the establishment of the principles and practice of immunization hailed a new era. In 1948, George Marshall, then US Secretary of State, proclaimed that the conquest of all infectious diseases was imminent. This optimism persisted for several decades. It later appeared that this optimism was not so much wrong, or even premature, as misconceived. Explain why this might be the case. Illustrate your explanation with a few examples.

Feedback

This misconception was related to a simpler view of the relationship between infectious agents and human beings than we hold today. Relationships between humans and the microbial world are hugely complex and dynamic. The milieus in which parasites and host operate are informed by political, cultural, institutional and environmental forces.

Examples that illustrate this misconception include the more recent emergence of newly identified infectious diseases such as the acquired immune deficiency syndrome (AIDS) and severe acute respiratory syndrome (SARS), the re-emergence of 'ancient' diseases such as tuberculosis or diphtheria, the recognition that infectious agents might play a role in the genesis of many diseases previously not considered infectious, and the increasing anxiety that biological weapons may pose a substantial threat to public health.

The global burden of infectious disease

Infectious diseases are a major cause of ill health and death, particularly affecting children. They cause 15 million deaths annually, accounting for about 16 per cent of total global mortality in 2004 (World Health Organization 2008). HIV/AIDS and TB together caused 3.5 million deaths in 2004. Half of the deaths in children under 5 years old are caused by communicable diseases. They also accounted for almost 30 per cent of the total disability adjusted life years (DALY) lost worldwide in 2002.

Activity 7.3

In this activity you will take a closer look at mortality and at the burden of disease due to communicable diseases.

Tables 7.1 and 7.2 give information on the main causes of death and disease burden by WHO region. Using data from these tables, answer the following questions.

1 Identify in which regions deaths from infectious diseases are highest. Take into account the total number of deaths from infectious diseases, mortality rates (go back to Chapter 3 if you don't remember how to calculate mortality rates), and the proportion of deaths due to infectious diseases.
2 Identify in which regions the burden of disease due to infectious diseases is highest (consider the total number of DALYs and the proportion of DALYs due to infectious diseases).

Feedback

1 Mortality from infectious diseases is clearly highest in Africa where we see the highest number of deaths in absolute terms and the highest mortality rate for infectious and parasitic diseases (837 deaths per 100,000 population). Mortality from infectious/parasitic diseases or respiratory infections affects one in a hundred persons in Africa (1003 deaths per 100,000 population). Deaths from infectious diseases are also relatively high in South-East Asia (mortality rates: 184 per 100,000 for infectious/parasitic diseases and 276 per 100,000 for infectious/parasitic diseases and pulmonary infections taken jointly) and the Eastern Mediterranean region (190 per 100,000 for infectious/parasitic diseases and 260 per 100,000 for infectious/parasitic diseases and pulmonary infections taken jointly). In comparison, the death rate from infectious/parasitic diseases is only 22 per 100,000 population in Europe (although this hides regional differences within Europe that are not shown in Table 7.1).

Table 7.1 Deaths by cause in WHO regions, estimates for 2002

	Total (thousands)	% total	Africa (thousands)	The Americas (thousands)	South-East Asia (thousands)	Europe (thousands)	Eastern Medit. (thousands)	Western Pacific (thousands)
Population (thousands)	6 224 985		672 238	852 551	1 590 832	877 886	502 824	1 717 536
Total number of deaths	57029	100	10664	5962	14657	9564	4152	11940
Infectious and parasitic diseases	10904	19.1	5625	397	2922	195	953	804
Respiratory infections	3963	6.9	1118	226	1474	288	354	498
Maternal and perinatal conditions	2972	5.2	785	191	1184	68	370	370
Nutritional deficiencies	485	0.9	143	61	189	12	53	27
Neoplasms	7270	12.7	419	1145	1178	1871	296	2347
Diabetes mellitus, nutritional/endocrine disorders	1354	2.4	116	303	306	290	118	219
Neuropsychiatric disorders	1112	1.9	90	240	267	256	89	167
Cardiovascular diseases	16733	29.3	1036	1928	3911	4927	1079	3825
Respiratory diseases	3702	6.5	257	398	874	404	155	1609
Digestive diseases	1968	3.5	157	284	502	389	152	480
Other non communicable conditions	1521	2.7	187	237	389	188	175	342
Injuries	5168	9.1	741	540	1467	792	392	1229

Source: World Health Report 2004. Geneva: World Health Organization.

Table 7.2 Burden of disease in disability-adjusted life years (DALYs) by cause in WHO Regions, estimates for 2002[1]

	Total	% total	Africa	The Americas	South-East Asia	Europe	Eastearn Medit.	Western Pacific
Population (000)	6224985 (thousands)		672238 (thousands)	852551 (thousands)	1590832 (thousands)	877886 (thousands)	502824 (thousands)	1717536 (thousands)
Total number of DALYs	1490125643	100	361376478	145586527	426572902	150321605	139079337	264879260
Infectious and parasitic diseases	350332571	23.5	187448845	11890388	88952900	5665026	32410088	23671157
Respiratory infections	94603349	6.3	35595347	3315928	33026019	3115191	10818791	8653688
Maternal and perinatal conditions	130966679	8.8	33104006	9319806	50542629	3554015	16654594	17602104
Nutritional deficiencies	34416632	2.3	9573867	2124420	12127757	1703909	4490404	4360317
Neoplasms	77293663	5.2	4914205	11405860	14070924	17445197	4183809	25151663
Diabetes mellitus & nutritional/endocrine disorders	24155400	1.6	2404904	5753643	5893601	3169056	2095680	4751614
Neuropsychiatric disorders	193278495	13.0	17897036	35787391	48313777	29348996	15019744	46533897
Cardiovascular diseases	148190083	9.9	10910418	15173288	42987030	34417792	12059668	32413230
Respiratory diseases	55153199	3.7	5482583	7968078	15630419	6735413	3719707	15535384
Digestive diseases	46475768	3.1	5103566	5543889	14205642	7396276	4031778	10111155
Other non communicable conditions	153268686	0	18138712	17440027	45275063	16825972	16113431	39121304
Injuries	181991119	12.2	30802990	19863809	55547140	20944762	17481643	36973747

[1] Figures computed by WHO to assure comparibility, they are not necessarily the official statistics of WHO Member States, which may use alternative rigorous methods.

Source: Adapted from World Health Organization (2004).

The proportion of all deaths due to infectious diseases is also highest in Africa where more than half of all deaths are due to infectious or parasitic diseases (52.7 per cent) and 63 per cent to infectious/parasitic diseases or pulmonary infections. This compares with only 2 per cent and 5.1 per cent respectively in Europe. A relatively high proportion of deaths from infectious/parasitic diseases is also found in South-East Asia (19.9 per cent) and the Eastern Mediterranean region (23.0 per cent).

2 A pattern similar to that described above is found when we look at the burden of disease due to infectious diseases. Over 187 million DALYs are lost yearly in Africa due to infectious or parasitic diseases and 35.6 million lost due to respiratory infections. This compares with only 5.7 million and 3.1 million respectively in Europe. The burden of disease due to infectious diseases is also relatively high in South-East Asia. In this region, almost 90 million DALYs are lost due to infectious or parasitic diseases and 33 million due to respiratory infections. The third region with the highest disease burden due to infectious diseases is, as expected, the Eastern Mediterranean region (32.4 million and 10.8 millions DALYs lost respectively to infectious/parasitic diseases and respiratory infections).

Results for the proportion of total DALYs lost due to infectious diseases are similar with the highest values observed in Africa (51.9 per cent for infectious/parasitic diseases and 9.8 per cent for respiratory infections), followed by South-East Asia (20.9 per cent and 7.7 per cent) and the Eastern Mediterranean region (23.3 per cent and 7.8 per cent). The lowest proportions are found in Europe where 3.8 per cent of total DALYs are accounted for by infectious/parasitic diseases and 2.1 per cent by respiratory infections. You may like to consult *Introduction to Epidemiology* (Carneiro and Howard 2011) in this series for more detailed account of the Global Burden of Disease project.

Emergent and re-emergent infectious diseases

The nature of infectious diseases is changing not only in terms of magnitude and the inability of science to provide all the answers but also for the following three reasons. First, 'new' diseases, most notably HIV/AIDS and SARS, resulting from apparently new organisms are occurring. Second, 'ancient' diseases such as tuberculosis and diphtheria are re-emerging as serious threats to public health (often having 'disappeared' only in affluent western societies). Third, novel agents are being newly implicated in the causation of a number of clinical syndromes (for example parvovirus, human T-cell lymphotropic viruses I and II, and a number of human herpes viruses).

Following a period of uncertainty, the causative infectious agent has been defined in some conditions, including Legionnaires' disease and Lyme disease. Progress in the identification of micro-organisms through advances in molecular biology and epidemiology have led to the discovery that infectious agents may be responsible for diseases previously considered non-transmissible, such as a number of cancers, peptic ulcer disease, reactive arthritis and atherosclerosis. Examples of pathogenic microbes and the diseases they cause are given in Tables 7.3 and 7.4.

The spectre of drug resistant organisms, unresponsive to anti-microbial agents, has emerged since the 1950s. Multi-drug resistance of infectious micro-organisms is a major global health problem. Strains of resistant *Mycobacterium tuberculosis* have been reported from all countries in the world. Outbreaks of resistant *Staphylococcus aureus*, including methicillin resistant *Staphylococcus aureus* (MRSA), threaten health care

Table 7.3 Examples of pathogenic microbes and the diseases they cause since 1973

Year	Microbe	Type	Disease
1973	Rotavirus	Virus	Infantile diarrhea
1977	Ebola virus	Virus	Acute hemorrhagic fever
1977	Legionella pneumophila	Bacterium	Legionnaires' disease
1980	Human T-lymphotrophic virus (HTLV1)	Virus	T-cell lymphoma/leukemia
1981	Toxin-producing Staphylococcus aureus	Bacterium	Toxic shock syndrome
1982	Escherichia coli O157:H7	Bacterium	Hemorrhagic colitis; hemolytic uremic syndrome
1982	Borrelia burgdorferi	Bacterium	Lyme disease
1983	Human Immunodeficiency virus (HIV)	Virus	Acquired Immuno-Deficiency Syndrome (AIDS)
1983	Helicobacter pylori	Bacterium	Peptic ulcer disease
1989	Hepatitis C	Virus	Parentally transmitted non-A, non-B liver infection
1992	Vibrio cholerae O139	Bacterium	New strain associated with epidemic cholera
1993	Hantavirus	Virus	Adult respiratory distress syndrome
1994	Cryptosporidium	Protozoa	Enteric disease
1995	Ehrlichiosis	Bacterium	Severe arthritis?
1996	nvCJD	Prion	New variant Creutzfeldt-Jakob disease
1997	HVN1	Virus	Influenza
1999	Nipah	Virus	Severe encephalitis
2003	Coronavirus	Virus	SARS

Source: Adapted mostly from English Department of Health (2002)

Table 7.4 Diseases associated with infectious agents

Disease/syndrome/disorder	Agent
Chronic gastritis	H pylori
Peptic ulcer	H pylori
Guillain-Barre syndrome	Campylobacter jejuni
Bell's palsy	Borrelia burgdorferi, Herpes simplex virus
Tropical spastic paraparesis	HTLV-1
Haemolytic uraemic syndrome	E coli O157
Throbotic thrombocytopenic purpura	E coli O157
Polyarteritis nodosa	Hepatitis B virus
Insulin dependent diabetes	Enterovirus
Atherosclerosis	Chlamydia pneumoniae, cytomegolovirus
Reactive arthritis	Salmonella spp., Yersinia spp., Chlamydia trachomatis
Human T-cell leukaemia	HTLV-1
Hairy cell leukaemia	HTLV-2
Hepatocellular cancer	Hepatitis B and C
Cervical cancer	HPV
Burkitt's lymphoma	EBV
AIDS-related CNS lymphoma	EBV
Kaposi's sarcoma	HHV8
AIDS-related body cavity lymphoma	HHV8
Castleman's disease	HHV8

provision with potentially huge economic costs. Resistant *Salmonella* species have arisen from excessive use of antibiotics in the food animal industry with serious consequences for human health. Other examples of drug resistant infectious agents are provided in Table 7.5. The IOM (US Institute of Medicine) estimated the economic costs of drug resistance to be $4–5bn per annum in 2001.

The costs of outbreaks of infectious diseases are high (Table 7.6). The epidemic of bovine spongiform encephalitis is estimated to have cost approaching $40 billion,

Table 7.5 Examples of drug-resistant infectious agents and percentage of infections that are drug resistant, by country or region

Pathogen	Drug	Country/Area	Percentage of drug-resistant infections
Streptococcus pneumoniae	Penicillin	United States	10–35
		Asia, Chile, Spain	20
		Hungary	58
Staphylococcus aureus	Methicillin°	United States	32
	Vancomycin	United States	0
Mycobacterium tuberculosis	Any drug	United States	13
		New York City	16
	INH + RIF*	United States	2
		New York City	5
Plasmodium falciparum malaria	Chloroquine	Kenya	65
		Ghana	45
		Zimbabwe	59
		Burkina Faso	17
	Mefloquine	Thailand	40
Shigella dysenteriae	Multidrug	Burundi, Rwanda	100

* Resistance to isoniazid (INH), rifampicin (RIF), and/or other drugs.

° >50% by 2010 (Institute of Medicine 2010)

Source: Institute of Medicine (1997)

Table 7.6 Examples of economic impact of major infectious disease outbreaks

Year	Country	Disease	Cost (US$)
1979–94	New York City	Tuberculosis	Over 1 billion
1990–8	Malaysia	Nipah virus	540 million
1991	United Kingdom	Bovine Spongiform Encephalopathy (BSE)	38 billion
1994	India	Plague	2 billion
1997	Hong Kong	'Bird flu'	22 million
1998	Tanzania	Cholera	770 million
1999	New York	West Nile Fever	Almost 100 million
1999	Russian Federation	Tuberculosis	Over 4 billion
2003	China, Hong Kong, Canada, others	Severe Acute Respiratory Syndrome (SARS)	10–30 billion

Source: Adapted from selected WHO reports

decimating the British beef industry. The financial cost of the epidemic of HIV is beyond comprehension.

The picture of infectious disease changes as effective therapeutic measures are developed and become adopted in practice. For example, the clinical picture of HIV has changed dramatically for those able to access HAART (Highly Active Anti-Retroviral Therapy) in ways analogous to the improvement in prognosis for diabetics with the introduction of insulin.

Experience of the first twenty-first-century pandemic

The 2009 'swine flu' pandemic was the first influenza pandemic of this century. While the world's media had been raising alarm at the supposedly impending pandemic of 'bird flu' (H5N1), what actually emerged in 2009 was the rapid spread of H1N1, which affected millions of people worldwide, but with a lower mortality rate than had been feared by politicians and public and public health specialists. Unlike seasonal influenza, it affected mainly children and young adults, many of whom had no underlying or predisposing factors, but it affected pregnant women disproportionately, in line with greater susceptibility, probably due to altered immune response during pregnancy. H1N1 showed characteristics of a re-emergent infection, in that it appeared that older people – those who had been exposed to influenza in the pandemics of the 1957/8 ('Asian flu' H2N2) and 1968/9 ('Hong Kong flu' H3N2) – were less likely to become seriously ill in this pandemic, although there were exceptions, and in the UK 457 people died as a result of the pandemic, of whom 70 were under 18 years old. There was international collaboration in managing the pandemic and in most countries the mass media were considered to have reported fairly, in the main. In England the government introduced a centrally led Flu Plan in line with its 'National Framework for responding to an influenza pandemic'. Antiviral agents were made available early with algorithms for their use disseminated to GPs and hospitals, and a vaccine was subsequently developed and rolled out to highest risk groups. In the early 'containment' stage all suspected cases were swabbed to enable tracking of the epidemic, a practice stopped when the pandemic occurred. In the post-pandemic phase, there was a stock of unused 2009/10 H1N1 vaccine in many countries, some of which was subsequently utilized in the 2010/11 flu season, although the anticipated resurgence of H1N1 did not occur. Reviews have been published on management of the pandemic in several countries (for England, see DH 2010; Hine 2010). One important theme of the reviews was the lack of respect for national boundaries, so that although the effective international collaboration involving ECDC, CDC and WHO was recognized, the lack of complete convergence within the four UK countries was noted. The economic costs of the pandemic have yet to be assessed.

Factors affecting the growth and spread of infectious diseases

As noted above, factors beyond the immediate relationship of microbe and pathogenic host defences influence the growth and spread of infectious diseases. For example international travel and commerce is known to be associated with the spread of malaria, cholera and pneumococcal pneumonia.

The WHO responded to the increasing risks to population health posed by international travel and trade, and by emergence and re-emergence of communicable diseases, by development of the International Health Regulations (IHR) (2005). They came into force in 2007. The stated purpose and scope of the IHR are 'to prevent, protect against, control and provide a public health response to the international spread of disease in ways that are commensurate with and restricted to public health risks, and which avoid unnecessary interference with international traffic and trade' (World Health Organization 2008a).

Factors that contribute to the global spread of infectious disease

Numerous other potential factors contribute to the growth and spread of infectious diseases worldwide. These can be classified into seven main groups:

1 Demographic changes and human behaviours

a) *Population growth* Despite falling birth rates in some developed countries and the dramatic impact of the HIV/AIDS epidemic in others, the world population is growing at a rate of approximately 1.5 per cent per annum. It is likely that by 2030 the world population will be 8 billion. Overcrowding will increase and this will promote the spread of infectious diseases, including dengue/dengue haemorrhagic fever and giardiasis.

b) *Poverty* Approximately one quarter of the world's population live in extreme poverty, surviving on less than $1 per day and most of these people live in Asia and sub-Saharan Africa. The share and number of people living on less than $2 per day – a more relevant threshold for middle-income economies such as those of East Asia and Latin America – is roughly similar. These figures translate into the stark fact that some 2 billion people suffer from under-nutrition or malnutrition and lack access to basic health care and to safe water. The links between poverty, malnutrition and infectious diseases are clear.

c) *Population movements* People who flee their home countries out of a fear of persecution join a larger stream of migrants who leave in search of opportunities for work, education, reunification with family members, or for other reasons. It has been estimated that at the end of the twentieth century some 150 million people were living outside the country of their birth, amounting to approximately 2.5 per cent of the world's population, or one out of every 40 people. Two million people cross international borders every single day, about a tenth of humanity each year, and of these, more than a million travel from developing to industrialized countries each week. Many of these migrants live in overcrowded conditions and, as in centuries before, epidemics result from transmission through rapid person-to-person spread among susceptible populations or through the carriage of vectors.

d) *Human behaviours* Changes in behaviour, including sexual behaviour and injecting drug use, are associated with changes in the incidence of several infectious diseases. Increases in sexually transmissible infections in eastern Europe has followed marked socioeconomic and behavioural changes. Most notably, since the 1980s HIV has spread across the world. Sexual, vertical, and parental transmission is devastating communities. Hepatitis B is similarly transmitted. 'Non-compliance' by health care workers, patients, drug producers, and health care systems is resulting in drug resistant organisms. For example, outbreaks of multi-drug resistant tuberculosis that emerged often resulted in non-compliance of one or more of the actors/ institutions.

2 Technological development

The epidemic of BSE, which by 2001 had affected over 179,000 cows in Great Britain, has been ascribed to technological changes in the animal and human food chain which dated from the 1980s. By October, 2001, 101 people had become sick and died from variant Creutzfeldt-Jacob disease (vCJD). Both vCJD and BSE are transmissible spongiform encephalopathies and it is likely that they are linked.

The development and application of new technologies may have deleterious effects. Another example is the link between air conditioning systems and legionella outbreaks. Other infections that have been associated with technological development include toxic shock syndrome, nosocomial (hospital-acquired) infections, and haemorrhagic colitis/haemolytic uremic syndrome.

3 Economic development and land use

These are associated with Lyme disease, malaria, plague, rabies, yellow fever, Rift Valley fever and schistosomiasis. Development projects such as the building of dams, irrigation schemes, hydroelectric power plants and roads, which are intended to improve social wellbeing, may have negative effects that include the displacement of people, chronic food deficiency and the development of new and more pernicious forms of poverty. The Nam Pong dam in Thailand resulted in substantial increases in local rates of liver fluke and hookworm morbidity – the result of poor waste disposal and poor living conditions of resettled people.

4 Microbial adaptation and change

Immunological responses of hosts may vary in response to changes in micro-organisms. An example is antigenic *drift* resulting from spontaneous mutations that result in minor changes in the amino acid sequence of proteins. The changes result in mutant strains of the virus then becoming selected in the population by their ability to infect partially immune hosts. By contrast antigenic *shift*, which occurs much less frequently, involves replacement of the main neutralizing antigen by a different protein acquired as a result of genetic change when some of the genetic coding of the micro-organism is exchanged for a code from another agent (for example, by transfer of plasmids, which are small fragments of DNA). Major epidemics often result from antigenic drift because the host has little immune protection, such as the 1918 influenza pandemic. (The SARS epidemic illustrated the frailty of global public health systems to meet the challenge of an emergent pathogen that readily crosses international borders – SARS is considerably less transmissible than influenza.)

5 Breakdown of health infrastructure or public health policy

In the 1990s a massive epidemic of diphtheria occurred throughout the countries of the former Soviet Union. Diphtheria had been well controlled in the Soviet Union for more than two decades after universal childhood immunization was initiated in the late 1950s. However from the mid-1980s changes in the immunization schedule to incorporate fewer doses of lower antigenic content, an increasing number of contraindications to vaccination and decreased public confidence in the vaccination programmes led to levels of vaccination coverage below 70 per cent in most areas. In 1990 epidemic diphtheria re-emerged in the Soviet Union with the highest incidence rates in adolescents and adults aged 40–49 years reaching a peak in 1994–95. Other infectious diseases associated with the breakdown of public health include rabies, tuberculosis, trench fever, whooping cough (pertussis) and cholera.

6 Climate change

Global warming over the next century will result in increases in food productivity in some areas and falls in others. Some low-lying areas will suffer flooding and loss of agricultural land and contamination of fresh water supplies. Migration of large populations is likely to result. Five hundred million people currently live at or near sea level. Changes in temperature will result in different distributions of vectors. Mosquitoes will survive in previously mosquito-free regions introducing diseases such as malaria and dengue, cholera and yellow fever. See Chapter 12 for more on this topic.

7 Warfare, terrorism and conflict

Wars and conflicts create environments that micro-organisms exploit. The movements of large numbers of people, unhygienic living conditions, malnutrition and the destruction of public infrastructures encourage diseases and their spread.

The pollution of water supplies and catapulting of diseased human corpses into besieged cities are early examples of biological warfare. In the eighteenth century, the British distributed smallpox-infected blankets to North American Indians. But it was not until the twentieth century that research and development of biological warfare activities increased. By the 1940s a joint programme between the United States, United Kingdom and Canada sought to produce an anthrax bomb. Through the cold war the Soviet Union maintained programmes to develop biological weapons, sometimes leading to accidental releases that caused many fatalities; by the 1980s advances in genetic engineering were being harnessed to produce, for example, strains of plague resistant to antibiotics.

Since the first Gulf War in 1991 there has been increasing concern about biological weapons. This has resulted in considerable investment in detection, identification and protection measures. The events of 11 September 2001 in the USA and the subsequent distribution of anthrax through the US postal service raised anxiety further. This is reflected in plans to immunize 500,000 key personnel in the USA against smallpox. (See Chapter 9 for more on this topic.)

Control of infectious diseases – the state and individual responsibilities

As can be inferred from the sections above, the variables that influence the relationship between man and infectious agents are interrelated. What remains largely unclear, however, is what should be the appropriate responses to the changing nature of infectious diseases. The core principles of infectious diseases control and the resources available may be inadequate to assert 'control' even if that were theoretically possible. The complexity of the interrelationships between variables demands responses that go beyond those that focus on the hosts and organism but encompass socioeconomic, cultural and political imperatives.

Indeed, notions of **globalization** challenge conventional responses to infectious diseases in ways that are now becoming apparent. The roles and responsibilities of states and their often limited ability to control infectious diseases that have the potential to cross borders and threaten populations resident in other states is a potential source of tension. This was seen during the SARS epidemic and has influenced the development of the international health regulations (international laws that aim to control **transnational** spread of disease).

The tension between the individual and society plays out in several arenas when we contemplate responses to infectious diseases. For example, the free movements of people across borders may be inhibited through the quarantine of migrants potentially carrying infectious micro-organisms (for example returning soldiers, economic migrants, refugees from epidemics) – powers to quarantine cities in the United States have been suggested in the event of biological threat. Compulsory immunization may be deemed an appropriate measure in countries where it is not already in place.

Likewise, compulsory treatment or isolation of those who pose a threat might be considered where individuals either decline treatment or are untreatable respectively. These issues are explored further in consideration of human rights and health in Chapter 9.

The following activity will help you to think about this perennial tension and contemplate the responsibilities of the state to provide for the wellbeing of individuals and of individuals to comply with measures to reduce the threat they might pose in the context of re-emergent tuberculosis.

Activity 7.4

Paul Farmer has been at the forefront of the campaign to see the emergence of infectious disease as a response to social inequity. Now read the following extract from one of his papers (Farmer 1996) and answer the following questions:

1 What, in Farmer's view, explains the relative lack of visibility of many infectious diseases?
2 Take one of the examples quoted by Farmer (Argentinian and Bolivian haemorrhagic fever) and sketch a chain of events that has led to its emergence as a problem.
3 Farmer quotes Anthony McMichael as saying 'Modern epidemiology is oriented to explaining and quantifying the bobbing of corks on the surface waters, while largely disregarding the stronger undercurrents that determine where, on average, the cluster of corks ends up along the shoreline of risk.' What do you understand by this statement?
4 Can you think of examples other than those mentioned by Farmer of global or regional policies that have had consequences for the pattern of infectious diseases?

Infections and Inequalities: The Modern Plagues
The past decade has been one of the most eventful in the long history of infectious diseases. The sheer number of relevant publications indicates explosive growth; moreover, new means of monitoring antimicrobial resistance patterns are being used along with the rapid sharing of information (as well as speculation and misinformation) through means that did not exist even 10 years ago. Then there are the microbes themselves. One of the explosions in question – perhaps the most remarked upon – is that of 'emerging infectious diseases'. Among the diseases considered 'emerging', some are regarded as genuinely new; AIDS and Brazilian

purpuric fever are examples. Others have newly identified etiologic agents or have again burst dramatically onto the scene. For example, the syndromes caused by Hantaan virus have been known in Asia for centuries but now seem to be spreading beyond Asia because of ecologic and economic transformations that increase contact between humans and rodents. Still other diseases grouped under the 'emerging' rubric are ancient and well-known foes that have somehow changed, in pathogenicity or distribution. Multidrug-resistant tuberculosis (TB) and invasive or necrotizing Group A streptococcal infection are cases in point.

In studying emerging infectious diseases, many make a distinction between a host of phenomena directly related to human actions – from improved laboratory techniques and scientific discovery to economic 'development', global warming, and failures of public health – and another set of phenomena, much less common and related to changes in the microbes themselves. Close examination of microbial mutations often shows that, again, human actions have played a large role in enhancing pathogenicity or increasing resistance to antimicrobial agents.

The study of anything said to be emerging tends to be dynamic. But the very notion of emergence in heterogeneous populations poses questions of analysis that are rarely tackled, even in modern epidemiology, which 'assigns a primary importance to studying interindividual variations in risk. By concentrating on these specific and presumed freerange individual behaviors, we thereby pay less attention to the underlying social-historical influences on behavioral choices, patterns, and population health' (McMichael 1995). A critical (and self-critical) approach would ask how existing frameworks might limit our ability to discern trends that can be linked to the emergence of diseases.

A critical approach pushes the limits of existing academic politesse to ask harder and rarely raised questions: What are the mechanisms by which changes in agriculture have led to outbreaks of Argentine and Bolivian haemorrhagic fever, and how might these mechanisms be related to international trade agreements, such as the General Agreement on Tariffs and Trade and the North American Free Trade Agreement? How might institutional racism be related to urban crime and the outbreaks of multidrug-resistant TB in New York prisons? Similar questions may be productively posed in regard to many diseases now held to be emerging.

Questions for a critical epistemology of emerging infectious diseases

Ebola, TB, and HIV infection are in no way unique in demanding contextualization through social science approaches. These approaches include the grounding of case histories and local epidemics in the larger biosocial systems in which they take shape and demand exploration of social inequalities. Why, for example, were there 10,000 cases of diphtheria in Russia from 1990 to 1993? It is easy enough to argue that the excess cases were due to a failure to vaccinate. But only in linking this distal (and, in sum, technical) cause to the much more complex socioeconomic transformations altering the region's illness and death patterns will compelling explanations emerge.

Standard epidemiology, narrowly focused on individual risk and short on critical theory, will not reveal these deep socioeconomic transformations, nor will it connect them to disease emergence. 'Modern epidemiology' observes one of its leading contributors, is 'oriented to explaining and quantifying the bobbing of corks on the surface waters, while largely disregarding the stronger undercurrents that determine where, on average, the cluster of corks ends up along the shoreline of risk' (McMichael 1995).

Research questions identified by various **blue-ribbon panels** are important for the understanding and eventual control of emerging infectious diseases. Yet both the diseases and popular and scientific commentary on them pose a series of corollary questions, which, in turn, demand research that is neither the exclusive province of social scientists nor bench scientists, clinicians, or epidemiologists. Indeed, genuinely transdisciplinary collaboration will be necessary to tackle the problems posed by emerging infectious diseases. As **prolegomena**, four areas of corollary research are easily identified. In each is heard the recurrent leitmotiv of inequality:

Social inequalities
Study of the **reticulated** links between social inequalities and emerging disease would not construe the poor simply as 'sentinel chickens', but instead would ask, What are the precise mechanisms by which these diseases come to have their effects in some bodies but not in others? What propagative effects might social inequalities per se contribute?

Social inequalities have sculpted not only the distribution of emerging diseases, but also the course of disease in those affected by them, a fact that is often downplayed.

Transnational forces
Travel is a potent force in disease emergence and spread, and the current volume, speed, and reach of travel are unprecedented. The study of borders qua borders means, increasingly, the study of social inequalities. Many political borders serve as semipermeable membranes, often quite open to diseases and yet closed to the free movement of cures.

Research questions might include, for example, What effects might the interface between two very different types of health care systems have on the rate of advance of an emerging disease? What turbulence is introduced when the border in question is between a rich and a poor nation?

The dynamics of change
Can we elaborate lists of the differentially weighted factors that promote or retard the emergence or re-emergence of infectious diseases? It has been argued that such analyses will perforce be historically deep and geographically broad and they will at the same time be processual, incorporating concepts of change. Above all, they will seek to incorporate complexity rather than to merely dissect it.

Critical epistemology
Many have already asked: What qualifies as an emerging infectious disease? More critical questions might include, Why do some persons constitute 'risk groups,' while others are 'individuals at risk'? These are not merely **nosologic** questions; they are canonical ones.

Finally, why are some epidemics visible to those who fund research and services, while others are invisible? In its recent statements on TB and emerging infections, for example, the World Health Organization uses the threat of contagion to motivate wealthy nations to invest in disease surveillance and control out of self-interest – an age-old public health approach acknowledged in the Institute of Medicine's report (date) on emerging infections: 'Diseases that appear not to threaten the United States directly rarely elicit the political support necessary to maintain control efforts'. If related to a study under consideration, questions of power and control over funds, must be discussed. That they are not discussed is more a marker of analytic failures than of editorial standards.

Feedback

1 Farmer suggests that infectious diseases that attract more attention are those that represent a threat for wealthier nations (for example the United States), thus stimulating investment in disease surveillance and control. Diseases that do not seem to represent such a threat – although they might be very important in other countries – do not lead to the same support and thus to a lack of visibility.

2 A possible chain of events leading to emergence of Argentinian and Bolivian haemorrhagic fever as a problem:

→ Increased national prosperity
  → Ecological changes and degradation of land and water resources
  → Increased transport and consumption of energy
  → Increased movement from rural to urban areas with resulting uncontrolled urban growth
  → Increased illegal housing and slums
  → Poor/unsanitary living conditions
  → Reduced access to health care
  → Increased vulnerability to diseases
  → Increased possibility of mosquito breeding in stored water and non-biodegradable trash
  → Increased risk of infection
→ Constant movement within the country/region helps spread the disease
→ Lack of resources for epidemiological and vector control programmes and for treatment

3 Epidemiology usually examines the more direct causes of diseases (as in Farmer's example: the fact that a lack of vaccination was explaining an excess in the number of cases of diphtheria in Russia from 1990 to 1993), disregarding the more distal complex causes of diseases (in the above example the complex socioeconomic transformations altering the region's illness and death patterns).

4 Other examples of global or regional policies that have had consequences for the pattern of infectious diseases might include the European Common Agricultural Policy providing agricultural subsidies to EU countries. Markets for some developing nation products are thus restricted, which leads to poverty, inequalities in health and accompanying infectious diseases. Economic policies advocated by the international community to create market economy in Russia lead to great inequalities, economic hardship for many, high unemployment among the young, drug use, alcoholism, crime, high incarceration rates and a rise in infectious diseases rates such as tuberculosis and HIV.

Summary

This chapter was concerned with the evolution of infectious diseases and the way we have confronted them over time. You were first introduced to the historical development of our understanding of what infectious diseases are and how they can be contained. You then looked at the importance of infectious disease on the world's health. The nature of the recent changes in infectious diseases and the factors that contribute to them were then discussed. Finally, you were invited to consider the balance between the role of the state and that of individuals to reduce the threat of infectious diseases.

References

DH (Department of Health) (2002) *Getting Ahead of the Curve: A Strategy for Combating Infectious Diseases (Including Other Aspects of Health Protection)*. London: Department of Health.

DH (Department of Health) (2010) *Pandemic Influenza Preparedness Programme*. London: Department of Health (available at http://www.dh.gov.uk/prod_consum_dh/groups/dh_digitalassets/@dh/@en/@ps/documents/digitalasset/dh_122754.pdf).

Farmer P (1996) Social inequalities and emerging infectious diseases. *Emerg Infect Dis* **2**: 259–69.

Gostin LO (2001) *Public Health Law: Duty, Power, Restraint* (California/Milbank Series on Health and the Public, 3). Berkeley, CA: University of California Press.

Hine D (2010) *The 2009 Influenza Pandemic: An independent review of the UK response to the 2009 influenza pandemic*. London: Cabinet Office (available at http://www.cabinetoffice.gov.uk/sites/default/files/resources/the2009influenzapandemic-review.pdf).

Institute of Medicine (1997) *America's Vital Interest in Global Health: Protecting Our People, Enhancing Our Economy, and Advancing Our International Interests*. Washington, DC: National Academy Press.

Institute of Medicine (2010) *Antibiotic Resistance: Implications for Global Health and Novel Intervention Strategies: Workshop Summary* (available at http://books.nap.edu/openbook.php?record_id=12925).

McMichael A (1995) The health of persons, populations, and planets: epidemiology comes full circle. *Epidemiology* **6**: 633–6.

World Health Organization (2008a) *International Health Regulations (2005) (IHR)*, 2nd edition. Geneva: WHO (available at http://whqlibdoc.who.int/publications/2008/9789241580410_eng.pdf).

World Health Organization (2008b) *The Global Burden of Disease 2004 Update*. Geneva: WHO (available at http://www.who.int/healthinfo/global_burden_disease/GBD_report_2004update_full.pdf).

Further reading

Coker R (2000) The law, human rights, and detention of individuals with tuberculosis in England and Wales. *Public Health* **22**: 263–7.

Farmer P (1999) *Infections and Inequalities: The Modern Plagues*. Berkeley, CA: University of California Press. The author provides a critique of economic and health care inequalities.

Garrett L (2000) *Betrayal of Trust: The Collapse of Global Public Health*. New York: Hyperion. This book discusses the impact of globalization of infectious agents and diseases risks throughout the world.

Institute of Medicine, Washington DC (2010) *Antibiotic Resistance: Implications for Global Health and Novel Intervention Strategies: Workshop Summary* (available at http://books.nap.edu/openbook.php?record_id=12925&page=3).

MacLehose L, McKee M and Weinberg J (2002) Responding to the challenge of communicable disease in Europe. *Science* **295**: 2047–50.

Mann JM and Tarantola DJM (eds) (1996) *AIDS in the World II: Global Dimensions, Social Roots, and Responses*. New York, NY: Oxford University Press. This book describes the gap between the pandemic and global response to AIDS.

World Health Organization's Infectious Diseases website (available at http://www.who.int/topics/ infectious_diseases/en/). This website will provide you with a description of the activities, reports, news and events, as well as contacts and cooperating partners in the various WHO programmes and offices working on infectious diseases.

8 Tobacco: still a global public health priority

Anna Gilmore, Martin McKee, Fiona Sim and Joceline Pomerleau

Overview

Tobacco is unique in being the only product that kills when used as intended. Because about half of all regular cigarette smokers will eventually be killed by their habit, and because the geography of smoking continues to shift from developed to developing countries, tobacco smoking needs to be treated as a major global public health issue. In this chapter you will learn about the health impact of tobacco use and the four-stage model of the smoking epidemic. You will then examine current debates around tobacco control policies and options for these policies. Finally, the chapter discusses how globalization represents a major challenge for tobacco control.

Learning objectives

By the end of this chapter, you should be able to:

- describe the health impact of tobacco use and its importance as a global and national public health issue
- have a broad understanding of the options for tobacco control
- outline the influence that powerful multinationals have in public health policy-making

Key terms

Addiction   Dependence on something that is psychologically or physically habit-forming.

Globalization   A set of processes that are changing the nature of human interaction by intensifying interactions across certain boundaries that have hitherto served to separate individuals and population groups. These spatial, temporal and cognitive boundaries have been increasingly eroded, resulting in new forms of social organization and interaction across these boundaries (based on Lee 2003).

International   Refers to cross-border flows that are, in principle, possible to regulate by national governments.

> **Tort** Legal term used to describe a wrongful act, resulting in harm or loss to another person or their property, on which a civil action for damages may be brought.
>
> **Transnational** (as opposed to international) Refers to transborder flows that largely circumvent national borders and can thus be beyond the control of national governments alone.

Introduction

Tobacco is causing a major public health disaster; the rising rate of tobacco consumption seen worldwide is set to harm global health on an unprecedented scale. By 2020, tobacco is expected to kill more people than any other single factor, surpassing even the HIV epidemic.

The study of tobacco and the control of its use are therefore warranted simply by virtue of tobacco's huge impact on public health. But tobacco also serves to illustrate many of the issues discussed in previous chapters in this book: it is a major cause of health inequalities and there have been ethical debates around the methods that can be appropriately used to control its use. In addition, tobacco illustrates some of the complex issues facing public health practitioners in the twenty-first century – it highlights the key challenges that globalization poses for public health, the complex relationship between trade and health, the potential conflicts of interest that tobacco control poses for governments and the difficulties of enacting effective public health policies that are opposed by powerful transnational companies.

The history of tobacco use stretches back to the first century AD amongst the Mayan people of Central America. From there, tobacco use spread through America and to the Caribbean islands, where leaves were presented to the invading Spaniards at the end of the fifteenth century. A few years later, tobacco was brought back to Spain and Portugal and from there its use gradually spread throughout Europe. Tobacco has subsequently been chewed and smoked in various forms. However, it was not until the late nineteenth century, when the introduction of the Bonsack machine (for rolling cigarettes) led to the mass manufacture of cigarettes, that its use really escalated. Since then, cigarette smoking has spread worldwide on a massive scale.

Health effects of smoking

The health impacts of tobacco use are daunting. It has been recognized as the single largest avoidable cause of premature death and the most important known carcinogen to humans. Half of all long-term smokers will eventually be killed by tobacco and of these, half will die during middle age, losing 20–25 years of life. Smoking is also associated with health inequalities by virtue of the social patterning of smoking. For example, international comparisons indicate that overall smoking prevalence is now higher in low- and middle-income countries than in high-income countries (Table 8.1). In high-income countries smoking is now much less common among the better off, although social-class patterns are less clear in middle-income and low-income countries (Bobak and colleagues 2000).

Table 8.1 Estimated smoking prevalence by sex and number of smokers aged 15 years and older, by World Bank Region, 1995

World Bank Region	Smoking prevalence, %			Total smokers	
	Males	Females	Overall	No. in millions	% of all smokers
East Asia and Pacific	62	5	34	429	38
Europe and Central Asia	53	16	34	122	11
Latin America and Caribbean	39	22	31	98	9
Middle East and North Africa	38	7	23	37	3
South Asia (cigarettes)	20	1	11	84	7
South Asia (bidis)	20	3	12	94	8
Sub-Saharan Africa	28	8	18	56	5
Low and middle income	49	8	29	919	82
High income	37	21	29	202	18
World	47	11	29	1121	100

Source: Jha et al. (2002)

The direct health effects of tobacco consumption can be considered under two headings, nicotine addiction and health problems.

Nicotine addiction

Experts conclude that nicotine is as addictive as hard drugs such as heroin and that smoking tobacco meets the criteria of substance dependence in both the fourth edition of the Diagnostic and Statistical Manual of Mental Disorders (DSM-IV) and the tenth revision of the International Statistical Classification of Diseases and Related Health Problems (ICD-10). Repeated exposure rapidly leads to physiological and psychological addiction, reinforced by marked withdrawal symptoms. These include irritability, anxiety, restlessness and poor concentration. It is likely therefore that the benefits smokers attribute to nicotine use such as stress relief, improved mood and enhanced cognitive performance are really just the relief of nicotine withdrawal symptoms. Yet the status of nicotine as a seemingly innocuous legal drug and attempts by the tobacco industry to equate addiction to nicotine with addiction to substances such as coffee or chocolate has diverted attention from the highly addictive nature of nicotine in cigarettes.

Health problems

The negative impact of tobacco on health was first reported over 200 years ago in relation to carcinoma of the lip but it was not until the 1950s with the publication of a number of case control studies that the relationship between smoking and lung cancer began to gain credence. Subsequent cohort studies including the pioneering work of Doll and Hill (Doll and Hill 1954) confirmed the enormous health impacts of tobacco and showed that overall mortality is twice as high in smokers as non-smokers and three times as high in middle age.

Activity 8.1 Diseases associated with smoking

Smoking has now been positively associated with over 40 diseases. Try to list as many of these diseases as possible. You can browse through the internet to help you.

Feedback

Smoking has been positively associated with over 40 diseases and negatively associated with eight or nine more. For most diseases the evidence is strong and the associations between smoking and mortality are causal in character. Findings have been confirmed in numerous studies in different populations, biological mechanisms are understood, the association is strong and a dose response relationship is seen. The diseases fall into three main categories, cancer, vascular diseases and chronic lung diseases, as described in Table 8.2, which is taken from the 2004 United States (US) Surgeon General's report on the health effects of smoking.

Table 8.2 Main diseases known to be associated with smoking

Main diseases	
Cancers	Bladder, cervix*, oesophagus, kidney*, larynx, acute myeloid leukaemia*, lung, oral cancer, pancreas*, stomach
Cardiovascular diseases	Abdominal aortic aneurysm*, atherosclerosis, cerebrovascular disease, coronary heart disease
Respiratory diseases	Chronic obstructive pulmonary disease, pneumonia*, respiratory effects in utero, respiratory effects on children and adolescents
Reproductive effects	Fetal deaths and stillbirths, infertility (in women), low birth weight, pregnancy complications
Other effects	Cataract*, diminished health status*, hip fractures, low bone density, periodontitis*, peptic ulcer disease

*Added as being 'causally associated with smoking' in 2004

Source: Adapted from United States Department of Health and Human Services (2004)

Recently it has been observed that the health effects differ between countries, with, for example, lower than expected incidence of lung cancer in some populations, notably Japanese men, despite high prevalence of smoking. This so-called 'smoking paradox' has not yet been explained fully, but may be linked with lower alcohol consumption and fat intake by Japanese men; lower levels of carcinogenic ingredients or better filters in Japanese cigarettes; and protective hereditary factors (Takahashi et al. 2008).

Health impacts of involuntary exposure

Tobacco is also a major cause of morbidity and mortality in those involuntarily exposed to secondhand smoke or environmental tobacco smoking. Since the 1980s a growing series of high profile reports have drawn attention to its health impact. These include the US National Research Council and the US Surgeon General reports in 1986, the National Health and Medical Research Council of Australia report in 1987 and the United Kingdom (UK) Independent Scientific Committee on Smoking and Health report in 1988. These reports concluded that environmental tobacco smoking can cause lung cancer in adult non-smokers and that the children of parents who smoke have increased frequency of respiratory symptoms and lower respiratory tract infections. In 1992, the US Environmental Protection Agency published a review that classified environmental tobacco smoking as a Class A (known human) carcinogen. This is a status afforded to only 15 other carcinogens (including asbestos, benzene and radon) and indicates that there is sufficient evidence that environmental tobacco smoking causes cancer in humans. Moreover, only environmental tobacco smoking has actually been shown to cause cancer at *typical* environmental levels. More recently, WHO and the UK Scientific Committee on Tobacco, among others, have published further major reviews. Jointly, these reports indicate that environmental tobacco smoking:

*   contains over 4,000 toxic chemicals;
*   is the largest source of particulate indoor air pollution;
*   has major health impacts that include: 1) in infancy: low birth weight and cot death; 2) in childhood: middle ear infection, bronchitis, pneumonia, induction and exacerbation of asthma; 3) in adulthood: heart disease, stroke, lung cancer, cervical cancer, nasal cancer, increased bronchial responsiveness, miscarriage;
*   causes about 600,000 premature deaths per year.

These impacts stand in addition to the irritant effect of environmental tobacco smoking on the eyes and airways and the major damage caused by fires from smoking.

Evidence of the health impacts of environmental tobacco smoking continues to grow. For example one study found that just 30 minutes of exposure to environmental tobacco smoking at levels similar to that experienced in venues such as bars compromised the coronary circulation of non-smokers (Otsuka et al. 2001). More recent work, using improved measures of exposure (measuring cotinine, a nicotine metabolite) has shown that the dangers of passive smoking are substantially greater than was previously thought (Whincup et al. 2004). It is now known that the tobacco industry engaged in a long-term secret programme to confuse and conceal the evidence on the dangers of secondhand smoke (Diethelm et al. 2005).

Despite this overwhelming evidence, it took a long time for many countries to implement measures to prevent exposure to environmental tobacco smoking. This can be attributed to a variety of factors. However, it is clear that the tobacco industry's attempts to distort the scientific debate about the interpretation of secondhand smoke studies, thereby delaying pressure for action in this area, has played a role. As early as 1978, the industry identified the health effects of passive smoking as 'the most dangerous development yet to the viability of the tobacco industry'. In the mid-1990s, in an attempt to create unwarranted controversy around the research on passive smoking, the industry arranged a series of advertisements in newspapers across Europe. These compared the risk of lung cancer from passive smoking with a variety of other apparent risks from everyday activities such as eating biscuits or drinking. Reports published in the medical literature also challenged the evidence but it later became apparent that many of these were funded by the tobacco industry. Internal industry documents have revealed that, while publicly denying the evidence – criticizing the methodology of published research and funding its own research to refute the existing evidence – the industry was privately more circumspect, admitting that 'we are constrained because we can't say it's safe'. Another attempt by the industry to fuel controversy over environmental tobacco smoking was its effort to undermine the largest European study (by the International Agency for Research on Cancer – IARC) on the risk of lung cancer in passive smokers.

By 2006, many European governments had accepted the evidence on environmental tobacco smoke. Whether or not to regulate became a matter of personal freedom, with which some states are loath to interfere. One of the first European governments to introduce a ban on smoking in restaurants, pubs and other workplaces was Ireland in 2004. In the UK, Scotland implemented legislation to control smoking in enclosed public buildings in 2006 and by 2011 Scotland was celebrating a 15 per cent drop in hospital admissions for asthma in children and a 17 per cent fall in heart attacks, although 25 per cent of adults were still smoking, with prevalence over 40 per cent in the most deprived areas. Wales, Northern Ireland and finally England introduced bans during 2007, despite several years of passionate advocacy from the public health lobby and by the then Chief Medical Officer for England, Sir Liam Donaldson. Smoking bans have now been implemented in many countries (see http://en.wikipedia.org/wiki/List_of_smoking_bans for an up-to-date list). The imposition and enforcement of bans on smoking in public places marks an important step on the way to reducing smoking to the minimum level possible (none: realistically, less than 5 per cent) but it is now recognized that further steps are necessary, in particular removing highly visible tobacco displays at point of sale, preventing smoking in cars, particularly when children are on board, the introduction of plain packaging, and controls on the growing, and largely unregulated use of social media by the tobacco industry. There is also growing pressure to act on the widespread use of product placement in films, given evidence that the tobacco industry pays large sums of money for its products to appear in films that appeal to young people and that exposure to smoking in films is strongly associated with rates of youth smoking (see http://www.smokefreemovies.ucsf.edu/).

The tobacco epidemic

Despite the huge body of evidence on the health impacts of smoking, few realize how hazardous tobacco really is. The industry has sought to subvert the evidence on the health impacts of passive smoking and to undermine public understanding of the health impacts of active smoking. It has denied the negative health impacts, promoted so-called 'light' cigarettes as 'healthier', dissuaded lay journals (via its huge advertising spend) from reporting on health risks, and sponsored biased scientific research. However, the lack of understanding may also arise from the delayed health impact of tobacco, illustrated best in the model of the tobacco epidemic shown in Figure 8.1. This figure shows the smoking epidemic using a four-stage continuum. This model is based on observations of trends in cigarette consumption and tobacco-related diseases in developed countries with the longest history of cigarette use.

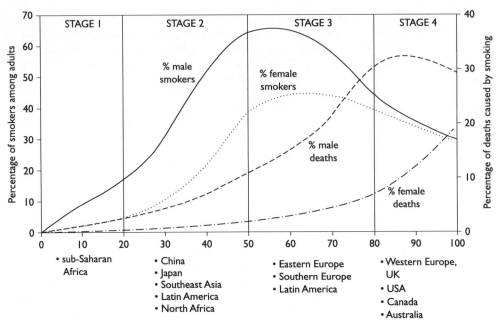

Figure 8.1 Four stages of the tobacco epidemic

Source: Lopez et al. (1994)

Activity 8.2 Stages of the smoking epidemic

Examine Figure 8.1 and describe what happens to smoking prevalence and mortality in males and females during each stage of the smoking epidemic.

Feedback

In Stage 1, there is a low prevalence (<20 per cent) of cigarette smoking in the population. Smoking is principally limited to males. There is yet no apparent increase in lung cancer or other chronic diseases caused by smoking. This stage applies to some countries in sub-Saharan Africa that have not yet been drawn fully into the global tobacco epidemic, but that are vulnerable to the growth and changing strategic initiatives of transnational tobacco companies.

In Stage 2, the prevalence of smoking increases to above 50 per cent in men and there is an early increase in women (there is a one to two decade delay between the increase in male and female smoking). There is also a shift towards smoking initiation at younger ages (not shown). The burden of lung cancer and other tobacco-attributable disease is increasing in men. Many countries in Asia (China, Japan, South East Asia), North Africa and Latin America are at this stage of the smoking epidemic. Now 30 per cent of the world's smokers live in China. Note that tobacco control activities are generally not well developed during this stage and that health risks of tobacco are not well understood. There is usually relatively low public and political support for the implementation of effective policies to control tobacco use.

In Stage 3, there is a marked downturn in smoking prevalence among men, a more gradual decline in women, and convergence of male and female smoking prevalence. In spite of this, the burden of smoking-attributable disease and death continues to increase. Between 10 and 30 per cent of all deaths are attributable to smoking, and about three quarters of these deaths are found in men. Thus the rise in mortality from tobacco mirrors the rise in smoking prevalence but occurs some three or four decades later. This stage applies to many countries in Eastern and Southern Europe and Latin America. Note that health education about the health problems caused by smoking begins to decrease public acceptance of smoking at this stage of the epidemic, especially among more educated population subgroups. Indeed, there is a shift in the social pattern of smoking as the epidemic advances: smoking is initially more common amongst the upper classes, but as the better educated quit, this pattern reverses accounting for the inequalities in health caused by tobacco.

The last stage of the epidemic is characterized by a marked downturn in smoking prevalence in both men and women. Deaths attributed to smoking among men peak at 30–35 per cent of all deaths (40–45 per cent in middle-aged men – not shown) and subsequently decrease. In women, smoking-attributable deaths increase to about 20–25 per cent of all deaths. Many industrialized countries in Northern and Western Europe, North America (US, Canada) and the Western Pacific region (Australia) are generally in or approaching this stage. However, there is considerable variation in the progress against tobacco even in these countries and in the ability of the countries to sustain national commitment to reduce tobacco use. An example of this risk of slipping backwards is the pressure in Scotland to lighten legislation to permit some smoking in pubs for what are presented, falsely, as 'economic reasons'. However, there have been relatively few reversals, largely because of the extent of popular support for measures against tobacco, which has been increasing steadily over time. Thus, where surveys have been done, support for smoking bans typically increases after they have been imposed, even among smokers.

Please note that not all countries in the world follow this four stage model in every detail. In China, for example, the prevalence of smoking among women has remained below 5 per cent despite a high prevalence of smoking among men for several decades, reaching 60 per cent by 2008. However, the general model does highlight the deadly course of the epidemic in most countries.

The global epidemic

The previous section described the development of the tobacco epidemic within individual countries. Worldwide there have also been shifts in the burden of disease from tobacco. As consumption declines in industrialized countries, the transnational tobacco companies have sought to maintain and expand their profits by seeking favourable markets elsewhere. They entered Latin America in the 1960s, Asia in the 1980s and more recently Africa and the former communist countries of Eastern Europe. As a result of this expansion to formerly closed or new markets, the decline in tobacco consumption in high-income countries has been more than balanced by an increase in low- and middle-income countries (Figure 8.2). This has in turn led both to a global increase in tobacco related diseases and deaths, and to a shift in the burden of disease from high- to low-income countries. In 2010, more than 80 per cent of the world's one billion smokers lived in low- and middle-income countries. According to the WHO, total tobacco-attributable deaths are projected to rise from 5.4 million in 2004 to 8.3 million in 2030, representing almost 10 per cent of all adult deaths globally.

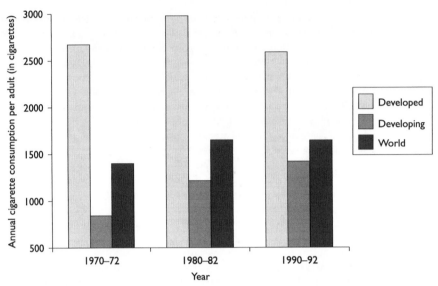

Figure 8.2 Trends in per capita adult cigarette consumption in the developing world
Source: World Health Organization (1997)

WHO therefore predicts that, unchecked, increasing levels of tobacco smoking in many middle- and low-income countries will contribute to increased deaths from cardiovascular disease, chronic obstructive pulmonary disease and some cancers (World Health Organization 2008), with 70 per cent of tobacco-related deaths occurring in low- and middle-income countries.

Tobacco control

Given the evidence presented above, it is clear that major action is needed to reduce the appalling health impact of tobacco. Tobacco control policies aim to reduce morbidity and mortality from smoking and to reduce inequalities by encouraging quitting, preventing uptake of smoking, reducing exposure to environmental tobacco smoking and reducing consumption among continuing smokers. Due to the delayed health impacts of smoking, policies that simply stop young people taking up the habit will not reap benefits for a few decades. To have an impact in the next few decades, policies need to get adult smokers to quit.

There is good evidence of the health benefits of quitting with the chance of survival depending on the age at quitting. Those who stop before 35 years of age have a life expectancy that does not differ significantly from that of non-smokers. For those who stop later, survival is intermediate between that of non-smokers and continuing smokers but there are still clear benefits. For example, those who stop smoking at age 30 avoid more than 90 per cent of their lung cancer risk, and even stopping at age 50 or 60 years avoids most of the subsequent risk. Smoking cessation has a substantial impact on life expectancy. The 50-year follow-up of the landmark British Doctors Study found that stopping at age 60, 50, 40, or 30 years of age led to a gain of about 3, 6, 9, or 10

years of life expectancy respectively (Doll and collaborators 2004). There is also growing evidence of the rapid benefits associated with preventing exposure to secondhand
smoke, with studies in several countries showing reductions in cardiovascular events
within a few months. Tailored help, in primary and secondary health care services, to
smokers wanting to quit thus can have major health impacts, and has been a mainstay
of NHS smoking cessation services in recent years (see Information Centre for
detailed account of NHS smoking cessation services).

Globally, the WHO Framework Convention on Tobacco Control (WHO FCTC)
was introduced in 2003 and implemented in 2005, with 168 signatory countries by
2011. The WHO FCTC 'was developed in response to the globalization of the tobacco
epidemic and is an evidence-based treaty that reaffirms the right of all people to the
highest standard of health' (World Health Organization 2011). However, progress has
been slow and the influence of industry continues to be very powerful.

Addiction and the ethics of public health interventions

The tobacco industry has long sought to portray control policies as controversial. It
frequently cites civil libertarians who argue that smoking is a matter for individual
choice, not state intervention and that measures that go beyond informing individuals of
the risks of smoking are paternalistic. It has similarly been argued that tobacco advertising bans constitute an infringement of commercial speech rights. Although there are
some people who hold these views as a matter of principle, the release of internal
tobacco industry documents as a result of litigation in the US has revealed the extent
to which these arguments have been hijacked and exploited by the tobacco industry.

Tobacco control experts oppose this position. They argue that addiction to nicotine
means that most smokers do not continue the habit through choice but because they
are addicted. Nicotine addiction makes it difficult for smokers to quit. Most smokers
start as teenagers and become addicted to nicotine at a young age (when they are
more vulnerable to industry advertising and marketing tactics). Later, when they want
to quit, only a minority succeed. In the UK for example, 70 per cent of smokers say
they would like to quit, about half tried to quit during the previous five years, yet only
about 2 per cent succeed (Brunnhuber et al. 2007). For these reasons, the population
(and some would argue, particularly the young) should be given greater protection via
more 'paternalistic' measures. The decrease in smoking prevalence and associated morbidity that has already been observed following smoking bans in indoor public places is
evidence of the effectiveness of such paternalistic control measures.

The growing interest of economists in tobacco control has also served to illustrate
the economic arguments for state intervention in the tobacco market. Economic theory assumes that consumer knows best and that privately-determined consumption
will most efficiently allocate society's scarce resources. This means that *if* smokers
know their risks and internalize all their costs and benefits, there is no justification (in
economic terms) for governments to interfere. However, these conditions do not hold
for three main reasons:

- inadequate information about the health impacts of tobacco smoking: consumers do
  not know well the health risks;
- inadequate information about addiction: there is good evidence that the young
  underestimate the risk of becoming addicted and therefore grossly underestimate
  the future costs of smoking. In high-income countries about seven in ten adult

smokers say they regret their choice to start smoking and two-thirds make serious attempts to quit;
• the external costs of smoking: these include physical externalities (risk of disease and death in non-smokers, nuisance of smell, physical irritation, risk of fire and property damage) and financial externalities which are seen in countries where non-smokers effectively subsidize smokers. This happens, for example, where there is a taxation based system of health funding and where few have pensions.

For these reasons, economists would argue that state intervention in the tobacco market is justified.

Policy options

Tobacco control policies are generally divided into those impacting on the supply of or demand for tobacco.

Activity 8.3 Examples and effectiveness of tobacco control policies

1 Give examples of control policies that can impact on the supply of tobacco, or on demand for tobacco.
2 Which policies do you think might be more effective at reducing smoking rates in a population? Explain why.

Feedback

1 Examples of policies that can impact on the supply of tobacco include:
• control of tobacco smuggling
• crop substitution
• tobacco subsidies
• youth access restrictions.

Examples of policies that can influence demand include:
• taxation
• workplace and public space smoking bans
• advertising and promotion bans
• counter-marketing campaigns
• information: health education and health promotion programmes (for example, population based media campaigns, school based health promotion campaigns), public reports, research and publication, labelling of tobacco products, bans on misleading descriptors such as 'light' and 'mild'
• smoking cessation services and access to nicotine replacement therapy.

2 There is not one perfect tobacco control policy and in order to have an effect on smoking rates, a comprehensive and sustainable package of measures is needed. However, it is generally agreed that most supply side measures other than the control of smuggling are generally ineffective. There is evidence that restrictions on youth access, if enforced, are effective in reducing teenage smoking rates. However, they are expensive to enforce and other evidence suggests that they may simply delay rather

than prevent recruitment into smoking. Indeed, they may even be counter-productive. Some tobacco control experts even argue that such measures, through highlighting that 'smoking is for adults', may increase the attraction of smoking for adolescents who aspire to be seen as adults and money spent on enforcement is better spent elsewhere. For these reasons, the focus of tobacco control policies is generally on demand side measures. Taxation, and bans on public smoking and on advertising and sponsorship are probably the most effective measures. A 10 per cent price increase reduces demand by approximately 4 per cent in high-income countries and 8 per cent in low- or middle-income countries, while raising revenues by approximately 7 per cent in the short to medium term. Young people and the poor are the most price-responsive. Thus, while tobacco taxation is regressive (has a greater impact on the poor) tax increases are not, and the overall effect may even be progressive because of the expenditure by the poor is deterred to a greater extent than among the rich.

Evidence from a meta-analysis of workplace bans suggests that total bans reduce the prevalence of smoking by approximately 3.8 per cent and reduce consumption amongst continuing smokers by 3.1 cigarettes per day, leading to an overall mean reduction in consumption of 29 per cent per employee (Fichtenberg and Glantz 2002). At population level, the impact of workplace bans will clearly depend on the number of workplaces that are already smoke free but it seems that such policies are at least as effective as a 10 per cent increase in price. Importantly, total work-place bans are twice as effective as bans that allow smoking in designated areas.

It should be noted however, that enacting smoking bans without public support is fraught with difficulties. For instance, despite attempts to introduce a smoking ban in public places in 2002 and again in 2003, which were largely ignored, Greece introduced a diluted ban in 2009, which permitted cafes to choose to serve smokers or non-smokers and larger restaurants to retain smoking areas, for example. It is also a good idea to introduce bans in summer, when smokers may not mind going outside to smoke, allowing those inside to get used to the fresh air.

Advertising bans are effective in reducing consumption as long as they are comprehensive. Partial bans simply allow a shift of advertising to other media.

The provision of information has been a vital component in tobacco control not least because it influences public opinion and hence the contexts in which policy decisions are made. This is illustrated by the gradual shifts in public understanding of the issues around tobacco: first the recognition that cigarettes were harmful to smokers, then that they were harmful to non-smokers and more recently, through the information released via litigation, that tobacco is an issue of corporate misconduct and fraud.

Many governments have been afraid to discourage smoking, because they fear that the economy might suffer. For example, some policy-makers fear that reduced sales of cigarettes would mean the permanent loss of thousands of jobs; that higher tobacco taxes would result in lower government revenues; and that higher prices would encourage massive levels of cigarette smuggling. These arguments have been pushed very strongly by the tobacco industry. A wealth of evidence shows that the economic fears that have deterred policy-makers from taking action are unfounded. Policies that reduce the demand for tobacco, such as a decision to increase tobacco taxes, would not cause long-term job losses as the savings made by those giving up smoking will be spent on other things. Nor would higher tobacco taxes reduce tax revenues; rather, revenues would climb in the short to medium term as the increase in tax income outweighs the loss from reduced consumption. Such policies could, in sum, bring unprecedented health benefits without harming economies.

Litigation

In the United States litigation against tobacco companies has also become a prominent aspect of tobacco control, albeit a somewhat unpredictable one. Litigation commenced in the mid-1950s but was unsuccessful until the 1990s, when fortunes changed for two reasons. First, internal industry documents, initially provided by whistleblowers, started to reveal the extent of corporate misbehaviour and turned public opinion against the industry. Second, litigators started to pursue new paths of action – class action tort suits, state health care reimbursement cases and environmental tobacco smoking cases. Since 2000 there has been a steady stream of successful cases. The most positive impacts on tobacco control have probably been indirect, that is, through the release of more highly damaging internal tobacco industry documents.

Tobacco control and globalization

The need for a regional and global response

Tobacco control can be performed at different levels: locally, nationally, regionally and globally. All levels are important. However, as a result of the processes of globalization, it has become clear that even the most comprehensive national control programmes can be undermined without collective regional and global responses. The lessons learned from tobacco control can also be applied to other major public health issues such as obesity and food (see Chapter 9).

Globalization poses a number of challenges for tobacco control, for example it:

- enhances tobacco industry access to markets worldwide through trade liberalization and specific provisions of multilateral trade agreements;
- increases marketing, advertising and sponsorship opportunities via global communication systems;
- leads to greater economies of scale which arise from the purchase of local cigarette manufacturers, improved access to ever larger markets, and the development and production of global brands;
- enables transnational corporations to undermine the regulatory authority of national governments; and
- facilitates the legal and illegal transfer of tobacco products worldwide and the transfer of tobacco industry policies and strategies from country to country.

As Yach says:

> The tobacco industry acts as a global force. As countries from the former Soviet Union, or in Asia and Africa start to embrace democracy it is often the tobacco companies who are there first selling their products as symbols of new freedoms. Globalization brings with it some very real threats to tobacco control. Tobacco is an issue at the center of contradictions inherent in the evolving process of globalization. It is where the goals of a particular set of multinationals are in conflict with public health and views of most governments.
>
> (Yach 1999)

Thus, not only do weak control policies in some parts of the world affect the capacity to control tobacco consumption elsewhere, highly lucrative operations in new markets enable the industry to remain a thriving concern worldwide despite declining profits elsewhere. As a profitable global industry, tobacco companies can sustain a strong presence and influence in all countries.

WHO recognized the need for global tobacco control measures and in July 1998 created the Tobacco Free Initiative to focus international attention, resources and action on the tobacco pandemic. The WHO Framework Convention on Tobacco Control, an international tobacco control treaty, forms the cornerstone of Tobacco Free Initiative policy. This world's first public health treaty was adopted unanimously by WHO's 192 member states during the 56th World Health Assembly which took place in May 2003.

Trade and health

The tobacco industry's penetration of new markets has been facilitated by multilateral trade agreements, which have liberalized trade in many goods including cigarettes. The removal of trade barriers leads to greater competition, lower prices and more advertising and promotion. In turn this leads to increased demand, sales and consumption of tobacco.

In the 1980s, for example, the US government cooperated with the US Cigarette Export Association (USCEA) to threaten trade sanctions against countries in Asia. In these countries, import quotas, high taxes or other restrictions were alleged (by USCEA) to unfairly limit the market to US tobacco products. In the face of US threats, Japan, Taiwan, South Korea and Thailand removed restrictions on tobacco imports. This led to a growth in cigarette trading in these markets, a 75 per cent increase in US cigarette exports to Asia and a rapid rise in smoking rates. The World Bank has estimated that in these four Asian economies, consumption of cigarettes per person was almost 10 per cent higher in 1991 than it would have been if these markets had remained closed. Evidence suggests that the removal of trade barriers has little impact on smoking in high-income countries and greatest impact in low-income countries.

The tobacco industry

In many areas of public health, policies can be enacted without any major opposition. In contrast, tobacco control faces a huge, powerful and politically well organized opposition in the form of the tobacco industry.

A useful comparison has been drawn between the EU response to tobacco and another recent health threat, bovine spongiform encephalopathy (BSE). The fear of mad cow disease led to several years of frenzied activity within the EU, producing a range of initiatives designed to minimize risk and protect the health of the public despite the fact that bovine spongiform encephalopathy has caused very few deaths compared to a yearly total of 500,000 deaths from tobacco. Yet, tobacco has not led to the same degree of activity. While public perceptions of risk from these two health threats (in part based on intrinsic understanding, but perhaps also influenced by industry attempts to confuse risk perception) are quite different, it has been suggested that lack of action on tobacco has resulted mainly for political reasons and, in particular, a failure to tackle the vested interests of farmers, producers, advertisers, distributors, retailers and governments.

In his book *The Smoke Ring* (1984), Peter Taylor usefully compares the political action taken against cholera at the end of the nineteenth century with the twentieth-century scourge of tobacco, reaching similar conclusions:

> The spread of lung cancer in the twentieth century and the subsequent identification of its major cause, is very similar to the history of cholera. But when cigarettes were shown to be the agent responsible, ... no parallel political action was taken because of the commercial and political interests which cigarettes involved.
>
> (Taylor 1984)

In 2000, the Institute of Policy Studies released a report on corporate power that examined the world's top 200 corporations. It concluded that these corporations are enjoying increasing levels of economic and political clout that are out of balance with the tangible benefits they provide to society. They found that of the largest 100 economies in the world, 51 are corporations and 49 countries. Philip Morris (the largest transnational tobacco company) was identified as the world's twenty-eighth largest company, more powerful economically than the governments of Pakistan, Peru, Czech Republic and New Zealand (incidentally, General Motors, Exxon Mobil, Ford Motor, and Daimler Chrysler were all in the top five, highlighting the difficulty of enacting effective environmental policies).

It will come as no surprise therefore to know that the tobacco industry lobbies extensively and effectively against tobacco control measures. The true nature of industry lobbying did not however become clearly apparent until the recent release of internal industry documents through litigation in the United States. These documents provide fascinating insights into industry behaviour and activities. As indicated above, they have shown how the industry has denied the health impacts of active and passive smoking, sown confusion over the addictive effects of nicotine and promoted civil libertarian debates.

Despite these complexities and the degree of powerful opposition to tobacco control, success is possible! A number of countries have now implemented effective and comprehensive tobacco control policies and seen a decline in tobacco consumption and enormous health benefits as a result. A variety of strategies including legislation, litigation and multi-institutional approaches to tobacco control are needed and great care must be taken to ensure that industry efforts to undermine tobacco control are recognized and counter-acted.

Activity 8.4

Think of the country in which you live. Who are the key stakeholders in relation to tobacco control? How well do you think they understand the issue, and what might be their greatest misunderstandings. Justify your answer.

Feedback

The answer will obviously depend on the country in question, but likely candidates include:

- Ministry of Health – likely to support tobacco control. However in some countries they will focus on activities of limited effectiveness, such as youth anti-smoking campaigns (with those funded by the tobacco industry actually increasing the probability of smoking) while failing to take the most effective measures.
- Ministry of Finance – may be concerned about what it wrongly believes to be adverse economic consequences.
- Ministry of Agriculture – especially if tobacco is grown in the country. This ministry is often a key target for the tobacco industry, which can exert a strong influence on it.
- Ministry of Education – often disengaged, even though it can do much to foster an anti-smoking climate.
- Entertainment and hospitality industry (hotels, bars, and so on) – often opposed to a ban on smoking in public places, arguing, wrongly, that it would affect sales. Many industry associations are actually fronts for the tobacco industry. Trade unions representing staff, once aware of the negative health impacts of secondhand smoke are often supportive of bans on smoking in public places.
- Mass media and advertising industry – often opposed to tobacco control, arguing that a ban on advertising would reduce revenue. Many advertising trade associations are fronts for tobacco industry.
- Associations of health professionals (such as medical or nursing associations) – these are often not engaged, focusing their efforts on issues such as pay and working conditions. However where they do take an interest, they can be very powerful.
- Other civil society groups including powerful non-governmental organizations such as, in the UK, Action on Smoking and Health (ASH UK).

Summary

In this chapter you learnt about smoking as a major global public health issue. You have read about the major negative health effects of smoking and of involuntary exposure to secondhand smoke, and examined how the lack of universal understanding of these effects can be related to the delayed impact of tobacco, as can be illustrated with the four-stage model of the smoking epidemic. You then looked into the different policy options available to intervene and impact on the supply and demand for tobacco, and were invited to consider how globalization (and the influence of multinational companies on public health policy-making) represents a challenge for tobacco control. See Chapter 9 for more on this in relation to human rights.

References

Bobak M, Jha P, Nguyen S and Jarvis M (2000) Poverty and Smoking, in P Jha and FJ Chaloupka (eds) *Tobacco Control in Developing Countries*. Oxford: Oxford University Press, pp. 41–61.

Brunnhuber K, Cummings KM, Feit S, Sherman S and Woodcock J (2007) Putting evidence into practice: smoking cessation, BMJ Group (available at http://clinicalevidence.bmj.com/downloads/smoking-cessation.pdf).

Diamond J (1997) *Guns, Germs, and Steel: The Fates of Human Societies*. New York: W. W. Norton & Company.

Diethelm PA, Rielle J-C and McKee M (2005) The whole truth and nothing but the truth? The research that Philip Morris did not want you to see. *Lancet* **366**: 86–92.

Doll R and Hill AB (1954) The mortality of doctors in relation to their smoking habits. *BMJ* **328** (7455): 1529. doi:10.1136/bmj.328.7455.1529 (available at http://www.ncbi.nlm.nih.gov/pmc/articles/PMC437141/?tool=pmcentrez).

Doll R, Peto R, Boreham J and Sutherland I (2004) Mortality in relation to smoking: 50 years' observations on male British doctors. *Br Med J* doi: 10.1136/bmj.38142.554479.AE.

Fichtenberg CM and Glantz SA (2002) Effect of smoke-free workplaces on smoking behaviour: systematic review. *Br Med J* **325**: 188–94.

Information Centre: NHS Stop Smoking Services (available at http://www.ic.nhs.uk/statistics-and-data-collections/health-and-lifestyles/nhs-stop-smoking-services).

Jha P, Ranson K, Nguyen, N and Yach D (2002) Estimates of Global and Regional Smoking Prevalence in 1995, by Age and Sex. *American Journal of Public Health* **92**(6): 1002–6.

Lee K (2003) *Globalization and Health. An Introduction.* London: Palgrave Macmillan.

Lopez AD, Collishaw NE and Piha T (1994) A descriptive model of the cigarette epidemic in developed countries. *Tob Control* **3**, 242–7.

Otsuka R, Watanabe H, Hirata K et al. (2001) Acute effects of passive smoking on the coronary circulation in healthy young adults. *JAMA* **286**: 436–41.

Takahashi I, Matsuzaka M, Umeda T et al. (2008) Differences in the influence of tobacco smoking on lung cancer between Japan and the USA: possible explanations for the 'smoking paradox' in Japan. *Public Health* **122**(9): 891–6.

Taylor P (1984) *The Smoke Ring: Tobacco- Money- & Multinational politics.* New York: Pantheon Books.

United States Department of Health and Human Services (2004) *The Health Consequences of Smoking: A Report of the Surgeon General's.* Atlanta: Centre for Disease Control.

Whincup PH, Gilg JA, Emberson JR, Jarvis MJ, Feyerabend C, Bryant A, Walker M and Cook DG (2004) Passive smoking and risk of coronary heart disease and stroke: prospective study with cotinine measurement. *Br Med J* **329**: 200–5.

World Health Organization (1997) *Tobacco and Health: A Global Status Report.* Geneva: World Health Organization.

World Health Organization (2008) Global Burden of Disease Project (available at www.who.int/gbd).

World Health Organization (2011) Framework Convention on Tobacco Control (available at http://www.who.int/fctc/en/index.html).

Yach D (1999) Nowhere to run, nowhere to hide – world community joins WHO in holding up mirrors to big tobacco. California Tobacco Control Project Director's Meeting Lake Tahoe, California, 1 November 1999. Geneva: World Health Organization.

📖 Further reading

Action on Smoking and Health (ASH UK): visit website http://www.ash.org.uk/ This website provides excellent information on tobacco and tobacco control policies and tobacco industry documents.

ASH (2010) The smoke filled room: how Big Tobacco influences health policy in the UK (available at http://ash.org.uk/files/documents/ASH_726.pdf).

Gilmore A and Collin J (2002) The World's first international tobacco control treaty: leading nations may thwart this major event. *Br Med J* **325**: 846–7. This provides some background on the political complexities involved in negotiating the WHO Framework Convention on Tobacco Control.

Gilmore A and McKee M (2002) Tobacco control policy: the European dimension. *Clinical Med* **2**: 335–42.

Recognizing contemporary determinants of public health: human rights, armed conflict and genetics

Fiona Sim, Robyn Martyn, Abie Longstaff,
Bayard Roberts, Daniel Swerdlow,
Michael Holmes and Martin McKee

Overview

This chapter considers a number of determinants of health that have become recognized as significant to public health practice. Whilst these are certainly not new, their relevance to public health research and practice has only relatively recently become acknowledged by mainstream practitioners. The determinants selected for inclusion in this chapter are considered especially pertinent to contemporary and future public health practice in the UK and globally, namely: human rights, armed conflict and genetics.

Overall learning objectives:

For each of these emerging determinants the reader will learn how the fundamental building blocks of public health may be applied in novel areas of knowledge, research and practice. By the end of this chapter you will have learned that basic public health principles and methods prove just as relevant in understanding these new contexts as in more traditional areas.

Further learning objectives are provided for each section in this chapter.

Key terms are also described in each section in this chapter.

HUMAN RIGHTS

Human rights as a tool for public health

Nineteenth-century public health interventions, and the emerging public health acts that underpinned those interventions, were predicated on the assumption that the public good justified infringement of individual liberties. Measures such as quarantine, detention, compulsory medical examination and vaccination were commonly employed weapons for disease control in the armoury of most states (see Chapter 1). Such powers were wide ranging; there were few obligations to review decisions or rights of appeal against them. However, with the emergence of a body of health ethics in the second half of the twentieth century, and the increasing prominence of the doctrine of human rights, the assumption that the public good always overrides individual rights and liberties came to be questioned. This section will examine how the recognition of human rights has influenced attitudes to public health interventions, and how public health legislation has been amended to reflect this growing recognition of human rights. It will also consider how the recognition of human rights might assist rather than constrain the exercise of public health practice.

Human rights are viewed as a tool for the better implementation of public health rather than as an obstacle to public health, because:

* human rights ensure that all public health measures are carried out with respect for the dignity and worth of communities and their members;
* by this, they encourage public confidence in, and increase the legitimate authority of, health measures;
* human rights recognize that to live in an environment conducive to public health is a fundamental right.

However, it might be argued that human rights can act contrary to public health. This tension is explored next.

Learning objectives

By the end of this section you will be able to:

* describe the emergence of human rights arguments in public health
* recognize and explain legal frameworks for protection of rights relevant to public health
* describe the public health measures that might potentially infringe acknowledged rights
* recognize ways in which compliance with human rights might benefit public health

Key terms

Human rights   The Universal Declaration of Human Rights states that:

'All human beings are born free and equal in dignity and rights. They are endowed with reason and conscience and should act towards one another in a spirit of brotherhood' (Article 1), and that:

Everyone is entitled to all the rights and freedoms set forth in this Declaration, without distinction of any kind, such as race, colour, sex, language, religion, political or other opinion, national or social origin, property, birth or other status. Furthermore, no distinction shall be made on the basis of the political, jurisdictional or international status of the country or territory to which a person belongs, whether it be independent, trust, non-self-governing or under any other limitation of sovereignty (Article 2).

The interrelationship of human rights and public health

The Universal Declaration of Human Rights, cited above, provides a basis for protection of human rights everywhere, although in a far from perfect world there are too many examples of states that violate these rights. The principles set out in the Declaration have been transposed into many national and international laws. In a single chapter it is not possible to look at the many nationally specific provisions; instead we illustrate the key issues by reference to one international legal instrument, the European Convention on Human Rights. First, however, we examine the evolution of public health law and how it has been informed by human rights issues in one typical country, England.

England's first national Public Health Act in 1848 provided a model for public health legislation around the world, not just in Britain and its colonies but in other countries, such as Japan. The Act provided powers to intervene in relation to both places (water supplies, sewerage, housing, rubbish, etc.) and people. In relation to people, the Act provided a range of compulsory powers including compulsory medical examination and compulsory detention in a hospital for an unlimited time, with no review or appeal procedures. Reforms were introduced in the 1936 version of the Public Health Act, providing protections for civil liberties, for example by establishing limits on the time people could be detained and the rights to seek a review of a detention order, but these protections were abandoned in 1968 when a range of public health measures were consolidated into a single Act. They were not reinstated in the Public Health Act of 1984.

The development of public health legislation took place against a background of legal provisions recognizing the rights of individuals against interventions by the state. The Universal Declaration of Human Rights was adopted and proclaimed in 1948, and the European Convention on Human Rights came into force in 1953. While several of the rights listed in these documents had relevance for public health interventions, it was some time before states and public health communities recognized that commonly accepted public health measures might be constrained by the provisions of these human rights instruments.

The revised International Health Regulations (IHR 2005), produced by WHO, have enshrined the importance of human rights in the exercise of public health. The requirement that WHO members states comply with the IHR has prompted countries around the world to revise their public health legislation.

In England and Wales, the Health and Social Care Act 2008, Part 3, amending the 1984 Public Health Act, introduces some human rights constraints on public health measures, particularly procedural protections against abuse of quarantine and isolation powers. For example, a public health measure imposed on an individual must now be proportionate to what it seeks to achieve (section 45D), compulsory medical treatment and vaccination are prohibited (section 45E), and there are provisions for review and appeals against compulsory power orders (section 45F).

The European Convention on Human Rights (ECHR) and how it might constrain public health measures

The ECHR lists rights that signatories, including all EU member states, must comply with the exercise of governmental powers. Some of the rights in the ECHR are 'qualified', which means that restrictive measures can be justified in certain circumstances.

Examples are Article 8 (right to respect for private and family life), Article 9 (freedom of thought, conscience and religion), Article 10 (right to freedom of expression) and Article 11 (freedom of assembly and association). Article 5 (the right to liberty and security) is a 'limited' right and restrictions can only be imposed in certain specified circumstances. The ECHR also sets out 'absolute' rights that cannot be interfered with under any circumstances, such as Article 3 (prohibition on torture, inhuman or degrading treatment), Article 4(1) (prohibition on slavery) and, arguably, Article 6 (right to a fair trial).

Compulsory vaccination, treatment or medical examination

Interventions such as compulsory vaccination, examination and treatment raise issues in relation to Article 3 (inhuman and degrading treatment), Article 8 (the right to private and family life) and Article 9 (freedom of thought, conscience and religion) of the ECHR.

If Article 3, an absolute right allowing for no exceptions, is to be invoked, it must first be determined whether the medial intervention in question amounts to inhuman and degrading treatment. Ill treatment must be of at least a minimum level of severity to fall within the scope of the Article and factors taken into account include the duration of the treatment, its physical or mental effects and the sex, age and state of health of the victim (Abdulaziz 2005). The European Court has in the past stated that there must be an element of humiliation to count as ill treatment (Labita 1995), going beyond the 'inevitable element of suffering or humiliation connected with a given form of legitimate treatment or punishment'. In the case of *Jalloh v. Germany* (Jalloh 2000) for example, the administration of emetics (to cause vomiting) against a patient's will was held to be a violation of Article 3.

The courts are generally quicker to rule that inhuman or degrading treatment has taken place where a citizen is detained by the state. 'Where a person is deprived of his liberty, the State must ensure that he is detained under conditions which are compatible with respect for his human dignity and that the manner and method of the execution of the measure do not subject him to distress or hardship exceeding the unavoidable level of suffering inherent in detention (A and others 2005). Concerns might arise where a citizen is detained under a compulsory quarantine power and, on the word of a single doctor, subjected to an invasive medical examination. Where a patient refuses to consent to invasive medical examination or treatment, there is often an underlying religious or cultural reason for doing so. In these circumstances forced medical examination could be seen as disrespectful and humiliating to the individual.

Where the intervention does not amount to inhuman and degrading treatment, Articles 8 or 9 could come into play and, as these are both qualified rights, the proposed infringement would be subject to the balances set out in the Convention. These balances consider whether the measure is in accordance with the law, in pursuit of a legitimate aim and necessary and proportionate in a democratic society. The doctrine of patient consent is a core value in medical law and the European Court is reluctant to interfere with a competent patient's decision to refuse treatment, even where such refusal might harm the patient (re AK 2001). However, the harm being considered in the context of disease control is harm not only to the patient him/herself, but also harm to the wider public.

There have been surprisingly few challenges to the use of compulsory powers in this way, perhaps because the diseases where such powers are most commonly exercised, for example in relation to tuberculosis, often arise in migrant, poor and insular communities who might have limited access to legal knowledge or assistance.

Quarantine and detention

These measures may potentially infringe Article 5: 'Everyone has the right to liberty and security of person. No one shall be deprived of his liberty save in the following cases and in accordance with a procedure prescribed by law.'

As Article 5 is a limited right, restrictions on liberty and security will only be lawful if they are for a purpose listed in the ECHR. One such purpose does relate specifically to public health: *(e) the lawful detention of persons for the prevention of the spreading of infectious diseases.*

In the case of *Enhorn v Sweden* (Enhorn 2000), an HIV positive man who had transmitted the virus to another was held in isolation by the Swedish public health authorities. He challenged his detention in the European Court of Human Rights, arguing that his ECHR rights had been breached (Martin 2006). The Court held that in order for a detention to be lawful:

- the measure must be proportionate;
- there must be an absence of arbitrariness;
- the detention must be a last resort measure;
- the detained person must be suffering from an infectious disease;
- the spread of disease must be dangerous to public safety *and*;
- the detention must have as its objective not only protection of the healthy but also care of the ill.

The Court found that the Swedish Government had failed to consider whether any lesser measures could have achieved the same outcome of protecting public health and thus the measure was not a last resort. Accordingly, there had been a breach of Article 5.

The legality of the quarantine or isolation, and in particular large-scale programmes envisaged in many national pandemic preparedness plans, would need to be judged under the conditions set out in the *Enhorn* judgement. It is important to note that HIV is not transmitted in the same way as influenza, which is spread considerably more easily and is usually airborne (Health and Safety 2009). The European Court, therefore, might be inclined to allow detention on health grounds more readily than in the *Enhorn* case. The counter argument is that the speed of transmission makes isolation almost redundant, as transmission may well have occurred before an infected person enters quarantine or detention.

It is likely that quarantine will be more difficult to justify than simple isolation. Although both measures potentially infringe human rights, there is a stronger public health argument for containing those infected in isolation. Article 12(1) of the *International Covenant on Economic, Social and Cultural Rights* recognizes 'the right of everyone to the enjoyment of the highest attainable standard of physical and mental health'. Isolation of people displaying symptoms is arguably necessary both for the health of the public at large and in the interests of society in controlling the spread of the virus (Boggio et al. 2008). Quarantine, however, envisages the detention of those not yet displaying symptoms, on the basis that some of those detained are at risk of developing the disease and thus may pose a risk to others. This can mean detaining those who might develop symptoms together with those who might not, putting the

health of some persons at risk for the benefit of others. Concerns were raised by the
Nuffield Council on Bioethics (2007) that quarantine might be implemented inappro-
priately or abused. At issue also is whether the measure is actually effective. In the
SARS outbreak some 1200 people were quarantined in Hong Kong and 131,000 in
Taiwan (Gostin and Berkman 2007). Quarantine was later considered of limited effect
due to the difficulty in diagnosing mild cases, the raised level of panic that the measure
created, and the number of violations of it (Rothstein et al. 2003).

Fear of quarantine can make people reluctant to seek diagnosis and can result in
stigmatization of groups or individuals (Murphy and Whitty 2009). If quarantine is not
considered effective, any benefit in terms of protecting the public will be reduced and
it will be harder to demonstrate proportionality. The WHO guidelines on preparedness planning state that the use of social distancing measures such as isolation and
quarantine 'must be carefully circumscribed and limited to circumstances where they
are reasonably expected to provide an important public health benefit' (World Health
Organization 2007) and that isolation should be voluntary to the greatest extent
possible.

Relevant factors would include whether the period of quarantine or isolation is time
limited and whether the detention is subject to regular review. Other considerations,
related to proportionality and arbitrariness, include the degree of due process (such as
whether the detained person is allowed a right of appeal) and whether plans are in
place to detain separately those displaying symptoms from those who might only
potentially be infected (Gostin and Berkman 2007).

Rights of review and appeal

Article 6 of the ECHR provides that, 'In the determination of his civil rights and obligations or of any criminal charge against him, everyone is entitled to a fair and public
hearing within a reasonable time by an independent and impartial tribunal established
by law.'

This is arguably an absolute right (Brown v Stott 2001), entitling citizens to a fair trial
including the right to take court proceedings to settle a civil dispute. The courts have
held that the right includes access to a court; adequate notice of a hearing and time to
prepare a defence; and a proper opportunity to present one's case (Dombo Beheer
1993). There is also an obligation on the state to provide legal assistance for persons
that have been isolated or put in quarantine, as they are not able to arrange adequate
defence for themselves (Megyeri v Germany 1992). Many states in Europe and elsewhere, including until recently England and Wales, do not provide procedures for
review or appeal of compulsory orders such as for quarantine or detention (Martin
et al. 2010).

Medical information sharing

Systems of surveillance to track the spread of infections and isolate those infected are
vital in containing disease (Gostin and Berkman 2007). However, such systems have
implications for the right to privacy under Article 8 of the ECHR. As with medical
interventions, an important consideration will be whether control could be achieved
by lesser means. The Home Affairs Select Committee in the United Kingdom Parliament
considered the issue of data collection in 2008 (Home Affairs Committee 2008) and
suggested a move towards 'data minimalization' – collecting only necessary data and
storing it for the shortest amount of time possible.

Human rights and non-communicable diseases

Issues of human rights are less likely to arise in the context of public health measures to prevent or control non-communicable diseases. Despite arguments by the pro-tobacco or pro-alcohol lobbies, there is no legally recognized right to smoke or to drink alcohol. What is at issue here are not *rights* but *freedoms* – individuals arguing that their freedom or autonomy is being constrained by tobacco or alcohol restrictions and taxes, or on controls on fast food advertising. The counter argument is that our freedom or autonomy to choose has been deliberately eroded by intensive advertising, and by the availability and use of addictive substances, such that public health interventions, for example, prohibition on advertising or protection of smoke-free public places, are necessary to restore our freedom to choose a healthy lifestyle rather than eroding it.

One issue that has raised human rights arguments is the fluoridation of water supplies. This is complex because someone living in an area where there is fluoridation does not have a realistic freedom to choose not to drink fluoridated water. In many countries, arguments based on public benefit and utilitarianism (the greatest benefit for the greatest number) have prevailed. There have also been claims that fluoridation is harmful to health (it is, but only at levels far higher than those in fluoridated drinking water), but if such arguments were true then human rights might become an issue in the context of fluoridation.

The 2005 International Health Regulations (IHR) and human rights

The revised IHR 2005 explicitly requires that human rights be taken into account in the exercise of public health measures, stating that 'the implementation of the IHR shall be with full respect for the dignity, human rights and fundamental freedoms of all persons.' The IHR make clear that states must recognize principles of human rights in that

- state responses must be appropriate;
- any measures taken must be no more intrusive than available alternatives;
- consent should be obtained for measures unless compulsory measures are warranted;
- there is an obligation to preserve the confidentiality of identifiable information.

These provisions place a responsibility on nations to ensure both that their public health laws incorporate human rights principles, and that public health practice is exercised in accordance with these principles.

Human rights recognition can benefit public health

The protection by the state of rights and freedoms is fundamental for public trust in government initiatives, and if the public is to cooperate with public health measures. Enforcement of measures is not always easy or practical. A population-wide refusal to comply with anti-smoking legislation or with prohibitions on public gatherings to control spread of disease, could severely damage public health objectives (although it is important to ascertain the true level of support, as one may argue that the tobacco industry, for instance, has under-played the widespread support for bans on smoking in public places – see Chapter 8 for more on this topic). This is especially so in circumstances of a disease pandemic. Indeed pandemic preparedness plans rely heavily on volunteers, on home nursing, on neighbours taking food to the sick and on care for the children of the sick. We can see this from the pandemic simulation exercises that have taken place for assessing the feasibility of plans.

The success or failure of disease control measures lies not with enforcement mechanisms but with the willingness of the population to behave responsibly and in accordance with communitarian values. Where the state fails to recognize either limits on its powers or the need not to sacrifice the rights of individuals for the public benefit, then trust and cooperation are less likely. The objective of public health practice is care and protection of the population against all threats to health. It is not law enforcement for the sake of it. Countries with the most draconian public health powers are rarely those with the highest level of public trust or the best population health. The recognition by the state of individual rights is a good starting point to creating the public trust necessary to achieve effective public health.

Of course the achievement of public support for public health initiatives is not just about rights. It is also about justice in the distribution of public health burdens, and about social justice in access to opportunities and goods. It concerns normative responsibilities to redress inequalities, to care for those most at risk of public health harms, and to redistribute goods so that all members of the population have an equal opportunity to survive a threat to public health. While rights documents often focus on what states must not do, rather than on responsibilities of states to take positive action for the protection of their populations, some human rights instruments have attempted to impose positive obligations on states to assist in the achievement of conditions for health. The Universal Declaration of Human Rights, for example, states the following in Article 25:

- Everyone has the right to a standard of living adequate for the health and well-being of himself and of his family, including food, clothing, housing and medical care and necessary social services, and the right to security in the event of unemployment, sickness, disability, widowhood, old age or other lack of livelihood in circumstances beyond his control.
- Motherhood and childhood are entitled to special care and assistance. All children, whether born in or out of wedlock, shall enjoy the same social protection.

And Article 12(1) of the International Covenant on Economic, Social and Cultural Rights recognizes 'the right of everyone to the enjoyment of the highest attainable standard of physical and mental health'.

One thing that can be achieved by an enforceable legal framework of human rights is to make clear that everyone has a right to the minimum conditions necessary to attain health, and that the state has an obligation to work towards the attainment of these conditions. This supports an expectation by the population of a healthy environment, and supports the work of individuals and lobby groups working to improve public health.

Activity 9.1

The following Open Access paper can be found at: http://medicine.plosjournals.org/perlserv/?request=get-document&doi=10.1371/journal.pmed.0040050

Singh JA, Upshur R and Padayatchi N (2007) XDR-TB in South Africa: no time for denial or complacency. *PLoS Med* **4**(1): e50.

Commenting on this paper, Coker et al. wrote (Coker R, Thomas M, Lock K and Martin R (2007) Detention and the evolving threat of tuberculosis: evidence, ethics and law. *J Law Med Ethics* **35**(4): 609–15, 512.

Singh et al.'s paper on the challenge posed by XDR-TB in South Africa stimulated afresh the debate around the use of detention in order to protect public health. The debate originated a decade earlier when New York City, responding to its epidemic of drug resistant tuberculosis in the early 1990s, passed laws facilitating the detention of non-infectious individuals and shifting the burden of proof from an assessment of risk posed to public health to an assessment of likely treatment compliance. In relation to XDR-TB in South Africa, the authors propose that under some circumstances individuals might be isolated whilst awaiting susceptibility results. They advocate initial voluntary isolation of patients with drug resistant tuberculosis, separating those with multi-drug resistance from those with extensive drug resistance, and recommend coercive measures where voluntary isolation is declined, acknowledging that the duration of isolation may potentially be indefinite or until death in some cases of XDR-TB. The authors conclude: 'Although such an approach might interfere with the patient's right to autonomy and will undoubtedly have human rights implications, such measures are reasonable and justifiable, and must be seen in a utilitarian perspective. Ultimately in such cases, the interests of public health must prevail over the rights of the individual.'

After reading the paper by Singh et al. consider the following questions in the context of Europe, where the European Convention on Human Rights applies:

1 What human rights issues arise in relation to involuntary detention of persons who have not yet been confirmed as having MDRTB or XDRTB?
2 Where an individual has been confirmed as suffering from multi-drug resistant tuberculosis, what human rights concerns might arise where a decision is made to detain that person on grounds that his/her personal or social circumstances suggest that he/she might not comply with a treatment regime?
3 Would it infringe a person's human rights to detain that person without specifying the length of the detention?
4 Could compulsory treatment of a person with MDR/XDR tuberculosis be justified on public health grounds?
5 Is it the case that, as Singh et al. suggest, 'Ultimately in such cases, the interests of public health must prevail over the rights of the individual'?
6 Should we take in to account, in considering the questions above, the differing disease context in Africa? Would it be justifiable to accept differing levels of human rights protection in different countries?

Feedback

1 There is a prima facie breach of the detained person's right to liberty and security, and right to family life, by them being detained. Detention is only justified if it is imposed for the purpose of protection of public health, if it is the least restrictive alternative measure, if the choice of whom to detain is not discriminatory, if the risk posed by the detained person outweighs the harm done by the detention, and if the place of detention is appropriate to the health of the detained person.

There is also a prima facie breach of the person's right to a fair trial if the decision to detain has not been made in accordance with the law, if the person has had no opportunity to challenge the detention, if there is no time limit given to the period of detention and if there is no appeal or review process.

The detention of someone who has not yet been confirmed as infectious is problematic as the person may pose no risk at all to public health. Quarantine procedures with time limits accompanied by regular medical examination to confirm infectiousness would be more appropriate.

2 A person suffering from MDRTB can potentially create a public health risk. Where that person complies with a treatment regime and with advice on limiting contact with others, there is no need to compulsorily detain. Hence it might be arguable that it is justified to take into account that person's capacity to comply. However such an assessment involves passing judgement not on the person's physical state of health but on psychological and social factors. Public health officials may not have the necessary skills to undertake these judgments. It would be easy for judgments to be made on social or racial stereotyping rather than on the attributes of the individual. The history of the exercise of public health powers tells us that attribution of irresponsible disease behaviours to particular sections of society has been common, especially in the context of disease epidemics and pandemics. Any such judgment must be made on concrete evidence of the person's previous health behaviours and not on an assumption of non-compliance based on ethnicity or socioeconomic status.

3 This would amount to a breach of the right to a fair trial. Wherever a person is detained, be it for the commission of a criminal offence or for the protection of public health, the infringement of the person's right to liberty cannot be indefinite or infinite. The person is entitled to know the proposed length of detention, and that time period must be justifiable on public health grounds and must be challengeable. The detention time need not be specified in terms of days or months, but could be predicated on an event, such as a confirmation that the person is no longer infectious.

4 Western legal systems support the notion of autonomy. Every person with capacity to make decisions about their health is entitled to choose whether to consent to, or refuse, medical treatment. The fact that someone is suffering from an infectious disease does not lessen that person's capacity to make an autonomous decision. However, refusal of treatment, and failure to treat, could result in the detention of a person indefinitely if the person continues to be infectious. Such a person would need to be monitored regularly to determine continued infectiousness, as continuation of detention must be justified on grounds that the risk of that person to the health of the public outweighs the infringement of their rights.

5 Singh's comments were made in the context of a different culture, with different beliefs, ethics and legal culture. Western health ethics, and laws, assume the autonomy of the individual and prioritize autonomy over other values such as communitarianism, family or tribal loyalty, etc. The African Charter on Human and People's Rights for example, unlike the European Convention on Human Rights, makes clear that individuals owe duties to their family and their community, and that rights do not prevail over the public good. Asian values based on Confucianism and Buddhist beliefs would take a similar approach. Hence the answer to this question will depend on the culture and ethics beliefs of the population of the state.

6 The level of disease risk in each state will be relevant to the assessment of risk. The compulsory detention or treatment of a person with disease must be justified by an assessment that on balance, the risk created by the infectious person outweighs the infringement of rights. So seriousness of the level of disease, access to medical resources, closeness of living quarters etc. will all input into the assessment of risk that person creates to the health of others. This is not to say there are differing levels of human rights. The rights remain the same, and the

principles for assessment of protection of those rights remain the same, but the facts on which those principles are to be determined differ. It is also the case that the culture and ethics of the society will be relevant in determination of the balance between public good and private right. Imposition of western interpretations of human rights on African and Asian states has been rejected as 'cultural imperialism'. African and Asian values, so long as they are debated and supported by the public, should be taken into account in the determination of how rights are to be protected and enforced.

ARMED CONFLICT

Armed conflict and public health

The deaths, injuries and illness attributable to armed conflict are major contributors to the global burden of disease (Murray et al. 2002). The discipline of public health plays a crucial role in mitigating the impact of armed conflict on health. In this section you will learn how conflict can have an impact on the health of civilian populations, and then examine key epidemiological approaches that should be used by humanitarian organizations to help understand the scale of health needs and the impact of the humanitarian response.

Learning objectives

By the end of this section you should be able to:

- describe how armed conflict can influence health
- explain the direct and indirect effects of armed conflict on health
- discuss the key epidemiological approaches used to measure the health status of conflict-affected populations

Key terms

Armed conflict There are various definitions of armed conflict, but a commonly used definition of major armed conflict is one that has over a 1,000 battle-related deaths in one year.

Household surveys Collection of information from a representative sample of households on health events.

Mortality rate The number of deaths occurring in a given population at risk during a specified time period. In conflict-affected settings, this is usually expressed as deaths per 10,000 persons per day.

Surveillance The systematic collection and analysis of information over time to regularly monitor changes in health.

Background on armed conflict

There was an overall rise in the number of armed conflicts globally since the 1950s, with the majority being protracted civil conflicts between a national government and irregular armed groups, rather than international conflicts between countries. Civil wars are extremely complex in nature and often have many causes. These include: grievances over exclusion from economic resources, the scope to gain from potential spoils of war; entrenched economic and social inequalities, extreme poverty, economic stagnation and high unemployment; environmental degradation and scarcity of resources; political exclusion, weak governance, high militarization and a history of conflict; and ethnicity and religion (often exploited by political leaders) (Stewart 2002).

Although international law provides legal protection for civilians in times of war (Box 9.1), many conflicts are characterized by the deliberate targeting of civilians who may be killed, raped, maimed and abducted (Bruderlein and Leaning 1999). Civilian populations may also be forcibly displaced from their homes by violence and insecurity. These forcibly displaced populations currently include around 27 million internally displaced persons (IDPs) who have fled their homes but remain within the national borders of their own country and around 15 million refugees who have fled across an international border into a neighbouring country.

Refugees and IDPs have most commonly lived in camp settings but a relative majority now reside in urban areas, a phenomenon that presents new challenges for the way in which health services are provided (Spiegel et al. 2010). Another sizeable proportion lives in rural areas. There are also many people in conflict zones who, though not displaced, have low access to essential health services, food and other basic needs due to surrounding insecurity.

Box 9.1 International law in conflict-affected settings

There are a number of international treaties that seek specifically to protect civilians and the humanitarian organizations providing relief services in times of war. International Humanitarian Law (notably the 1949 Geneva Conventions and their two 1977 Additional Protocols) includes the obligation for all parties to collect and care for the sick and the wounded, as well as the obligation to respect and protect hospitals, ambulances, and medical personnel, and to provide protection against rape and indecent assault. However, many instruments within International Humanitarian Law are primarily intended to cover international wars and their application and enforcement in civil wars is limited. This increases the challenge of providing health care in civil wars.

Refugee Law (The 1951 Refugee Convention and related 1967 Protocol) addresses the specific rights of refugees. The Convention requires participating countries to provide refugees protection and social support, including for their health. It also created the post of United Nations High Commissioner for Refugees to manage protection and support services for refugees. However, Refugee Law does not cover IDPs. Although IDPs are guaranteed certain basic rights under the Geneva Conventions, ensuring these rights is often the responsibility of those national governments that were responsible for their displacement in the first place. As a result, protection and support provided for IDPs can be severely lacking, including access to health care.

The influence of armed conflict on health

The ways in which armed conflicts influence health are specific to the individual contexts. Hence, it is necessary to take account of the underlying pre-conflict conditions, the characteristics of the conflict, and the impact of the conflict itself (Figure 9.1). The underlying pre-conflict risk factors include poverty and socioeconomic vulnerability ('distal' factors) which reduce the ability to withstand the impact of the conflict. The underlying epidemiological conditions are also critical, with younger populations living in areas with a high burden of communicable disease (mainly sub-Saharan Africa and Asia) generally at higher risk. Weaker health systems are also less able to withstand conflict than stronger systems, further reducing the availability of health services during the conflict.

Conflicts where there is a high intensity of violence towards civilians inevitably have a profound impact on health. Civilians may be attacked directly, forcibly displaced from

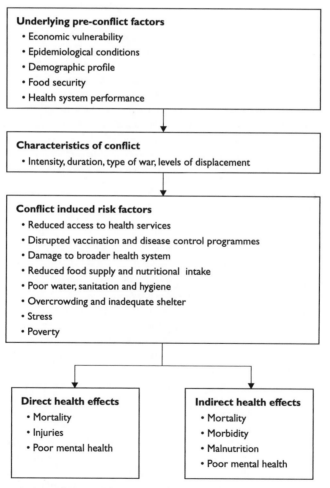

Figure 9.1 Ways in which conflict can influence health

their homes, and suffer from destruction of health facilities. Similarly, longer durations of conflict increase the impact on population health. Civil conflicts are frequently characterized by little adherence to human rights principles and International Humanitarian Law by combatants (see Box 9.1), leading to targeting of civilians and humanitarian organizations. Entrapped populations may be particularly vulnerable to such violence and loss of access to health services. Forced displacement can also have extremely detrimental consequences for health, particularly for IDPs living in very overcrowded camp conditions (for example, the camps in northern Uganda, Darfur and Somalia in the 2000s), and refugees who move into areas where support services are not yet available (for example, about ten per cent of the 500,000 to 800,000 Rwandan Hutu refugees who fled into Goma, Zaire in 1994 died within one month – mainly due to cholera). However, it should be noted that long-established and well-organized refugee camps are generally characterized by good health outcomes with mortality rates usually well below those of even the surrounding host community.

Armed conflict influences the risk factors for ill health in a number of ways. It can delay or prevent access to health services due to the insecurity involved in travelling to health facilities, destruction of health facilities, health workers being forced to flee, and vital medicine and supply chains being disrupted. Importantly, it frequently disrupts vaccination and disease control programmes resulting in outbreaks of infectious disease. Already poor nutritional status may worsen due to inability to grow or purchase food because of insecurity, displacement and impoverishment. Rising malnutrition increases vulnerability to infection, especially among children and elderly people. Conflict and displacement commonly result in worsening living conditions as people are forced to flee into makeshift settlements which are often characterized by limited access to clean water, adequate sanitation and thus poor hygiene (increasing the risk of diarrhoeal diseases, such as cholera and typhoid), inadequate shelter (increasing the risk of diseases such as pneumonia and other respiratory infections) and overcrowding (increasing the risk of diseases such as measles, acute respiratory infections and tuberculosis).

Direct and indirect health effects

Civil conflicts are often extremely protracted (lasting on average for ten years) and so have extremely long-term effects on health, both during the war and long after it. These health effects can be divided into direct effects sustained in the fighting, such as deaths and injuries, and indirect effects resulting from an increase in the risk of infectious and non-infectious disease and poor nutrition. As noted above, the majority of indirect deaths occur among children and elderly people, and arise from preventable communicable diseases such as acute respiratory infections, diarrhoeal diseases, tuberculosis and malaria (with malnutrition, measles and HIV as common underlying conditions).

The ratio between direct and indirect effects depends on the timing and context of the conflict. It is common for the direct effects to predominate in the early stages of conflict as people die from the violence (particularly young men), but indirect effects take over as living conditions, health services and nutritional status deteriorate.

The burden of indirect effects is substantially higher in conflict-affected populations living in tropical and very poor settings because of underlying endemic communicable diseases and limited access to health services, food, and income. It is estimated that between 70 and 98 per cent of war-related mortality in nine major conflicts in sub-Saharan Africa since 1945 was due to the indirect effects of preventable and treatable diseases (Human Security Centre 2005).

Armed conflict also affects reproductive health because of the lack of access to health services, impoverishment and exposure to violence. Extremely high rates of sexual violence by combatants against civilians have been reported during wartime but also increasingly by civilians against other civilians in long-term chronically insecure situations such as those in the eastern part of the Democratic Republic of Congo. High rates of mental illness have also been recorded among conflict-affected populations as a result of exposure to violent and traumatic events, poor living conditions, insecurity, impoverishment, disrupted social norms, and the loss of livelihoods (Miller and Rasmussen 2010). There is also growing awareness of the impact of conflict on chronic diseases such as diabetes and heart disease among displaced persons in middle-income settings, such as IDPs in Georgia (Spiegel et al. 2010). The damage caused to health by civil conflicts extends well beyond the period of active warfare, with women and children the most affected by their prolonged effects (Human Security Centre 2005).

The role of public health in conflict-affected settings

There is broad consensus on the types of public health interventions required in conflict-affected situations. This consensus is formalized in the Sphere Guidelines and Handbook which provide the main standards for humanitarian interventions (see Box 9.2).

Box 9.2 Sphere Guidelines – key health interventions

- Initial assessment
- Sufficient and safe water, adequate sanitation facilities
- Sufficient food and nutrition supplements
- Mass vaccination
- Disease surveillance, outbreak preparedness and control
- Primary health care and referral hospital services for severe cases
- Shelter and site planning
- Reproductive health services
- Mental health and psycho-social care

Public health disciplines are essential in guiding decision-making to prioritize optimal activities within the agreed interventions outlined in Sphere and to ensure they are: (i) addressing the main health problems (e.g. high risk diseases); (ii) providing adequate coverage to meet health needs; and (iii) effective (and cost-effective) in addressing health needs. However, a fundamental challenge in quantifying the health impacts of conflict is that health information systems, particularly registration systems that record deaths and the causes of death, often cease to function in conflict-affected areas (indeed in many low-income conflict-prone countries they may not have been functioning before the conflict). In the absence of functioning standard health information systems, the methods commonly used to obtain health information to guide decision-making are rapid assessments, surveillance and surveys. This data collection is commonly carried by humanitarian organizations.

Rapid assessments

Rapid assessments provide a quick means of informing decision-making at the onset of a crisis. Types of information include: the characteristics of the conflict, such as general levels of insecurity and targeting of civilians; demographic and socioeconomic characteristics of the affected populations; health profiles of the affected area, in terms of endemic and epidemic-prone diseases; availability and functionality of health services; and living conditions and availability of food and clean water. Potential sources of information include:

- existing situational reports;
- media reports;
- databases and maps of global distribution of specific diseases;
- records of past disease outbreaks in the affected area or similar areas;
- past reports from health information system.

However, rapid assessments do have limitations due to the quantity and quality of available data and the trade-off between rapidity and quality of data collection. These reports are unlikely to provide accurate data on mortality rates, prevalence or incidence of diseases and acute malnutrition, or the impact of health interventions.

Surveillance systems

Surveillance systems provide the most important means of monitoring population health effectively in crisis-affected settings, providing trends in mortality, prevalence of acute malnutrition and enabling detection of epidemics (i.e. monitoring the burden of disease and the impact of interventions). Surveillance systems in conflict-affected settings may include: (i) health-facility based surveillance of epidemic-prone diseases, either from an exhaustive list of facilities or a few sentinel sites; (ii) demographic surveillance to monitor trends in mortality rates, by collecting information on births and deaths from all households by means of home visitors; and (iii) more specialized systems consisting of repeat surveys to monitor HIV at risk behaviours and prevalence, acute food insecurity and malnutrition prevalence. Surveillance systems should be established in the affected area as soon as is possible.

Household surveys

Cross-sectional household surveys are commonly used to collect data at a single point in time on crude and under-5 mortality rates (see Box 9.3) and on prevalence of acute malnutrition, in places where functioning surveillance systems do not exist. Follow-up surveys can then be used to identify any changes in these outcomes (so indicating the possible impact of interventions). A range of other health outcomes are also measured by household surveys (albeit far less frequently) such as maternal mortality, mental health conditions such as post-traumatic stress disorder and depression, HIV-related behaviour, and experience of sexual and gender-based violence. Surveys are also used to provide essential information on the coverage of interventions (e.g. vaccinations, therapeutic feeding, water and sanitation, and access to health care).

Box 9.3 Mortality data in conflict-affected settings

The primary goal of any comprehensive humanitarian programme should be to reduce loss of life. Crude and under-5 mortality rates are therefore crucial indicators to understand the nature and severity of the crisis, and the Sphere Guidelines use mortality rates to categorize whether there is an emergency or not (stating that a doubling of pre-conflict baseline mortality can be considered an emergency situation). Mortality rates are also essential in understanding the impact of humanitarian relief (i.e. in reducing the loss of life).

The difference between the observed mortality rate during the conflict and the mortality rate in the pre-conflict baseline period represents the excess mortality rate caused by the conflict. The excess mortality rate can be applied to the population and period it refers to in order to estimate the absolute number of excess deaths caused by the conflict. For example, it was estimated that there were 5.4 million war-related excess deaths (the vast majority from disease) in the Democratic Republic of Congo between 2000 and 2007. This represents a catastrophic combination of elevated mortality rates for a very large population over a long period of time (Coghlan et al. 2007).

Very approximate causes of mortality (e.g. disease, violence, pregnancy-related) can be collected by home visitors and lay data collectors. More specific and accurate causes of death can be recorded by using verbal autopsy questionnaires administered by trained clinical personnel.

Challenges for public health

Despite general agreement on the key interventions required in humanitarian settings, there has often been a failure to deliver them (United Nations 2005). Recent measures seek to strengthen coordination and accountability within the global humanitarian community, including the development of sectoral guidelines for the health sector (IASC 2009); a major obstacle to effective delivery of appropriate services remains the lack of detailed knowledge of health needs in particular contexts. This is largely due to a failure of humanitarian organizations (and country governments where they are still functioning) to conduct surveillance and surveys. As a result, essential information on health needs and the impact of interventions is missing. This also impedes global comparisons on the extent of humanitarian need, so risking inequitable targeting of aid and other resources. Instead there is a tendency for humanitarian organizations to collect process information (e.g. the number of health services provided) rather than information on outputs (e.g. coverage of interventions) or impact (e.g. changes in mortality rates). Even when surveillance and surveys are conducted, many are of a poor standard, often with low sensitivity for deaths that may have occurred. Household surveys very frequently feature inadequate sampling and insufficient sample sizes as well as multiple other biases, which can result in erroneous findings and imprecise results, and lead to potentially ineffective humanitarian responses (Prudhon and Spiegel 2007; Working Group for Mortality Estimation in Emergencies 2007).

There are several reasons for the failure to collect adequate surveillance and survey data. Insecurity and logistical challenges inhibit data collection, particularly for surveillance systems among dispersed populations. Donor agencies tend to favour process rather than impact indicators and are reluctant to pay for resource-intensive surveillance systems. Donors may be reluctant to fund collection of data that do not relate specifically to the activities they are undertaking. Importantly, there is limited capacity within many humanitarian organizations to conduct field epidemiology to a sufficiently rigorous standard, sometimes coupled with a failure to recognize its value. These reasons need to be addressed so that the quantity and quality of data collected among conflict-affected populations can be improved (Roberts and Hofmann 2004).

Activity 9.2

Figure 9.2 shows crude mortality rates (CMR) (per 10,000 persons per day) over a 12-month period in a conflict-affected population in sub-Saharan Africa. What factors do you think may explain the changes in the crude mortality rate?

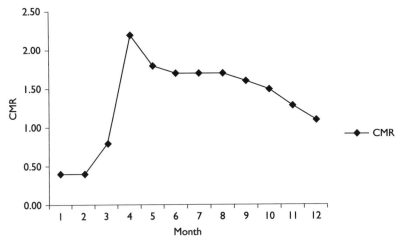

Figure 9.2 Mortality rates over a 12-month period in a conflict-affected population in sub-Saharan Africa

Feedback

Months 1 to 2 show a stable baseline rate fairly typical of the region (i.e. pre-conflict). Months 3 to 4 show a substantial increase in CMR, well above the baseline rate (therefore an emergency according to Sphere Guidelines). This increase could be attributable mainly to the direct effects of an outbreak of armed conflict (i.e. violence-related deaths). The slight fall in month 5 could be as violence reduces. The continuation of the high CMR in months 5 to 8 could be attributable to the indirect effects of the conflict such as increases in communicable diseases. The decrease in CMR in months 9 to 12 could be due to improved security and humanitarian interventions resulting in better access to health services, food, shelter, clean water and sanitation. However, the CMR in month 12 remains above double the baseline rate and so it should still be considered an emergency situation and further interventions are required to continue reducing the CMR.

Conclusion

In this section you have learnt about the ways in which armed conflict can influence health and key public health priorities in conflict-affected settings. You also learnt about the essential need for good epidemiological research in conflict-affected settings.

GENETICS

The emerging relevance of public health genetics

By its nature, our genome has influenced the health of the human population since the origins of mankind. Predisposition to, or causation of disease spanning all aetiologies and organ systems is, to varying degrees, mediated by our genes. Whilst the most potent effects of genetic variation on human health (Mendelian diseases such as Huntington's chorea or cystic fibrosis) were among the first to be recognized, these are rare and a comprehensive examination of the more subtle genetic influences on common diseases has taken decades to develop. In recent years, knowledge of the human genome sequence has permitted a much wider and more detailed investigation of genetic determinants of disease.

Here we illustrate some ways in which genetic information has influenced population health, and the wide range of opportunities for intervention to improve public health emerging from this rapidly developing area.

Learning objectives

By the end of this section you should be able to:

- understand key concepts in genetic epidemiology and how the unique features of the genome make it a valuable tool for investigating and influencing population health
- appreciate the importance of the human genome sequence to recent developments in genetic epidemiology and how it has facilitated research that has implications for population health
- understand the role of contemporary genetic research in identifying novel opportunities for improving population health and the potential for incorporating genetics into mainstream clinical care, therapeutics and prevention
- appreciate differences in the implications of genetics and genomics for the health of individuals and of populations

Key terms

Complex disease Conditions occurring frequently in the population, often with multi-factorial aetiologies (thus there is often an interplay between genes and environment). Examples are coronary heart disease and type II diabetes.

Genome The sum of all of an individual's genetic information.

Genome-wide association study (GWAS)   Large epidemiological study comparing frequencies of SNPs across the entire genome between groups with, and without a particular phenotype (e.g. type II diabetes or a circulating biomarker, e.g. blood cholesterol).

Genotype   The composition of an individual's DNA at a particular point (locus) or area of the genome.

Linkage study   Epidemiological study designed to identify sequences of DNA shared by individuals with a common phenotype, often a disease.

Locus   A defined point in the genome, which may be a single base (e.g. a SNP), a whole gene, a cluster of genes or another, larger area that may or may not contain any genes.

Mendelian disease   Diseases where a single mutation gives rise to a major, deleterious phenotype and is inherited in a Mendelian pattern through a family. Examples include Duchenne muscular dystrophy and some familial hyperlipidaemias.

Mutation   Usually refers to a larger change in genotype with more substantial phenotypic consequences, such as a large insertion or deletion of nucleotide bases.

Phenotype   The physical, biological manifestation of a gene, which may be simple (e.g. the concentration of a protein in the bloodstream) or complex (a personality or behaviour). Phenotype is also determined by environment.

Polymorphism   A small change in an individual's DNA sequence, usually limited to a few nucleotide bases, that may or may not influence the individual's phenotype: for example, a single nucleotide polymorphism (SNP).

Single nucleotide polymorphism (SNP)   A change from one nucleotide base to another at a particular location in the genome; SNPs accounts for the majority of genetic variation between individuals.

The pre-genome era

A key question in investigating the genetic architecture of disease is the degree to which risk of developing that disease (e.g. coronary heart disease, CHD) or variation in a risk factor associated with it (e.g. blood pressure, BP) is determined by genetic variation. Much of the research has used studies of identical (monozygotic) twins, who have the same genes but, especially where separated at birth, may have been exposed to different environments. The resulting heritability estimates vary considerably between traits (e.g. 50 per cent for CHD, 80 per cent for height). Scientists have gone on to try to identify the individual genes underlying this genetic component of disease, with results being harnessed for interventions in population health, including (i) improved disease prediction; (ii) elucidating novel pathogenic pathways and uncovering potential therapeutic and preventive targets; (iii) so-called 'personalized' medicine.

Before today's technological capacity to genotype many thousands of genetic variants rapidly, genetic studies to investigate disease causation in humans were typically performed using either linkage or candidate gene studies. Linkage analysis involves the investigation of an individual with a disease (e.g. familial hypercholesterolaemia) and their close relatives, both affected and unaffected by the disease, in order to identify DNA sequences shared by the affected individuals. Candidate gene studies investigate variation at a single genetic locus, typically in a case-control study design. However, this approach requires an *a priori* hypothesis that the genetic variant is implicated in disease, yielding several potential sources of error. First, genetic variation underpinning disease that is not already known – and which may yield important information about previously unknown aspects of a disease – will not be detected. Second, candidate gene studies are prone to bias in study design, which has led to many years of inconsistent results.

Identifying the majority of genetic determinants of disease required an approach for identifying variants without an *a priori* hypothesis. This hypothesis-free approach (the genome-wide association study, GWAS) performs multiple tests of association between several hundred thousand genotyped single nucleotide polymorphisms (SNPs) and disease status and employs statistical techniques to minimize false positive associations (Type I errors) likely to arise from such a large number of tests.

Sequencing the genome

Completed in 2003, the sequencing of the entire human genome was a task of unprecedented size. Composed of over 3 billion base-pairs and containing around 25,000 genes, the genome took a large, international collaboration 13 years to construct and laid out for the first time the full blueprint of the human body, providing opportunities for insights into its function in health and disease. Since 2003, technological advances have been a major catalyst in exploiting and applying the genome sequence data. Identification of SNPs across the genome and their cataloguing by the International HapMap Project have permitted a large-scale, quantitative approach to assessing genetic associations with many diseases and other traits, notably in the form of genome-wide association studies (GWAS).

Although many new loci have emerged from the growth of GWAS (catalogued at www.genome.gov/gwastudies), the resulting biomedical revolution predicted by some has not fully materialized. Expectations of the potential of GWAS to provide ground-breaking insights into the pathophysiology of the world's great diseases have been disproportionately high and several features limit their direct translation into clinical use. SNPs identified by GWAS studies appear to account for only a small amount of the heritability of traits estimated from monozygotic twin studies and the inference has been drawn that we have yet to discover all of the genetic determinants of many diseases. However, given the influence of natural selection on the genome, whereby the most harmful genetic variants are least likely to persist across generations (unless their effects only manifest after reproductive age, for example, Huntington's disease), genetic variants causing large differences in disease susceptibility are unlikely to be found commonly in the population. The most likely variants to be found by a method such as GWAS are common ones with modest effects. Although this may be seen as a limitation of GWAS, SNPs of modest effect can have a substantial effect on population health.

The post-genome era

Much research using the genome sequence has examined genetic determinants, identified by GWAS studies, of pathophysiology, therapeutics and prevention in a range of disorders. Identification of variants associated with a complex disease such as type II diabetes has propelled investigation of the role of these genes in disease aetiology; the translational potential of this investigation for population health is substantial. Mendelian randomization (MR) is a tool that exploits genetic information (often from GWAS) to this end, permitting causal inference that minimizes confounding and obviates reverse causation – two major limitations of traditional epidemiology (Figure 9.3). For example, using Mendelian randomization, the causal role of alcohol consumption in oesophageal cancer has been confirmed. Previous non-genetic observational studies were limited by confounding – since alcohol consumption is strongly correlated with smoking, and smoking is strongly associated with oesophageal cancer, it had been difficult to disentangle the role of alcohol using only non-genetic observational data. Furthermore, a randomized controlled trial of alcohol exposure would be difficult and perhaps unethical to implement. Using the *ALDH2* gene as an instrumental variable of alcohol exposure, because different variants of the gene influence an individual's tolerance, and thus consumption of alcohol, researchers were able to demonstrate that gene variants associated with higher alcohol intake were also associated with greater risk of oesophageal cancer, providing evidence of the causal role of alcohol that was free from confounding by tobacco.

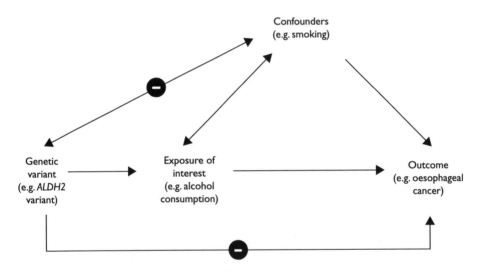

In MR analysis, polymorphisms are used as proxies for a risk factor or exposure and their association with risk of a disease is estimated. Robust causal inference from MR analysis is used to evaluate the 'true' causal impact of established and emerginig risk factors in disease and to evaluate potential targets for prevention and therapy.

Figure 9.3 The use of Mendelian randomization in epidemiology

Activity 9.3

List three examples of potentially causal exposures in common disease that could be investigated through Mendelian randomization. List the benefits of MR over (i) observational (non-genetic) research and (ii) randomized controlled trials, which are both conventional sources of evidence for causality in such conditions.

Feedback

Large numbers of putative risk factors are frequently reported by the lay press for conditions such as cancers. Examples are easily found in national daily newspapers. You might have included the following examples, although there are many other possibilities:

(i) coffee and cancer
(ii) artificial sweeteners and heart disease
(iii) aluminium and Alzheimer's disease

Advantages of MR over

(i) observational studies
   • MR minimizes confounding.
   • MR eliminates reverse confounding.
   • The genetic 'exposure' in MR studies is very robustly characterized, whilst exposures in observational epidemiology may be more difficult to measure. For example, a gene associated with intolerance to a particular food may influence intake over a lifetime, providing a better measure than a food diary kept for a week several decades earlier.
(ii) Randomized controlled trial
   • MR studies cost less and take less time than RCTs.
   • MR studies can easily be performed on a very large scale (i.e. not limited by the number of individuals recruited to a RCT).
   • Using a genetic 'exposure' may prevent exposure to a potential drug or therapy.
   • Large amounts of available data in MR studies allow investigation of a wide range of phenotypic associations with the genetic variant in question.
   • Genetic studies avoid ethical difficulties of exposing individuals to potentially harmful exposures.
   • Genetic variation reflects lifetime exposure to the phenotype altered by the genetic variant. In contrast, most randomized trials have durations of weeks or months, and, very rarely, years. Hence, through MR studies, differences in disease risk arising from lifetime exposure to phenotypes can be measured.

Predicting risk of common disease

Predicting which individuals in a population will develop a serious disease has long been a goal in individual and population health care, so as to be able to intervene to prevent cases from developing (primary prevention). Coronary heart disease (CHD) is a good candidate for prediction, since it is a common condition with a long preclinical phase, and well-established evidence for the causal roles of high blood pressure and elevated levels of circulating blood lipids. Moreover, effective behavioural and pharmacological interventions allow these risk factors to be modified early to reduce the risk of future disease.

At present, physicians calculate an individual's absolute risk of developing CHD within 10 years using models like the Framingham Risk Equation (Score) that take into account familiar risk factors such as smoking, cholesterol levels and age. The predicted risk from these models is used to decide whether, and how, to reduce a person's risk of developing CHD, based on agreed thresholds. However, these non-genetic risk equations are not perfect predictors of disease risk. It is well recognized that genes influence risk of disease, thus it may be possible to incorporate genetic information into risk scores. Furthermore, genotype is becoming increasingly cheap to measure and, in comparison to non-genetic risk factors (e.g. smoking), it is fixed at conception. However, whilst genotype appears a panacea for prediction, its clinical translation has been hampered for several reasons. First, genetic variation accounts for only a small proportion of the variance of the risk of diseases like CHD, and the effects of commonly measured variants on disease risk are modest. Second, since the architecture of genetic variation differs between ethnic groups, a variant predicting disease in one group may be unusable in another. Furthermore, and most importantly, Geoffrey Rose's **'Prevention Paradox'** (Rose et al. 2008) extends to genetics – because risk **alleles** are inherited independently (under Mendel's law), most individuals with a common disease such as CHD are exposed to average, and not markedly unusual, risk alleles (Figure 9.4). Hence, setting a threshold for high-risk genotype (as one might in conventional risk prediction) to distinguish people likely to develop CHD from those that are not, is unlikely to be very helpful. Indeed, epidemiological studies that have incorporated genetic information into established risk equations have reported only very small or no improvement in predicting disease events. It is possible that emerging technologies will uncover rarer alleles that have greater effect estimates though their rarity

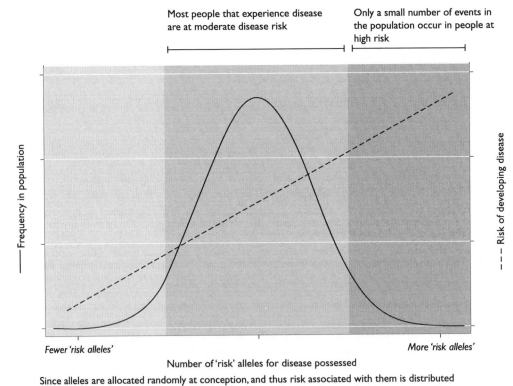

Since alleles are allocated randomly at conception, and thus risk associated with them is distributed approximately normally in a population, the majority of individuals in that population are at moderate risk. Most of the cases of disease therefore occur in individuals with average levels of risk alleles. This is analagous to Roses' 'prevention paradox'.

Figure 9.4 The prevention paradox analogy

may render population screening to detect them inefficient. Nonetheless, as more loci are associated with disease development, genetic information may gain utility when incorporated in disease prediction.

Activity 9.4

List the characteristics of an ideal predictive test for a chronic disease, such as CHD, that has a major impact on population health. Briefly, browse the literature available online to find any currently available or proposed tests that fit your criteria. What are the benefits and limitations of genetics for predicting diseases like CHD?

Feedback

Ideal features of a predictive test include the examples below. Many of these characteristics also apply to conventional screening tests.

- The test should be cost-effective to perform and must be able to be used on a large, population scale.
- The marker measured by the test should not change markedly with time.
- Measurement of the marker should not be operator-dependent (which can introduce error).
- The test should accurately designate individuals as high or low risk, or as cases or non-cases of the outcome in question (i.e. perfect discrimination – this is only rarely possible).
- A treatment for the condition in question should be available that is acceptable to patients, efficacious (i.e. prevents recurrence or occurence of disease), has no major adverse effects and is cost effective in the prevailing health care system.
- Treatment of those identified as 'at risk' reduces risk of disease to nil (NB this is unlikely at present for most genetic disorders).
- The test should be acceptable to the individual.
- The disease has a major impact on public health.
- The natural clinical course of the disease is well understood.

Pharmacogenomics

One of the most widely anticipated applications of genetic information is to predict response to treatment or prevention interventions – an example of 'personalized medicine'. A person's genotype may influence how they respond to therapeutic substances. You can identify whether your genes code for the fast of slow variants of the enzyme that breaks down drugs by acetylation in the liver by whether coffee at night keeps you awake (slow) or not (fast). Such a response could be either an intended effect (for example, the degree to which a statin reduces cholesterol) or an undesired, harmful effect. Pharmacogenetics is growing rapidly, with a surge in research articles published since the 1990s. However, only a few pharmacogenetic tests – predominantly in cancer medicine – are currently used, owing principally to an inadequate evidence base. Here we briefly contrast two pharmacogenetic tests that have shown different utility for clinical use: abacavir and *HLA-B*5701* and warfarin and *CYP2C9/VKORC1*.

Abacavir – a drug used in the treatment of HIV – is effective in controlling HIV infection but can cause a life-threatening hypersensitivity reaction in some individuals. A variant has been identified in the *HLA-B*5701* gene that predisposes individuals to this adverse reaction and consequently abacavir is not prescribed to people with the high-risk genotype in order to avoid this serious side effect – a pharmacogenetic success story.

Warfarin, a widely prescribed anticoagulant (blood-thinning agent) used in treating cardiovascular disease, presents a contrasting scenario. Warfarin is only effective in preventing harmful blood clots at a narrow range of doses, which is close to the range of drug levels that cause harm. Polymorphisms in the *CYP2C9* and *VKORC1* genes have been associated with the therapeutic response to warfarin. However, the studies concerned mostly investigated surrogates for warfarin efficacy rather than major clinical events associated with it and the real utility of genotype in predicting warfarin treatment response is, therefore, still uncertain.

Activity 9.5

What would be the key benefits to population health of an effective pharmacogenetic test?

Feedback

Key benefits include:

*   substantial reductions in the incidence of adverse drug reactions;
*   optimization of the intended effects of therapy; together, these will increase the therapeutic and preventive benefits of drug therapy, minimize the burden of disease caused by drugs, thus reducing costs to health care systems, maximizing cost-efficacy and optimizing the benefit of the intervention in the population;
*   increased drug concordance (i.e. with knowledge that the drug prescription is 'personalized' to an individual, they may be more likely to take it as prescribed).

A substantial, and familiar, limitation of pharmacogenetics is that common genetic variants are unlikely to explain much of the variability in drug response in a population. Many non-genetic factors such as drug dosing, concomitant drug use and the degree to which patients take their medications as prescribed by their doctor (concordance) are likely to play a role. If we are to use genetic information to predict therapeutic response more accurately, it will probably need to be incorporated with non-genetic information. As with risk prediction, an ability to predict response to a preventive or therapeutic intervention has important consequences for the efficacy of prevention and treatment strategies in the population.

Population genomics vs personal genomics

It is important to distinguish between the applications of genetic research for individuals and for populations. Common genetic variants tend to have small effects, which are, consequently, only detectable in very large samples; indeed, it is not uncommon for collaborative genetic studies to include hundreds of thousands of participants. The identification of a genetic variant associated with increased risk of myocardial infarction in such a study is likely to be of greater value in influencing the health of a whole population than of an individual since it may suggest a novel risk factor or an opportunity for pharmacological or behavioural prevention. Nonetheless, the vogue for personal genetic testing for such variants is growing. Marketed principally by commercial companies at prices that are falling rapidly, personalized genetic tests for a range of SNPs identified by GWAS studies for their association with many common, and several rarer conditions are offered to consumers. At present the clinical value of these tests to either the individual or the population has not been demonstrated, although future research may increase their utility in risk assessment and drug prescription. However, there is ongoing debate about the need to 'protect' the public from direct-to-consumer advertising of genetic tests, as their utility is not known.

The entry of genomics into public consciousness may, it has been suggested, have important implications for public health and health behaviours. As more associations between genes and common risk factors emerge, such as obesity, physical inactivity and smoking, and those findings become increasingly newsworthy, it is possible that obese individuals or smokers may begin to attribute risk factors increasingly to their genotype, believing them to be outside their control and therefore not amenable to modification for risk reduction. Important questions are therefore raised about appropriate marketing and publicity surrounding genetic information, particularly in an increasingly health-literate and information-driven society.

Genetics offers many powerful tools for investigating how common diseases develop and how they might be prevented or treated. While the field of population genomics is moving rapidly, it has yet to have a material impact on the population's health. The potential it holds, however, in risk assessment, risk factor identification and better targeting of prevention and treatment is great and is likely to eventually bear fruit.

Activity 9.6

Use the Internet to identify two direct-to-consumer genetic testing services. Consider the ethical implications of this type of marketing and service provision. List the advantages and disadvantages of direct-to-consumer genetic testing in general, paying particular attention to:

- benefits to individual health;
- benefits to public health;
- cost-effectiveness;
- viability for use in mainstream health care.

Feedback

Several companies, including 23andMe (https://www.23andme.com) and deCODEme provide such services, offering information on risk of around 95 diseases, and providing genetic information to predict drug response; the cost of testing your genome is currently approximately US$400. Table 9.1 illustrates the main advantages and disadvantages of direct-to-consumar testing.

Table 9.1 Advantages and disadvantages of direct-to-consumer genetic testing

	Advantages	Disadvantages
Individual health	• Knowledge of one's genome can aid motivation in adopting risk-reducing behaviours	• Genomic futility (rather than motivate lifestyle modification, individuals with 'bad' genes may decide such action is futile) • Most SNPs have small effect and therefore individually will not yield much information
Public health	• Can be incorporated into a prediction model • Individuals who pay for genetic testing may subsequently participate in research studies	• Widening the spectrum of inequality (at least initially, it is likely that only the well-off will pay for their genome sequence)
Cost-effectiveness	• Cost is relatively low, and decreasing	• Is the genetic information of sufficient clinical value to yield value-for-money?
Mainstream health care	• Rapid, low cost testing for a large number of genetic markers may, in the future, yield more information more quickly than conventional laboratory tests. • Patients may hold their genetic data indefinitely, compared to time-limited conventional test results.	• Superiority over conventional testing and prediction methods may take some time to be proven. • Health care workers will need extensive training in the application and interpretation of many genetic testing techniques.

Summary

This chapter introduced you to three of the newest areas of public health research and practice, which are doubtless going to become more prominent in the years to come. You are encouraged to keep up to date with the emerging evidence from each of these areas, regardless of where your public health career takes you, as a reminder of the ever-expanding role of public health and its importance to the future of mankind and of civilization.

References

Human rights

A. and Others v the United Kingdom Application no. 3455/05.
Abdulaziz, Cabales and Balkandali v UK [1985] Application nos. 9214/80; 9473/81; 9474/81.
Boggio A, Zignol M, Jaramillo E et al. (2008) Limitations on human rights: are they justifiable to reduce the burden of TB in the Era of MDR and XDR-TB? **Health and Human Rights 10**(1): 121–6.
Brown v Stott [2001] 2 WLR 817.
Dombo Beheer BV v Netherlands [1993] 18 EHRR 213.

Enhorn v Sweden Application no. 56529/00.

Gostin L and Berkman B (2007) Pandemic influenza: ethics, law, and the public's health. *Administrative Law Review* **59**: 121.

Health and Safety (2009) *Health and Safety Laboratory Annual Report & Accounts 2008/2009.*

Home Affairs Committee Publications (2008) 'A Surveillance Society'. Fifth Report of Session 2007–2008 8 June.

Jalloh v Germany Application no. 54810/00.

Labita v Italy Application no. 26772/95.

Martin R (2006) The exercise of Public Health Powers in cases of infectious disease: human rights implications. *Medical Law Review* **14**(1): 132–43.

Martin R, Conseil A, Longstaff A et al. (2010) Pandemic influenza control in Europe and the constraints resulting from incoherent public health laws. *BMC Public Health* **10**: 532.

Megyeri v Germany [1992] 15 EHRR 584.

Murphy T and Whitty N (2009) Is human rights prepared? Risk, rights and public health emergencies. *Medical Law Review* **17**(2): 219–44.

Nuffield Council on Bio-Ethics (2007) *Public Health: Ethical Issues.* London: Nuffield Council on Bio-Ethics.

Re AK [2001] 1 FLR 129.

Rothstein M, Alcalde M, Elster R et al. (2003) Quarantine and isolation: lessons learned from SARS. Unpublished report to the Centers for Disease Control and Prevention, November 2003. (available at http://www.louisville.edu/medschool/ibhpl/.../.../fig/pdf/SARS REPORT.pdf, last visited

World Health Organization (2007) *Ethical Considerations in Developing a Public Health Response to Pandemic Influenza.* Geneva: World Health Organization.

Armed conflict

Bruderlein C and Leaning J (1999) New challenges for humanitarian protection. *BMJ* **319**: 430–5.

Coghlan B, Ngoy P, Mulumba F et al. (2007) *Mortality in the Democratic Republic of Congo: An Ongoing Crisis.* New York/Melbourne: International Rescue Committee/Burnett Institute.

Human Security Centre (2005) *Human Security Report 2005: War and Peace in the 21st Century.* Vancouver: University of British Columbia.

IASC (2009) *Health Cluster Guide: A Practical Guide for Country-level Implementation of the Health Cluster.* Geneva: Inter Agency Standing Committee/World Health Organization.

Miller KE and Rasmussen A (2010) War exposure, daily stressors, and mental health in conflict and post-conflict settings: bridging the divide between trauma-focused and psychosocial frameworks. *Soc Sci Med* **70**: 7–16.

Murray CJ, King G, Lopez AD et al. (2002) Armed conflict as a public health problem. *BMJ* **324**: 346–9.

Prudhorn C and Spiegel PB (2007) A review of methodology and analysis of nutrition and mortality surveys conducted in humanitarian emergencies from October 1993 to April 2004. *Emerg Themes Epidemiol* **4**: 10.

Roberts L and Hofmann CA (2004) Assessing the impact of humanitarian assistance in the health sector. *Emerg Themes Epidemiol* **1**: 3.

Spiegel PB, Checchi F, Colombo S and Paik E (2010) Health-care needs of people affected by conflict: future trends and changing frameworks. *Lancet* **375**: 341–5.

Stewart F (2002) Root causes of violent conflict in developing countries. *BMJ* **324**: 342–5.

United Nations (2005) *Humanitarian Response Review.* Geneva: United Nations.

Working Group for Mortality Estimation in Emergencies (2007) Wanted: studies on mortality estimation methods for humanitarian emergencies, suggestions for future research. *Emerg Themes Epidemiol* **4**: 9.

Genetics

Rose G, Khaw K-T and Marmot M (2008) *Rose's Strategy of Preventive Medicine*. Oxford: Oxford University Press.

 Further reading

Checchi F and Roberts L (2005) *Interpreting and Using Mortality Data in Humanitarian Emergencies: a Primer for Non-epidemiologists*. London: Overseas Development Institute.

Checchi F, Gayer, M, Freeman Grais R and Mills E (2007) *Public Health in Crisis-affected Populations: A Practical Guide for Decision-makers*. London: Overseas Development Institute.

European Convention on Human Rights [1950, as updated 2010] Convention for the Protection of Human Rights and Fundamental Freedoms (accessed at www.echr.coe.int/NR/rdonlyres/D5CC24A7-DC13-4318-B457-5C9014916D7A/0/ENG_CONV.pdf)

Hingorani A and Humphries S (2005) Nature's randomised trials. *Lancet* **3;366** (9501): 1906–8.

Hingorani AD, Shah T, Kumari M, Sofat R and Smeeth L. (2010) Translating genomics into improved health-care. *BMJ* **341**: c5945.

Holmes MV, Shah T, Vickery C et al. (2009) Fulfilling the promise of personalized medicine? Systematic review and field synopsis of pharmacogenetic studies. *PLoS One* **4**(12): e7960.

Human Security Centre (2005) *Human Security Report 2005: War and Peace in the 21st Century*. Vancouver: University of British Columbia.

Leaning J, Briggs S and Chen L (eds). (1999) *Humanitarian Crises: The Medical and Public Health Response*. Cambridge, MA: Harvard University Press.

McCarthy MI, Abecasis GR, Cardon LR et al. (2008) Genome-wide association studies for complex traits: consensus, uncertainty and challenges. *Nature reviews* **9**(5): 356–69.

Online Resource: The use of epidemiological tools in conflict-affected populations: open-access educational resources for policy-makers (http://conflict.lshtm.ac.uk/page_02.htm).

Pearson TA and Manolio TA (2008) How to interpret at Genome-wide Association Study. *JAMA* **299**(11): 1335–44.

Rose G (1985) Sick individuals and sick populations. *International Journal of Epidemiology* **14**(1): 32–8.

SMART (2006) Measuring Mortality, Nutritional Status, and Food Security in Crisis Situations: SMART Methodology (Version 1). Standardised Monitoring and Assessment of Relief and Transitions Programme (SMART) (available at www.smartindicators.org).

Food, trade and health 10

Tim Lang, Joceline Pomerleau, Fiona Sim and Martin McKee

Overview

This chapter will introduce you to nutrition and health. Since the 1960s, there has been a shift from an emphasis on macro-nutrients and quantity of food to micro-nutrients and non-nutrient components of food – such as contaminants and adulterants. The growing realization of food's complexity has been added to by an appreciation of the human and ecological health consequences of food production. The new health thinking includes concepts such as **food miles**, environmental degradation, fair trade and sustainable development. This chapter puts such notions into the context of the mechanisms and burdens of disease that are linked to nutrition. It argues that four foci emerge in modern thinking: food safety, nutrition, sustainable development and **food security**. Food is clearly a major factor in the unfolding global epidemic of obesity. Obesity is one of the most rapidly growing public health problems facing mankind globally (Roth et al. 2004). This global challenge is considered alongside potential interventions to tackle it at different levels. Finally, the chapter discusses the relationship between food and public policy. It raises the question that, given the evidence base for public health interventions, why is progress still so patchy and slow?

Learning objectives

By the end of this chapter you should be able to:

- describe some key features in the evolution of thinking about the importance of diet on health
- assess various social forces affecting changes in dietary behaviour
- map the key strengths and weakness of arguments about the impact of social change on nutrition and health
- understand that food illustrates the links between human and environmental health
- recognize obesity as a global public health phenomenon and describe different levels of intervention
- suggest some policy pointers for the future

Key terms

Food miles Distance that foods travel from where they are grown to where they are ultimately purchased or consumed by the end user.

Food security Physical and economic access for everyone and at all times to enough foods that are nutritious, safe, personally acceptable and culturally appropriate, produced and distributed in ways that are environmentally sound and just.

Nutrition transition Process of change in which populations shift their diet from a restricted diet to one higher in saturated fat, sugar and refined foods, and low in fibre; as a result, diet related ill health previously associated with affluent Western societies takes root in developing countries.

The debates about diet and health

From the 1950s, evidence mounted from epidemiological studies that dietary composition was a key factor in patterns of disease. As a result, in the last quarter of the twentieth century, food became the subject of heated policy debate in many countries. Arguments raged about what and how much particular factors matter. Was it fats? Which fats? What ratio of different types of fat? Was it micro-nutrients? Was it the overall dietary balance? And latterly, what was the role of physical activity in the obesity epidemic? Does genetic inheritance play a role in pre-disposing humans to disease from mal-consumption? Can diet counteract the cards that genetic fate deals us?

Work by a number of diet and disease pioneers suggested that a pattern of eating – characterized by high fat consumption and polyunsaturated/saturated ratios, with high added sugars, low fibre and high salt, low in fruit and vegetables – was coinciding with a rise in the degenerative diseases. The importance of fat was noted by Prof Ancel Keys in the Seven Nations study, where Keys and co-workers showed how Finland and the UK had high CHD rates while Japan and Greece (Crete) had low levels (Menotti, Keys et al. 1989).

The emerging consensus from such studies has been summarized in numerous reports. The 1990 WHO document entitled *Diet, Nutrition, and the Prevention of Chronic Diseases*, is a good assessment of the consensus towards the turn of the century; an updated version was published in 2003. In 2000, the Sub-Committee on Nutrition of the UN produced another major statement with the *4th Report on the World Nutrition Situation: Nutrition Throughout the Life Cycle*. These reports proposed that trends in global diet – first noted in affluent societies but now emerging in developing societies – are followed by the emergence of clear patterns of chronic disease, particularly: cardiovascular disease (CHD, high blood pressure, cerebrovascular disease); some cancers (including stomach, colorectal, breast, prostate); diabetes and obesity. They proposed that the world was experiencing these effects as the result of a nutrition transition, a shift from a restricted diet to one with more choices.

While this evidence grew, the application of earlier insights from food science and technology was showing how controls on food production could reduce the risk of the spread of contaminants, toxins and microbiological threats to human, plant and animal safety. By the 1970s, food technologists felt that they had developed answers to the old policy fears of waste (spoilage), hunger and mal-distribution. Yet within two decades this promise had unravelled. Although progress in raising agricultural output was considerable, the absolute numbers of people experiencing famine remained stubbornly high. Food poverty and the lack of access to an adequate quantity of food had dominated international food and agricultural policy since the 1950s.

By the turn of the new millennium, although global public policy – for example from WHO and the Food and Agriculture Organization (FAO) – was still largely framed by concern about hunger and population growth, the new evidence about the co-existence of under-consumption, over-consumption and mal-consumption required policy responses. The WHO and FAO worked together and in 2004, the WHO produced a new Global Strategy on Diet, Physical Activity and Health, approved at the World Health Assembly in May 2004. By 2008, WHO was able to report that more than 30 countries had implemented policy options recommended by the Global Strategy (World Health Organization 2008).

Thus, a new paradigm was emerging for food and health policy, in which thinking was increasingly framed by four distinct discourses on food and health, each giving priority to different aspects of what could better be seen as a whole. These discourses centred on food's role in: ecology and the environment; food safety; nutrition; and food security.

Activity 10.1

Give examples of how population health can be influenced by (1) the environmental conditions of food supply, (2) food safety, (3) the nutritional content of food and its impact, and (4) having adequate food supplies.

Feedback

There are many examples that can be given for all four. A few are listed below:

Ecology and the environment:

- Some foods (and water) are contaminated by environmental chemical pollutants such as lead, mercury, polychlorinated biphenyls (PCBs), dioxins and radionuclides with potentially important health effects. Intoxication with lead, for example, leads to neurological impairment in children.
- Globalization and increasing food trades mean that foods travel longer distances before reaching our plates, thus leading to a greater environmental cost (higher use of non-renewable fossil fuels) including higher pollution rates with their associated potential long-term deleterious health effects.
- With improved trade routes, populations with limited reach to diverse food supplies can increase their available food. They can move from a diet restricted by local terrain and growing conditions to one where they have access to other land.

Food safety:

- Infection with *Listeria monocytogenes* has a mortality rate of 20–30 per cent.
- It is estimated that 10 per cent of patients (particularly children) with haemorrhagic colitis caused by verotoxin-producing *Escherichia coli* later develop the lifethreatening complication haemolytic uraemic syndrome.
- Bovine spongiform encephalopathy (BSE) and avian and swine flu (linked to chickens and pigs respectively) have become a new concern among both the public and decision-makers.

Nutrition:

- Inadequate vitamin A intake leads to high rates of vitamin A deficiency and blindness in many developing countries, particularly in children.
- High intake of energy, fat and sugar have been associated with overweight, cardiovascular disease and some cancers.
- Sub-clinical deficiency of vitamin D may increase the risk of bone fractures if osteoporosis is already present.

Food security:

- The pattern of consumption of fruit and vegetables is still seasonal in many countries (for example, annual cycle of seasonal excesses and out-of-season shortages in the less economically developed countries of the former Soviet Union), with evidence that seasonal shortage may contribute to cardiovascular disease.
- Poverty is generally associated with reduced access to adequate food supplies.
- In 1995/1997, the prevalence of undernourishment was 18 per cent in the developing world (17 per cent in Asia and the Pacific region, 11 per cent in Latin America and the Caribbean, 9 per cent in the Near East and North Africa, and 33 per cent in Sub-Saharan Africa). In comparison it is less than 2.5 per cent in industrialized countries, but it reaches 7 per cent in countries of the former Soviet Union.

Some of these issues will be developed further in the next section.

Nutrition, food security, safety and the environment

The greatest burden of disease over the last half century was premature death from hunger and malnutrition. But epidemiological evidence mounted about the toll from inappropriate nutrition and not just under-consumption. Specifically, from the 1950s, the issue of diet-related degenerative diseases emerged. In the European Union (EU), for instance, by the turn of the twentieth century the number of deaths due to poor food safety could be measured in the low thousands, while annually 1.5 million people died prematurely due to heart disease. Despite this evidence, even into the 1990s, policy discourse in rich, developed countries was largely dominated by the other two concerns – food safety and to a lesser extent the environment – and by food security (that is, under-consumption and poor availability of supplies) in the developing world.

At the end of the twentieth century, although the environmental aspects of food production such as pesticides and genetic modification attracted considerable global attention from the public and from policy-makers, it was food safety that had greater impact on the architecture of governance. New food agencies and laws were rushed through the legislatures of many developed nations, under pressure from consumers and industry alike. Developing countries, seeking export markets, had to create parallel institutions or expertise. Consumer confidence in the food supply chain demanded change. Industry introduced risk-based approaches to hazards, particularly by application of the two management approaches; the first being Hazards Analysis Critical Control Point (HACCP), which sought to identify any weak points in the processing system; and the second being new systems of traceability. Both were designed to improve trust and confidence in complex supply chains.

These concerns remind us that the relationship between policy and evidence is not simple. Even though millions may die prematurely from preventable diseases (think of the weak response to the annual toll from road traffic injuries or smoking), this situation can somehow be accepted as 'normal'. Yet, the return of communicable diseases was not seen in this way. In the 1980s, food poisoning figures began to rise in most affluent societies (they were always higher in developing countries), even in societies with processing industries that prided themselves on being modern, clean and run to high technical standards. The monitoring of food-borne illness suggested that existing controls were not sufficient. Explanations included: new varieties of existing diseases (for example new phage types of *salmonella*); new opportunities for diseases due to production changes; changing food handling in the home; and poor training and skills in food service industries. Outbreaks of comparatively rare diseases due to organisms such as *E coli* or *Listeria* became world news, with the emergence of new types, in the case of *E coli 0157*, and new opportunities, in the case of *Listeria monocytogenes*. The emergence of food-borne health problems in rich societies followed the emergence of new systems of food handling, sometimes associated with changes in women's roles in the home. New technologies such as packaging, cook-chill (pre-made 'TV dinners') and changes in cooking technology (microwaves) gave greater choice to affluent consumers. 'Cook chill' meals, for instance, are preserved at 0–3 degrees Celsius, but provide opportunities for *Listeria* (which survives in this temperature range) to survive if reheated inadequately. Further, these meals are frequently not eaten straight after purchase, but stored in domestic refrigerators at temperatures above 3°C.

After promising that its modern 'clean' products were more wholesome, as well as giving consumers (particularly mothers) greater choice, this evidence was deeply embarrassing to the food industry, particularly the meat sector. Faced with evidence of rising food-borne pathogens, food manufacturers initially tended to put the onus on consumers to protect themselves, blaming consumers for poor handling, particularly in the case of poultry products, which were and are high risk foods. Despite a high percentage of poultry coming to market with detectable levels of contamination (for example *salmonella*), the publicity about food safety suggested that all would be well if only the 'housewife' stored, de-frosted and cooked 'her' bird correctly. Consumer groups argued a public health position, namely that, while consumer management of food post-purchase is of course important, there is little justification for selling food that is contaminated in the first place! Such levels of risk and faulty goods would be unacceptable in cars and most other consumer products, for instance. Yet in the UK, in the early 1980s, the Public Health Laboratory Service suggested that more than 60 per cent of poultry was contaminated. It took a decade of scandals and exposés to shake up UK food supply chains, creating a Food Standards Agency in 2000 and legislation. Similar changes occurred throughout Europe.

Whilst food safety brought public health issues right into everyone's homes, environmental arguments around food and health took longer, perhaps because they seemed initially more distant in their relevance. From the 1960s, a rising tide of evidence emerged about the environmental 'downside' of agricultural and food modernization. Specific questions emerged about residues from pesticides or fertilizer run-off, as well as general policy and philosophical questions about the earth's carrying capacity and cycles of pollution: what sort of lifestyle can the planet sustain? Can populations be healthy if the environment is not? Which social groups are to blame for 'mining' the world's ecology? Such environmental questions raised questions for public health about equity, which has been explored in Chapter 4.

We should recognize, however, that global resources are not unlimited (Brown 1996), and there may be better ways of redistributing those that exist (Dyson 1996). For health gains to be won for everyone, policies and structures need to be different (McMichael 2001). In fact, there could be a new ecological wealth for all nations. See Chapter 12 for more about this.

To meet projected population growth and consumer demand, global food production must double between 2004 and 2020. The FAO is optimistic that food supplies can and will grow faster than the world population. Even with eight billion people by 2030, the FAO suggests that: 'they can expect to be better fed with more people having an adequate access to food than in earlier times.... Growth in agriculture will continue to outstrip world population growth of 1.2 per cent up to 2015 and 0.8 per cent in the period to 2030' (Food and Agriculture Organization 2000). This optimism is welcome, but a note of caution is due. It is based on total food supplies, and takes little account of distribution or of ecological constraints.

Food security is the phrase used in policy circles to refer to the goal of having countries able to feed themselves or at the household level everyone being confident that they can be fed. In the post Second World War period, food security was deemed to be a national concern. Countries aimed for self-reliance, that is, to feed themselves from their own resources. The over-arching policy goal of under-consuming countries was to increase production. By the end of the twentieth century, the goal of food security had been redefined – to mean not necessarily producing food within borders, but to produce enough economic output to be able to afford to buy food on world or regional markets. This shift of definition represented the triumph of neo-liberal approaches to managing economies, supported by global institutions such as the World Bank and the FAO, which had encouraged developing countries to build export markets in preference to promoting self-reliance. Transporting food long-distance to earn foreign currency is a fragile policy; it depends on commodities retaining their value when, as many export-dependent developing countries have found, they may not. Public health in the twenty-first century will require more coordination between environmental and public health: notions such as the concept of food miles, which refers to the distance that food travels before it gets to consumers, are in common use. Although the majority of food is still produced regionally, if not locally, food trade has been encouraged by liberalization measures. An estimated 90 per cent of the world's food consumption occurs where it is produced (McMichael 2001). For food that is traded, food miles continue to rise between and within countries.

Note that in developing countries, where there has been a shift away from heart-protecting diets rich in vegetables and fish, towards a diet rich in carbohydrates, sugar and fat, we observe the 'double jeopardy' of undernutrition together with increasing prevalence of obesity and the health-related consequences of both. So, as we have seen above, there are high levels of undernourishment in many developing nations, but alongside that, escalating levels of obesity: for example, over 39 per cent of women are obese in Egypt, 14 per cent in Congo, and 5 per cent in Mali, one of the world's poorest nations (IASO 2011).

Policy shift?

During the 1980s and 1990s the inadequacy of policy to address the new complexities of health and environment in policy areas such as food, became ever clearer. It has been argued that, by the end of the twentieth century, the entire post Second World War policy framework had begun to unravel. That policy framework had a number of key characteristics and goals:

- intensification of production;
- price reduction and cost control;
- labour-shedding;
- application of food science and technology throughout the supply chain, but especially in agriculture;
- emphasis on raising output and quantity (to tackle the spectre of hunger);
- choice as the key driver of consumer behaviour;
- concentration and specialization.

This policy package had been successful until the 1990s. By then, its legitimacy/relevance was being questioned. For instance, the rate of increase of crops yields was slowing down. The opposition to environmental consequences of some of the inputs to intensive agriculture (for example pesticides, fertilizers) was growing. The evidence of harm to health countered the claims of capital efficiency. The food sector is sensitive to such criticism. However it can be also highly resistant to change: there was furious opposition from some large vested interests – for example the sugar, soft drinks, and dairy industries – to the proposals in the 2004 WHO Global Strategy on Diet, Physical activity and Health. But by then, there had been over a decade of food crises throughout the world which had heightened political sensitivity, public health commitment and public attention, a combination which perhaps prompted conflict but also change.

The four public health discourses concerning food – ecology, safety, nutrition, food security – had come together in a politically explosive manner with the emergence of bovine spongiform encephalopathy (BSE), popularly known as mad cow disease. First noted in cows in the early/mid-1980s, by 1996, this disease was proven to have 'jumped' to humans as variant Creutzfeld-Jakob Disease (vCJD). First occurring in the UK, the impact of BSE went worldwide and altered public concerns about risk, evidence and confidence in decision-makers. The aetiology of BSE is still unclear but it is presumed either to have jumped species or to have spontaneously mutated and to have been spread by human-created cannibalism among cows (Dudas et al. 2010). Although comparatively few people have died from vCJD in the UK (170 cases by the end of 2010 – source: www.cjd.ed.ac.uk), the disease was hugely influential in policy terms. The UK was effectively put into quarantine despite being a member of the European Union with its single market. BSE reminded policy-makers, who had for decades prioritized trade and industry liberalization over other policy considerations, that public health cannot be taken for granted. For practitioners in public health in developed countries, BSE was a reminder that the era of contagious diseases had not ended.

Interventions to reduce food-related ill health

The range of public health interventions to reduce food-related ill health is potentially considerable and includes:

- prevention – on an individual and/or population basis;
- health education and promotion;
- composition regulation;
- labelling and product information;

- production controls and monitoring;
- product traceability;
- product development and specification of niche markets such as low-fat spreads, fortification or other technological change;
- genetic screening (if and where possible).

In the UK, since 2004, there have been a number of initiatives aimed at tackling obesity, with recognition of the need for policy change as well as individual behaviour change. Despite recognition of the need for policy change, in practice, the government has tended to rely upon individual behaviour change, with little appetite for major policy shift that would require substantial changes in its relationship with the food sector. Of major importance in setting the scene for policy-makers was the Foresight Report (Foresight 2007), which described a 'complex web of societal and biological factors that have, in recent decades, exposed our inherent human vulnerability to weight gain'. This was closely followed by the report on public health from the Nuffield Council on Bioethics (2007), which, using obesity as a case study, started from the premise that the UK has the highest prevalence of obesity in Europe. This report introduced the concept of a 'ladder of intervention', pointing out the possible roles of government and other stakeholders in tackling public health issues, including obesity – which has subsequently been adopted by the coalition government in England in its Public Health White Paper in November 2010 (DH 2010). Alongside these policy initiatives, we have seen guidance published by the National Institute for Health and Clinical Excellence (NICE 2006) for tackling obesity in adults and children, through both behaviour change and wider public health, including health promotion, interventions.

One reason that food safety crises can be so devastating politically is that they undermine consumer responsibility. No label warns consumers that food is or may be contaminated or unsafe, for instance, and food is presumed to be safe at source. In the case of nutrition, however, there is ongoing debate about consumer choice and information. Even where scientific evidence is strong, for example in relation to obesity, consumers regularly ignore information about fat contents of processed foods or appear unable to act on it. Nesle (Nesle and Jacobson 2000) showed how, if agriculture is producing high levels of fat, somehow it will end up 'down consumers' throats'. Producers' invention of 'low fat' products is accompanied by a plethora of other products replete with hidden fats. In 2002, preliminary legal steps were begun in the United States to confront food industry responsibility for hidden fats and the lack of industry warnings about the potential harm from excessive consumption. In the UK, successive governments have established mostly voluntary agreements with the industry to improve both labelling and contents, with mixed results.

With regard to the impact of poor nutrition on health, strategic emphasis has been largely on health education and promotion. More recently emphasis has been on social marketing, with appeals for individuals to take personal responsibility for behaviour change. Table 10.1 draws out some distinctions between individualist and population approaches to food and health.

Two exceptions to the general domination of individualism in modern food and health policy shine out of the policy literature: Thailand and Finland. Both are strongly commended by the UN Sub-Committee on Nutrition (SCN). Finland achieved major changes in mortality from coronary heart diseases, accounted for mainly by dietary changes (operating through lowering plasma cholesterol and blood pressure levels) that were achieved through community action and the pressure of consumer demand on the food market. In Thailand, since the mid-1970s nutrition has been an

Table 10.1 Individual and population approaches to food and health

Policy focus	Individualist public health approach	Population public health approach
Relationship to general economy	Trickle down theory; primacy of market solutions; inequality is inevitable	Health as economic determinant; public-private partnerships; inequalities require societal action
Economic direction for health policy	Individual risk; personal insurance; reliance on charity	Social insurance including primary care, welfare and public health services
Morality	Individual responsibility; self protection; consumerism	Societal responsibility based on a citizenship model
Health accountancy/costs	Costs of ill health not included in price of goods	Costs internalized where possible
Role of the State	Minimal involvement; avoid 'nanny state' action; resources are best left to market forces	Sets common framework; provider of resources; corrective lever on the imbalance between individual and social forces
Consultation with the end user	As consumer; dependent on willingness to pay	Citizenship rights; authentic stakeholder
Approach to food and health	The right to be unhealthy; a medical problem; individual choice is key driver; demand will affect supply; niche markets	The right to be well; entire food supply geared to deliver health

Source: Adapted from Lang and Caraher (2006)

integral element of both primary health care and community development, each seeking to improve food and nutrition security within households; this provides a strong infrastructure, extending beyond government services to ensure community participation.

The core message is that degenerative disease can be tackled even in developing countries, but there has to be concerted action, for which the precondition is political will. If a country wishes to reduce its toll of diet-related disease, a population approach rather than just individualism or technology is essential. The policy challenge is to meet health objectives not just through choice but by generating a health-enhancing culture, where the objective is health. It is worth noting the rise in interest in the USA and UK of a 'third way' that may permit a state to be both paternalist and libertarian, which is known as the nudge theory. Coined by Thaler and Sunstein in the US (Thaler and Sunstein 2008), the dearth of an evidence base is met with scepticism by public health (Bonell et al. 2011), but it has the interest of contemporary politicians, including the UK Coalition Government.

Despite the potential for population-based approaches and interventions, policy to tackle diet-related ill health remains predominantly at the individual level and the explanation is clear: governments and companies are more comfortable offering a combination of exhortation, advice and individual appeals than in setting out to re-frame food culture. They are frightened of accusations of 'nanny state-ism', an ethic set by the neo-liberal consensus in the face of public health evidence. There has been rapid market concentration (domination by fewer giant companies). They vie for market share and compete in the tough market where tens of thousands of food products jostle for consumer attention; they are uncomfortable with a population approach. The prevailing logic is to appeal to consumers to choose particular products and to take responsibility for themselves. In the corporate world, health is a matter of appealing to people to change diet to make themselves more beautiful, to be culturally positive, to seek sexual advantage, to follow role models, to fit social marketing norms, to respond to advertising, to be targeted by advice leaflets, and so on, a rather different set of values from those held by public health.

The prognosis

Progress in the policy areas continues to be mixed. Progress in respect of food safety has been poor, particularly in the developing world. Environmental externalities are only just being appreciated. Hunger is proportionately declining but static in absolute numbers as population growth continues. In all countries, obesity and diabetes are escalating. In many affluent societies the incidence of heart disease is declining. Of great concern is how, with the rapid rise in child obesity, a new second wave of diet-related ill health associated with affluence may be expected. CHD may be contained by statins (a class of drugs that lowers the level of blood cholesterol by reducing the production of cholesterol by the liver), but as yet there is no equivalent strategy for controlling diabetes.

The integrated approach to food and health described here is threatening and awesome in its implications. Some sections of the food processing and farming industries – particularly those producing fats, using salts and sugars and making/selling refined foods – are troubled by the new analysis and evidence. Tactics familiar to the tobacco and health discourse have emerged (see Chapter 8). These range from denial to stonewalling defensive tactics. This has led some people to wonder if the spread of obesity worldwide means that diet and food are the 'new tobacco' (Daynard 2003). In 2002, financial analysts (for example JPMorgan and UBSWarburg) began to audit food companies to assess how exposed their product ranges were to accusations that they contributed to obesity. In many countries, including the UK, voluntary agreements have been sought by government with the food industry, resulting in several examples of reducing saturated, fat, salt or sugar content, and improved front or back of pack labelling, including the government preferred 'traffic light system' adopted by some manufacturers. The Coalition government in the UK has also engaged in Responsibility Deals with industry to encourage commercial participation in shaping policy, alongside government officials and representatives from professional organizations and NGOs. It is too early to assess the impact of such relationships, but they are proving highly contentious – the WHO model of involving the commercial sector in implementation, only after policy has been developed is, perhaps, rather less likely to be subject to commercial conflicts of interest.

Activity 10.2

List tactics that some food processing and farming industries can use to reject any integrated approach to food and health.

Feedback

There are several tactics used. They include:

* denial that there is an issue;
* refusal to accept evidence;
* employment of dissident scientists to cast doubt;
* *ad hominem* and personalized attacks on opponents;
* strategic company and political alliances;
* appeals to Government to consider the economic consequences of constraint;
* advertising to 'drown' health messages;
* revised marketing;
* development of niche products that can offer 'choice';
* preparation of 'escape routes' (diversification of whole industries);
* and so on.

The food sector is famously powerful but it went through a period of remarkable change in the late twentieth century creating considerable internal tensions. The interests of farming, processing, retailing, food service, advertising, and so on are rarely identical. In many countries, a number of major companies emerged dominating each sector. There was also considerable cross-border activity in mergers and acquisitions. Food manufacturing internationalized first but food retailing (supermarkets), food service (restaurants and hotels) and cultural industries (advertising and marketing) followed. This adds complexity to the public health challenge. Diet-related problems may be manifest at the national or local level but significantly framed by powerful forces at the regional or global level.

Food – where science and politics mix

When considering the new public health agenda on food, it can be helpful to recognize that arguments about food are not new. Modern food policy might have to juggle quality, production efficiencies, prices, ownership, education, public health, food security, cultural messages, and more, but these have their equivalents in governmental debates in earlier centuries. Nevertheless, we can note some important policy shifts over the last century. For instance, the mid-twentieth century concern with quantity has now shifted to quality; similarly, attention has moved from macronutrients to micronutrients. Unravelling this history reminds us how public health is socially constructed. The roots of nutritional science are just such an example.

Dr James Lind, although not the first to note the connection between diet and ill health, is often credited with beginning to put it on a scientific basis in the eighteenth century (although his results were ignored for several decades). With the viability of European/British trade routes dependent upon maintaining the health of ships' crews, the problem of scurvy was a major threat to European expansionism. Scurvy amongst the crew could devastate ships' efficiency. In 1753, Lind published the results of the first controlled study, showing conclusively that scurvy could be prevented and cured by eating citrus fruit (such as oranges and lemons) (Lind 1753). This was an early demonstration of how the science of nutrition could contribute to economic and even military wellbeing, although in this case the main driver was to facilitate trade. State interest in nutrition tends to rise in times of war. Napoleon Bonaparte is famously stated to have said that an army marches on its stomach; in the late eighteenth century he initiated the search that delivered canning, the means to perfect, portable and long-lasting food (and also the French sugar beet industry!). Moving to the present day, one key reason for the global policy concern about obesity is not only its cost to advanced economies, but its emerging even greater cost to economies with less well resourced health care systems. Box 10.1 demonstrates the impact of obesity in Europe.

Box 10.1 Impact of obesity: European region

Health burden
- ~ 80% of cases of type 2 diabetes
- ~ 35% of ischaemic heart disease and
- ~ 55% of hypertensive disease among adults
- > 1 million deaths and 12 million life-years of ill health each year.

Economic burden
- Direct: up to 7% of health care costs
- Indirect: ~ 3–4% of health care costs
- Intangible: underachievement in education, reduced social activity and discrimination at work

---

Two and a half centuries since Lind, nutrition now covers a vast field ranging from social nutrition (for example studying at risk social groups), nutritional epidemiology (plotting the contribution of diet to diseases), biochemistry (the study of the biochemical interaction of nutrients and the body), sports nutrition (optimizing physiological performance), animal nutrition (ditto) and psychophysiology (including the study of attitudes and food choice).

Partly fuelled by huge pharmaceutical and food industry research funds, it is biochemistry that dominates nutrition research today, with researchers seeking the holy grail of a discovery that can be turned into a profitable food ingredient, technology or product. This pursuit began with Sir Gowland Hopkins' discovery in 1901 that the human body could not make the essential amino-acid *tryptophan*, and later established that it could only be derived from the diet. He demonstrated a principle that without a proper diet, bodily function could be impaired or deficient. Hopkins proved the existence of what he called food hormones or 'vitamines' (sic). The 'e' was dropped and they are now called vitamins. Most were discovered by the end of the 1930s.

Despite increasing scientific sophistication, nutrition – like any subject based on the study of humans – is inevitably framed by social assumptions. Is the pursuit of better nutrition a social duty or a right? Or is it a tool for national efficiency? Throughout the twentieth century, nutrition was a battleground with some forces seeing and using nutrition as an opportunity for social control and others arguing that it could either constrain or liberate human potential. This tension between social control and democracy – 'top down' science versus people-oriented science – still characterizes the world of food.

Although the recent history of public health and food policy has been stormy, it seems reasonable to hope that a new integrated policy approach might emerge. The success or otherwise of the WHO's 2004 Global Strategy and of moves to develop and implement solutions which integrate food policy with other policy areas such as environment and social justice will be important to watch in coming years.

Activity 10.3

'A burger with fries and a packet of cigarettes please' – industry, corporate responsibility and health

A news item in *The Lancet* (10 August 2002) reported that a group of New Yorkers had filed a lawsuit against four large fast food chains, alleging that their restaurants had knowingly served meals that cause obesity and other diseases. One of the plaintiffs claimed that the marketing efforts by the restaurants misled him into thinking the meals were good for him. In contrast, the representative of the National Restaurant Association said that the claims were 'senseless, baseless and ridiculous'.

In a paper published in the same issue, Ebbeling and collaborators (2002) mounted a serious criticism of the role that the food industry has played in the rise of childhood obesity. Read the extract from their paper below and perform the following task:

You are a special adviser on nutrition policy to a health minister in a country of your choice in which childhood obesity is increasingly recognized as a problem. Your minister has a distinguished record of effective action against the tobacco industry and has asked you to prepare a brief setting out the lessons that might be learned from anti-smoking campaigners in their actions against the tobacco industry in tackling the issue of fast food. Describe the arguments that you would include in such a document.

Childhood obesity: public health crisis, common sense cure

Prevention and treatment

Prevention and treatment of obesity ultimately involves eating less and being more physically active. Though this sounds simple, long-term weight loss has proven exceedingly difficult to achieve. The relative intellectual and psychological immaturity of children compared to adults, and their susceptibility to peer pressure, present additional practical obstacles to the successful treatment of childhood obesity. For this reason, most efforts to reduce obesity in children have used either family-based or school-based approaches, though pharmacological and surgical treatments are also available.

Limitations of current approaches

Although a few family-based studies produced significant long-term weight loss in motivated individuals, the overall success of non-surgical approaches has been disappointing, leading some specialists to conclude that treatment of obese children, which aims to establish a normal bodyweight, is unrealistically optimistic. Why is substantial long-term weight loss so difficult to achieve? One explanation is that the dietary and physical activity prescriptions used in family-based and school-based programmes might not be particularly efficacious. Indeed, most dietary interventions focus on reduction of fat intake, even though dietary fat might not be an important cause of obesity. Remarkably few paediatric obesity studies have sought to ascertain the effect of dietary composition on bodyweight, controlling for treatment intensity, physical activity, and behavioural modification techniques. With respect to physical activity, many studies have used conventional programmed exercise prescriptions, although increasing lifestyle activity or reducing sedentary behaviours might be better for long-term weight control. A second explanation for the difficulty in obtaining long-term weight loss is that adverse environmental factors overwhelm behavioural and educational techniques designed to reduce energy intake and augment physical activity.

The toxic environment

Battle and Brownell (1996) wrote, 'it is hard to envision an environment more effective than ours [in the USA] for producing ... obesity'. This statement probably applies to much of the developed world and, increasingly, to some developing countries. Several pervasive environmental factors promote energy intake and limit energy expenditure in children, undermining individual efforts to maintain a healthy bodyweight.

Food quality, policy, and advertising

In the late 1970s, children in the USA ate 17 per cent of their meals away from home, and fast foods accounted for 2 per cent of total energy intake. By the mid-1990s to late-1990s, the proportion of meals eaten away from home nearly doubled to 30 per cent, and fast food consumption increased five-fold, to 10 per cent of total energy intake. From 1965 to 1996, per capita daily soft drink consumption among 11–18-year old children rose from 179 g to 520 g for boys and from 148 g to 337 g for girls. There are 170 000 fast food restaurants in the USA alone. These trends have been driven, in part, by enormous advertising and marketing expenditures by the food industry, including an estimated US$12·7 billion directed at children and their parents. Marketing campaigns specifically target children, linking brand names with toys, games, movies, clothing, collectibles, educational tools, and even baby bottles. By contrast, the advertising budget for the US National Cancer Institute's '5-A-Day' programme to promote consumption of fruits and vegetables was $1·1 million in 1999. Large meals, often containing a child's total daily energy requirements, can be purchased for little additional cost over smaller portions, whereas fresh fruits and vegetables tend to be less readily available and comparatively more expensive. Furthermore, fast-food and soft-drink vending machines pervade schools. That US children overconsume added sugar and saturated fat, and underconsume fruits, non-starchy vegetables, fibre, and some micronutrients, is therefore not surprising.

Sedentary lifestyle

Availability of sedentary pursuits, including television, video games, computers, and the internet, has risen greatly. Children in the USA spend 75 per cent of their waking hours being inactive, compared with remarkably little time in vigorous physical activity; estimated at only 12 min per day. Opportunities for physical activity have decreased for various reasons. Physical education, typically considered less important than academic disciplines, has been eliminated in some school districts. In schools that do offer physical education, large class size and lack of equipment present barriers to successful programme implementation. After-school participation in unstructured activities can be limited, because of absence of pavements (sidewalks), bike paths, safe playgrounds, and parks in many neighbourhoods. Moreover, our culture places a premium on convenience: the car is preferred to walking, the lift to stairs, and the remote control to manual adjustment. These cultural forces arguably culminate in the drive-through window of fast-food restaurants, where a maximum of energy can be obtained with a minimum of exertion.

Barriers to change

Many special interests contribute to this problem of obesity, actively or passively, for financial reasons. The food industry, which generated almost $1 trillion in sales in 2000, spends enormous amounts of money to promote consumption of high calorie processed foods of poor nutritional quality. Underfunded school districts make money by establishing pouring rights contracts with soft drink companies, allowing them to place vending machines on school property and to sell beverages at school events. To save money, schools have subcontracted lunch programmes to corporate food services, encouraging the sale of high profit, low quality foods, including fast food. At the same time, budgetary pressures have led to reduction or elimination of physical education classes. Many communities do not adequately invest in urban environments that encourage physical activity, and instead pursue policies that favour real estate development to open space. Parents, for various socioeconomic reasons, work excessively long hours, leaving little time to prepare home-cooked meals and supervise non-sedentary activities. Professional nutritional societies maintain lucrative relations through sponsorships and endorsement with the food industry, creating a potential conflict of interest. According to the Center for Responsive Politics, candidates for the US Congress and presidency received more than $12 million between 1989 and 2000 from the sugar industry. Might these political contributions have a corrosive effect on regulatory efforts to revise national nutritional policy? Finally, the US health insurance industry reimburses poorly, if at all, for medical treatment of childhood obesity. However, all these short-term financial incentives are trivial when compared with the long-term costs to individuals and society. Annual hospital costs alone related to paediatric obesity in the USA approximate $127 million, and the effect of obesity on individuals is incalculable. Sadly, 10 per cent of children with type 2 diabetes develop renal failure, requiring dialysis or resulting in death by young adulthood, according to a preliminary report.

Conclusion

Almost three decades ago, an editorial in *The Lancet* called for efforts to prevent obesity in childhood. Since then, the worldwide prevalence of childhood obesity has risen several-fold. Obese children develop serious medical and psychosocial complications, and are at greatly increased risk of adult morbidity and mortality. The increasing prevalence and severity of obesity in children, together with its most serious complication, type 2 diabetes, raise the spectre of myocardial infarction becoming a paediatric disease. This public health crisis demands increased funding for research into new dietary, physical activity, behavioural, environmental, and pharmacological approaches for prevention and treatment of obesity, and improved reimbursement for effective family-based and school-based programmes. However, because this epidemic was not caused by inherent biological defects, increased funding for research and health care, focusing on new treatments, will probably not solve the problem of paediatric obesity without fundamental measures to effectively detoxify the environment (Figure 10.1).

A common sense approach to prevention and treatment of childhood obesity

Home	Set aside time for
	Healthy meals
	Physical activity
	Limit television viewing
School	Fund mandatory physical education
	Establish stricter standards for school lunch programmmes
	Eliminate unhealthy foods – eg, soft drinks and candy from vending machines
	Provide healthy snacks through concession stands and vending machines
Urban design	Protect open spaces
	Build pavements (sidewalks), bike paths, parks, playgrounds, and pedestrian zones
Health care	Improve insurance coverage for effective obesity treatment
Marketing and media	Consider a tax on fast food and soft drinks
	Subsidise nutritious foods – eg, fruits and vegetables
	Require nutrition labels on fast-food packaging
	Prohibit food advertisement and marketing directed at children
	Increase funding for public health campaigns for obesity prevention
Politics	Regulate political contributions from the food industry

Figure 10.1 Suggested approach to prevention and treatment of childhood obesity

Source: Ebbeling and collaborators (2002)

Although these measures require substantial political will and financial investment, they should yield a rich dividend to society in the long term.

Feedback

Possible points include:

- It is extremely important to tackle head on the issue of individual responsibility versus collective/environmental action – 'healthy choices need to be the easy choices'.
- Evidence of harm is necessary but not sufficient to motivate policy change – we already have sufficient knowledge to act on fast foods, rather than using the call for research as a means of delaying action. Some countries, correctly, took action to control tobacco when we still had much to learn about the harm it caused. Action on fast foods has begun, but mainly slowly. For example, in the US, fast food chains have agreed to display nutritional information on their menus and this is also being introduced in the UK; marketing food for children has been addressed differently around the world [IASO 2011]. The existence of fast food outlets in hospitals and of vending machines selling sugar-laden soft drinks in schools continues in many countries.
- Decisions to act need not wait for evidence of the effectiveness of interventions – Initial tobacco control interventions were not evidence based but represented sound judgment at the time: we know now what has worked for tobacco and can adapt some elements immediately.

- We need to look at the wider issues involved in food production, for example concerns of farmers. For tobacco control, this meant addressing all forms of tobacco use and not just cigarettes; and considering the concerns of tobacco farmers and providing convincing evidence that their livelihoods were not under threat in the mid-term. For the diet/nutrition area this will be more complex and require that close interaction be sought between those working to address hunger, micronutrient deficiencies and under-nutrition in general and those working to develop policies for overweight and chronic disease prevention. The goal should be to promote the optimal diet for all.
- We have learned from tobacco that the more comprehensive the package of measures considered, the greater the impact.
- Media-savvy individual and institutional leadership is extremely important.
- Change in support for tobacco control took decades of dedicated effort by all, so we should not expect immediate results.
- Modest, well-spent funds can have a massive impact. But without clear goals they may not be sustainable.
- Rules of engagement with the tobacco and food industries may need to be different but there is scope for those involved in promoting healthy lifestyles in both areas to learn from each other.

These points draw on a report on lessons from tobacco control compiled for Oxford Vision 2020, a movement dedicated to tackling the growing tide of chronic diseases globally. We should also note continuing efforts at national levels to produce comprehensive multi-sectoral approaches to obesity, a symbol of the challenges facing food and health practitioners (see for example the report by Nesle and Jacobson (2000) for an American example).

Summary

In this chapter you learnt about the development of thinking on nutrition and health and the need for a new integrated approach to improve dietary intake and health. The chapter described the key features in the evolution of thinking about the importance of diet on health and the four foci in modern thinking (food safety, nutrition, sustainable development and food security). It discussed the social forces affecting changes in dietary behaviour, and the key strengths and weakness of current arguments about the impact of social change on nutrition and health. It introduces the emerging obesity pandemic and some of the challenges facing public health in tackling it. Finally, it examined how food illustrates the links between human and environmental health and suggested some public policy pointers for the future. The next chapter, on the environmental determinants of health and disease, includes more about food in that context.

References

Battle EK and Brownell KD (1996) Confronting a rising tide of eating disorders and obesity: treatment vs prevention and policy. *Addict Behav* **21**, 755–65.
Bonell C, McKee M, Fletcher A, Haines A and Wilkinson P (2011) The nudge smudge: the misrepresentation of the 'nudge' concept in England's public health White Paper. *The Lancet* 2011; 377: 2158–9.
Brown LR (1996) *Tough Choices: Facing the Challenge of Food Scarcity*. London: Earthscan.

Daynard RA (2003) Lessons from tobacco for the Obesity Control Movement. *J Public Health Policy* **24**: 291–4.

DH (Department of Health) (England) (2010) *Healthy Lives, Healthy People*. London: DH (available at http:// www.dh.gov.uk/en/Publichealth/Healthyliveshealthypeople/index.htm).

Dudas S, Yang J, Graham C et al. (2010) Molecular, biochemical and genetic characteristics of BSE in Canada. *PLoS ONE* 5(5) e10638 (available at http://pubget.com/search?q=authors%3A%22Michael%20B%20 Coulthart%22#).

Dyson T (1996) *Population and Food: Global Trends and Future Prospects*. London: Routledge.

Ebbeling CB, Dorota DT and Ludwig DS (2002) Childhood obesity: public health crisis, common sense cure. *The Lancet* **360**: 473–82.

Food and Agriculture Organization (2000) *Agriculture: Towards 2015/2030 Technical Interim Report April 2000*. Rome: Food and Agriculture Organization Economic & Social Department.

Foresight (2007) Report: Tackling Obesities, Future Choices, 2nd edn, chair D King. Foresight, 2007 (available at http://www.bis.gov.uk/assets/bispartners/foresight/docs/obesity/17.pdf).

IASO (2011) International Association for the Study of Obesity (available at http://www.iaso.org/policy/ marketing-children/policy-map/).

Lang T and Caraher M (2006) Influencing international policy, in D Pencheon, C Guest, D Melzer and J Muir Gray (eds) *Oxford Handbook of Public Health Practice*, 2nd edn. Oxford: Oxford University Press, pp. 364–71.

Lind J (1753) *A Treatise of the Scurvy*. Edinburgh: Kincaid and Donaldson.

McMichael P (2001) The impact of globalisation, free trade and technology on food and nutrition in the new millennium. *Proc Nutr Soc* **60**: 215–20.

Menotti A, Keys A, Aravanis C, Blackburn H, Dontas A, Fidanza F, Karvonen MJ, Kromhout D, Nedeljkovic S, Nissinen A, et al. (1989) Seven Countries Study: First 20-year mortality data in 12 cohorts of six countries. *Annals of Medicine*. 21(3): 175–9.

Nesle M and Jacobson MF (2000) Halting the obesity epidemic: a public health approach. *Public Health Rep* **115**: 12–24.

NICE (2006) *Obesity: The Prevention, Identification, Assessment and Management of Overweight and Obesity in Adults and Children* (available at http://guidance.nice.org.uk/CG43/Guidance/Section).

Nuffield Council on Bioethics (2007) *Public Health, Ethical Issues* (available at http://www.nuffieldbioethics. org/public-health).

Roth J, Qiang X, Marban SL, Redelt H and Lowell B (2004) The obesity pandemic: where have we been and where are we going? *Obesity Research* **12**: 88S–101S; doi: 10.1038/oby.2004.273.

Thaler R and Sunstein C (2008) *Nudge: Improving Decisions about Health, Wealth, and Happiness*. New Haven, CT: Yale University Press.

World Health Organization (2004) *WHO Global Strategy on Diet, Physical Activity and Health*. Geneva: WHO (available at http://www.who.int/dietphysicalactivity/strategy/eb11344/strategy_english_web.pdf).

World Health Organization (2008) *WHO Action Plan for the Global Strategy for the Prevention and Control of Noncommunicable Diseases*. Geneva: WHO (available at http://whqlibdoc.who.int/ publications/2009/9789241597418_eng.pdf).

 Further reading

Food Standards Agency (UK) – for policy issues on food safety and healthy eating. Visit: http://www.food. gov.uk/

International Association for the Study of Obesity. Visit: http://www.iaso.org/ Information and science for professionals, policy-makers and the public.

Lang T and Heasman M (2004) *Food Wars: The Global Battle for Mouths, Minds and Markets*. London: Earthscan. This book discusses the impact of the growth of a single global market on what we eat, with corresponding implications for public health.

Mathers C and Loncar D (2006) Projections of global mortality and burden of disease from 2002 to 2030. *PLoS Med* **3**(11): e442. doi:10.1371/journal.pmed.0030442, 2006 (available at http://www.plosmedicine.org/article/info:doi/10.1371/journal.pmed.0030442).

National Obesity Observatory, England. For information about obesity in the UK, including data, evaluation and evidence for interventions, and results of the National Child Measurement Programme (available at http://www.noo.org.uk/).

Nestle M (2002) *Food Politics*. Berkley CA: University of California Press. This book offers a critique of the role of the food industry in shaping our diets, and by extension our health.

Obesity Learning Centre. For advice and information for people working on obesity, the site is hosted and maintained by the National Heart Forum (available at http://www.obesitylearningcentre-nhf.org.uk/).

Puska P, Tuomilehto J, Nissinen A and Vartiainen E (eds) (1995) *The North Karelia Project: 20 Year Results and Experiences*. Helsinki: National Public Health Institute of Finland. This book will introduce you to the different measures used in Finland to help improve population health.

The Commission on the Nutrition Challenges of the 21st Century (2000) Ending malnutrition by 2020: an agenda for change in the millennium. *Food and Nutrition Bulletin (United Nations)* **21** (3, Suppl). This report proposes major new initiatives to speed up the aid process to eradicate malnutrition.

World Health Organization (2003) *Diet, Nutrition and the Prevention of Chronic Diseases*. WHO Technical Report Series No. 916. Geneva: World Health Organization. This report examines the science base of the relationship between diet and physical activity patterns, and the major nutrition-related chronic diseases.

Drains, dustbins and diseases

Giovanni Leonardi, Martin McKee, Fiona Sim and Joceline Pomerleau

Overview

Environmental issues, in particular the potential health effects of pollution, are a growing cause of concern among populations around the world. For centuries, man has recognized the link between common pests, such as rats, living in the drains and around the rubbish of our cities and towns, and diseases. In contemporary times, while that 'traditional' environmental threat to our health has not gone away, people have pointed an accusing finger at motor vehicles and fuel combustion in residential, commercial and industrial heating and cooling and coal-burning power plants. However, the potential health hazard of commonly adopted waste disposal systems such as landfill and incineration is also examined more closely nowadays. In addition, indoor air pollution is now recognized as a major contributor to disease burden, particularly in developing countries. Health protection being a key element of public health, the protection of the population from toxic chemical substances coming from all sources of pollution needs to be closely examined as it links with other aspects of public health practice. This chapter will discuss the environmental and health aspects of waste disposal systems. You will also be introduced to the health impacts of indoor and outdoor air pollution. Other examples such as water management would also be relevant but are not discussed here. See Chapter 12 for a more detailed account of climate change and public health.

Learning objectives

By the end of this chapter you should be able to:

- describe local health impacts of landfill and incineration
- describe global ecological impacts of waste disposal activities
- discuss the health impacts of outdoor and indoor air pollution for different groups of people in developed and developing countries

Key terms

Ecological footprint Accounting tool for ecological resources developed by the Task Force on Healthy and Sustainable Communities at the University of British Columbia (Canada). It corresponds to the area of productive land and aquatic ecosystems required to produce the resources used, and to assimilate the wastes produced, by a defined population at a specified material standard of living, wherever on Earth that land may be located.

Environmental or occupational exposure   Any contact between a substance in an environmental medium (for example water, air, soil) and the surface of the human body (for example skin, respiratory tract); after uptake into the body it is referred to as dose.

Exposure assessment   Is the study of distribution and determinants of substances or factors affecting human health (Nieuwenhuijsen 2003).

Precautionary principle   This principle states that when there is reasonable suspicion of harm, lack of scientific certainty or consensus must not be used to postpone preventative action to avoid serious or irreversible harm.

Waste and health: an overview

The composition of manufactured goods is very complex. Think, for example, of a computer, microwave oven, or television set. You can easily imagine that each of these goods is made of a vast number of components, each in turn made of a vast number of substances. In order to have a better idea of how these products could affect the health of a population, you could decide to analyse their specific chemical composition and the health aspects of their production and disposal, taking into account the accompanying environmental and social impacts.

Activity 11.1

Consider a specific example: think about two different consumer goods: a Ferrari and a personal computer. List some hazardous materials coming from them.

Feedback

A car is a heap of waste. Raw materials for a Ferrari come from all continents, are packaged in Italy, and get dispersed in the environment usually, but not always, in the country where it has been purchased. Many hazardous materials come from cars and are dispersed in the environment. These include for example:

- headlight bulbs and anti-lock braking systems which contain mercury;
- anti-corrosion coating which contains some hexavalent chromium and cadmium;
- the battery which contains lead;
- the catalytic converter, which contains platinum.

Other substances include arsenic, polyvinyl chloride, and polychlorinated biphenyls, while electronic and hybrid cars also include a range of rare earth metals.

A particular problem is posed by compound substances, such as tyres and plastics included in cars: they are more difficult to recycle than the steel and metals.

Electronic and electrical equipment is responsible for an increasing proportion of all hazardous waste produced in developed societies. Examples of hazardous materials in a personal computer include:

- plastic which contains brominated flame retardants (they produce dioxins when burned);
- cathode ray tubes (in the monitor) which contain lead;
- the switches and gas discharge lamps which contain mercury.

The EU's Waste Electrical and Electronic Equipment (WEEE) Directive is its mechanism for achieving better environmental protection and encouraging resource efficiency. The Directive sets targets for the collection, reuse and recycling of electrical and electronic equipment.

In England and Wales, the Environment Agency's principal aims are to protect and improve the environment, and to promote sustainable development. It uses traditional regulation, and increasingly voluntary agreements and local levies to achieve its aims. Its Modernising Waste Regulation Panel considers and makes recommendations on environmental issues concerning waste.

Local health impacts of landfill and incineration

Landfill and incineration are the most commonly adopted waste disposal options. Unfortunately, both options result in the dispersal in the environment of materials hazardous to health.

Landfill

Activity 11.2

Figure 11.1 shows a schematic representation of a landfill, with its sources, pathways and receptors. Describe the fate of the waste materials disposed in it.

Feedback

We can see that gases and odours are emitted from the surface and go into the air. Contaminated rainwater infiltrates the landfill and leachate (water seeping from the waste) is produced. Unfortunately it contains a mixture of the landfill materials and can amount to thousands of litres per day. Rainwater also leads to the production of contaminated surface water which runs off from the landfill to contaminate ditch and river water. The leachate and seepage in the landfill site infiltrates groundwater and migrates through the soil in unsaturated zones, potentially affecting the quality of the water supplied by the borehole. Methane is also produced by the landfill; it migrates through fissures or permeable zones.

In the UK, as in many other countries, landfill has been the most popular option for waste disposal. A study by the Small Area Health Statistics Unit (SAHSU) (Elliott and colleagues 2001) found that over 80 per cent of the UK population lives within 2 km of a landfill site. In the past, highly hazardous materials have often been disposed of in

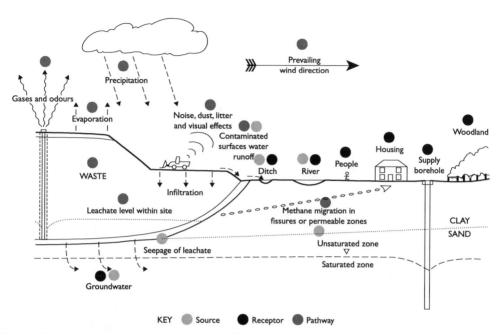

Figure 11.1 Schematic representation of a landfill

the same sites as municipal solid waste, in so called co-disposal sites, however this practice is being phased out.

Indeed, due to concerns across Europe, a case-control study – the EUROHAZCON STUDY – was conducted to look at the risk of birth defects in the vicinity of hazardous waste sites (Dolk et al. 1998). The study showed an increasing risk of congenital malformations with increasing vicinity to a site, having controlled for socioeconomic status. The public concern from these results persuaded the relevant government department (now the Department for the Environment, Farming & Rural Affairs, DEFRA) in England to review research priorities in relation to waste disposal and to consider funding a national case-control study of landfills and malformations. In addition, the Department of Health (England) decided to commission further research on this topic. One of the outputs was a review on the potential teratogenicity (potential to cause birth abnormalities) of substances emanating from landfill published in 2001 (Sullivan and colleagues 2001). This review classified substances according to their potential teratogenicity. The substances for which animal and/or human data demonstrate clear teratogenic potential (or potential for other important reproductive effects) at relatively low doses/ exposures (thus being the most likely candidates for teratogenic effects of landfill waste) include:

- Benzene
- 1,3 Butadiene
- Carbon disulphide
- Chloroform
- 1,2-Dichloroethylene
- Ethylbenzene

- Formaldehyde
- Methyl chloride
- Tetrachloroethylene
- Trichloroethylene
- Vinyl chloride

Cancer is the other main health concern for people resident near landfills. Evidence is equivocal but cannot be entirely dismissed. Since 2000, more studies have suggested that proximity to domestic waste landfill is not associated with increased cancer risk (Jarup et al. 2002; Goodman et al. 2010) than the contrary. Population mobility means that making an association between living near landfill and the occurrence of cancers whose latent period may be 20-20 years is very difficult. Mutagenicity (potential to cause cancer) tests conducted on leachate show a higher mutagenic activity of leachate than various types of surface water. However more long term, rigorous research is needed before reliable conclusions can be reached about the risk of cancer in the vicinity of municipal landfill sites.

Incineration

Though cancer has also been a concern in the vicinity of incinerators, dioxin and its dispersal via the food chain has been more prominent among the concerns of local residents. Another aspect, on which public health authorities have been asked to comment, is the potential health hazard represented by incinerator ash. This has a very high concentration of metals and dioxins. A group of experts on incinerator ash reviewed different types of disposal practice. The preferred disposal practices are either leachate containment and collection, or controlled contaminant release. The latter option means that disposal should be supported by a monitoring programme to allow control of the disposal of the hazardous components of the material.

In summary, direct impacts from landfill and incineration have not been demonstrated clearly by epidemiological studies, however there are many potential areas where health impacts are plausible and community concerns cannot be ignored based on the evidence currently available.

Ecological impacts of waste

We depend on nature for the supply of our food and energy, the absorption of our waste products, and for other life-support services. But in order to preserve this situation, we must ensure that nature's productivity is not used more quickly than it can be renewed, and that waste is not discharged more quickly than nature can absorb it. The impacts of waste production on the ecosystem create many hazards and they are considered by some to be more worrying than the direct health impacts of waste. The overall quantity of waste generated by humans continues to rise, a result of the more prosperous lifestyles of the developed world. By 2020, the OECD estimates, we could be generating 45 per cent more waste than we did in 1995. So the strategies of preventing waste, recycling and improving its disposal are together important for human health.

In order to find out whether nature provides enough resources to secure good living conditions, the Task Force on Healthy and Sustainable Communities at the

University of British Columbia has developed an accounting tool for ecological resources: the **ecological footprint**. It is a measure of how sustainable our lifestyles are and is calculated as the area of productive land and aquatic ecosystems required to produce the resources used, and to assimilate the wastes produced, by a defined population at a specified material standard of living, wherever on Earth that land may be located.

An example of the application of the concept of ecological footprint is offered by a study in Liverpool, England (Barrett and Scott 2001). This study examined the ecological sustainability of the city and concluded the following:

- The average Liverpool resident requires 4.15 hectares of land (compared with 4.9 hectares for the UK average) to supply him or her with all the necessary resources, transportation needs, and use and disposal of those resources. In comparison, 80.3 per cent of the world's population has an ecological footprint less than 4 hectares, and their total share of the world's footprint is 38.3 per cent, with an average footprint of 1.36 hectare.
- For the city of Liverpool, waste had the highest impact (1.6 hectare/person), followed by the provision of resources (1.1 hectare/person), transport of passengers and freight (0.7 hectare/person), utilities (0.63 hectare/person), biodiversity protection (0.3 hectare/person), and buildings and land (0.1 hectare/person).
- A sustainable ecological footprint is 2 hectares/per capita. This could be achieved by working on three key areas: energy (reduction of energy consumption, domestic waste, and water (reduction of leakage and domestic use consumption)). With regard to domestic waste, recycling alone would not be sufficient (the city will need to recycle 93 per cent of domestic waste by 2021) and waste minimization schemes are essential.

A similar study but applied to the whole planet (Wackernagel and colleagues 2002) suggested that the Earth as a whole has used more than the total capacity of its ecological services (water, soil capacity) for over a decade, and that we run the risk that the capacity of soil and water systems to regenerate themselves may be overcome. This conclusion was based on several assumptions, including the fact that it is possible to keep track of most of the resources we use and the wastes we generate, that most of the resource and waste flows can be measured according to the biologically productive area needed to maintain them, that the planet can be assessed in terms of 'global hectares' (representing the average productive hectare on Earth for that particular year), that natural supply of ecological services can be measured in the same way, and that area demand can exceed area supply, a phenomenon called ecological overshoot. The ecological overshoot described in this study could have public health as well as environmental impacts. This topic is considered further in Chapter 12.

A waste management hierarchy thus conveys the idea that waste reduction and minimization should be considered a higher priority than recycling, and recycling a higher priority than either landfill or incineration. This appears justified based on consideration of both (local) health and ecological effects of waste production and disposal. However, recycling rates in Europe remain variable, with some countries achieving 50 per cent recycling of household waste. At a regional level, the community of Flanders (Belgium) had achieved 70 per cent recycling of domestic waste by 2010 (see Figure 11.2). Since statutory recycling targets were set in England in 2000, many local authorities recycling services have improved. Some have achieved household waste recycling rates of over 40 per cent. The *Household Waste Recycling Act* was introduced in

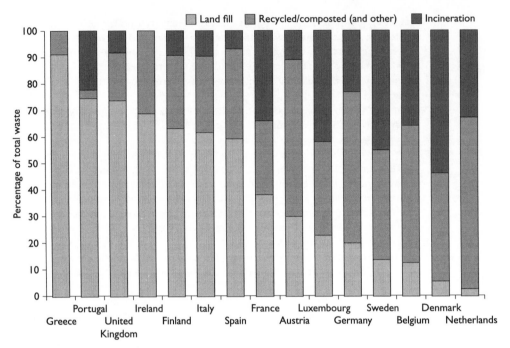

Figure 11.2 Waste disposal (%) in selected European countries

Source: Eurostat

2003. But policy in England has been criticized for focusing on domestic waste, which comprises only 10 per cent of all waste, while neglecting other, arguably more important waste from industry (EFRA 2010).

From the local public health point of view, waste is an issue that is not going to go away, with many communities dissatisfied with the passive approach of many official agencies. There are examples in the UK of new housing applications having received planning permission adjacent to landfill sites, inevitably leading to complaints and concerns about odour and health effects.

The possible contributions that public health professionals can make to waste management, locally, nationally and internationally, involve policy change and local action. They include:

- surveys and models of exposure in the vicinity of landfills;
- meetings with communities and health protection teams;
- health surveys;
- advice on the health impacts of proposed waste management activities (landfill and incineration) under the Integrated Pollution Prevention and Control (IPPC) legislation of the European Union (EC, updated 2007);
- contribution to regional and local waste strategies, including health impact assessments (see Chapter 6).

Public health professionals who would like to contribute to waste management in the contexts both of health protection and sustainability, can also collaborate with several agencies outside the health system, including environment ministries, academic units, and others, including non-governmental advocacy organizations active in this area, to develop their work in this difficult area.

Indoor and outdoor pollution

Air pollution, both indoor and outdoor, is a major environmental health problem affecting developed and developing countries alike. It comes from sources of dust, gases and smoke and is generated mainly by human activities. Air pollution has numerous adverse health effects starting from modest transient changes in the respiratory tract and impaired lung function, continuing to restricted activity and reduced performance, emergency room visits and hospital admissions, and to mortality (World Health Organization Regional Office for Europe 2004). Globally, outdoor air pollution is estimated to be responsible for about 3 per cent of mortality from cardiopulmonary disease, about 5 per cent of mortality from cancer of the trachea, bronchus, and lung, and about 1 per cent of mortality from acute respiratory infections in children under 5 yrs, with the burden falling predominantly on developing countries (Cohen and Anderson 2005).

Since the 1970s, attention has focused mainly on pollutants in outdoor air (for example particulate matters, ozone, nitrogen dioxide) or on indoor hazards, such as asbestos or environmental tobacco smoke. However, it is often forgotten that more than two billion people worldwide continue to depend on solid fuels, including biomass fuels (wood, dung, agricultural residues) and coal, for their energy needs. Using these on open fires or traditional stoves (for cooking or heating) results in high levels of indoor air pollution that contains a variety of health-damaging pollutants such as small particles and carbon monoxide. Overall, indoor air pollution was estimated to be responsible for 2.7 per cent of the global burden of disease (World Health Organization 2002), with substantially greater levels occurring once again in developing countries.

Recent research has linked outdoor air pollution with risk of myocardial infarction (heart attack), concluding a similar order of risk as alcohol or physical exertion, when the high prevalence of exposure is taken into account (Nawrot et al. 2011). Our dependence on solid fuels for energy can also have a major negative impact on the environment, for example if it leads to deforestation (for example in areas where wood fuel is scarce and the demand for wood outweighs nature re-growth) which can be associated with soil erosion and serious mud slides (such as those observed in Haiti in the summer of 2004 following tropical storm Jeanne) or to greenhouse gas emissions (for example because biomass stoves used in developing country homes typically have a low efficiency, thus leading to the lost of a large percentage of the fuel energy as products of incomplete combustion with an important greenhouse effect).

Activity 11.3

A non-governmental organization working in the developing world has argued that international agencies are paying too much attention to outdoor air pollution at a time when many millions of people in poorer countries are exposed to high levels of indoor air pollution. They argue that indoor air pollution may be more easily addressed in the short term than some of the problems of outdoor pollution. You have been invited by the United Nations Environment Programme to prepare a short briefing paper setting out the arguments that might be used to give priority to each of the two sources of pollution. What would be the key points that you would consider? As a guide you can use the papers from Bruce and collaborators (2000) and from McMichael (2000), and others, as well as documents on the World Health Organization website (2011) – all freely accessible on the Internet.

Feedback

- burden of disease attributable to each type of exposure – mortality, morbidity/DALY;
- understanding of causal pathways leading from exposure to disease;
- availability of effective interventions;
- feasibility of interventions;
- impact on for health of each type of exposure;
- potential to intervene;
- unequal burden of pollution by social class/environmental equity/justice/poverty;
- unequal burden of outdoor/indoor pollution by development stage of country;
- precautionary principle and approach, what influence on setting standards;
- process of setting standards for air quality, influence of scientific, policy, public/ societal factors in framing the question and the solutions.

Summary

In this chapter we discussed the health and environmental aspects of waste, as well as air pollution. We examined the local health impacts of landfill and incineration as well as the global adverse impacts of waste disposal activities and some strategies for impact reduction. We also discussed the health impacts of outdoor and indoor air pollution for different groups of people in developed and developing countries.

References

Barrett J and Scott A (2001) *An Ecological Footprint of Liverpool: Developing Sustainable Scenarios. A Detailed Examination of Ecological Sustainability.* Stockholm: Stockholm Environment Institute.

Bruce N, Perez-Padilla R and Albalak R (2000) Indoor air pollution in developing countries: a major environmental and public health challenge. *Bull World Health Org* **78**: 1078–92 (available at http://whqlibdoc.who.int/bulletin/2000/Number%209/78(9)1078–1092.pdf).

Cohen AJ and Anderson HR (2005) The global burden of disease due to outdoor air pollution. *Journal of Toxicology and Environmental Health*, Part A, **68**:1–7; ISSN: 1528–7394 print/1087–2620 online; DOI: 10.1080/15287390590936166.

Dolk H, Vrijheid M, Armstrong B et al. (1998) Risk of congenital anomalies near hazardous-waste landfill sites in Europe: the EUROHAZCON study. *The Lancet* **352**: 423–7.

EFRA Environment, Food & Rural Affairs (2010) *Select Committee Report,* House of Commons, London (available at http://www.publications.parliament.uk/pa/cm200910/cmselect/cmenvfru/230/23002.htm).

Elliott P, Briggs D, Morris S et al. (2001) Risk of adverse birth outcomes in populations living near landfill sites. *Br Med J* **323**: 363–8.

European Commission – Environment (2007) Intergrated pollution prevention and control (IPPC) regulations, updated 2007 (available at http://ec.europa.eu/environment/air/pollutants/stationary/ippc/ippc_revision.htm).

Goodman J, Hudson TC and Monteiro RJ (2010) Cancer cluster investigation in residents near a municipal landfill. *Human and Ecological Risk Assessment: An International Journal* 1549–7860, **16** (6): 1339–59.

Jarup L, Briggs D, de Hoogh C et al. (2002) Cancer risks in populations living near landfill sites in Great Britain. *British Journal of Cancer* **86**: 1732–6. doi:10.1038/sj.bjc.6600311www.bjcancer.com

McMichael AJ (2000) The urban environment and health in a world of increasing globalization: issues for developing countries. *Bull World Health Organ* **78**: 1117–26 (available at http://whqlibdoc.who.int/bulletin/2000/Number%209/78(9)1117–1126.pdf,).

Nawrot TS, Perez L, Künzli N, Munters E and Nemery B (2011) Public health importance of triggers of myocardial infarction: a comparative risk assessment. *The Lancet*, **26**: 377 (9767): 732–4.

Nieuwenhuijsen M (ed.) (2003) *Exposure Assessment in Occupational and Environmental Epidemiology.* New York: Oxford University Press.

Sullivan FM, Barlow SM and McElhatton PR (2001) *A Review of the Potential Teratogenicity of Substances Emanating from Landfill Sites.* London: Department of Health.

Wackernagel M, Schulz NB, Deumling D et al. (2002) Tracking the ecological overshoot of the human economy. *Proc Natl Acad Sci* **99**: 9266–71.

World Health Organization (2002) *World Health Report 2002.* Geneva: World Health Organization.

World Health Organization (2005) *Indoor Air Pollution: National Burden of Disease Estimates.* Geneva: World Health Organization, updated 2007 (available at http://www.who.int/indoorair/publications/indoor_air_national_burden_estimate_revised.pdf).

World Health Organization Regional Office for Europe (2004) *Health Aspects of Air Pollution. Results from the WHO project 'Systematic Review of Health Aspects of Air Pollution in Europe'.* Copenhagen: World Health Organization Regional Office for Europe.

📖 Further reading

Department of Agriculture, Food, and Rural Affairs. Waste Stratey for England 2007, DEFRA (available at http://www.defra.gov.uk/environment/waste/strategy/strategy07/documents/waste07-strategy.pdf).

Environment Agency (available at http://www.environment-agency.gov.uk/aboutus/default.aspx).

European Commission – Environment. A rich source of information on all aspects of the environment, with data from EU member countries as well as aggregated data (available at http://ec.europa.eu/environment/waste/index.htm).

McMichael A (2001) *Human Frontiers, Environments and Disease: Past Patterns, Uncertain Futures.* Cambridge: Cambridge University Press.

Milton J and Brahic C (2010) Track that trash, *New Scientist*, **206** (2756): 44–5.

National Research Council (2000) *Waste Incineration and Public Health. National Research Council, Committee on Health Effects of Waste Incineration, Board on Environmental Studies and Toxicology, Commission on Life Sciences.* Washington, DC: National Academy Press.

Vrijheid M (2000) Health effects of residence near hazardous waste landfill sites: a review of epidemiologic literature. *Environ Health Perspect* **108**(Suppl 1): 101–12.

12 Sustainable development and climate change – the 'new' determinants of health

Fiona Sim, Jenny Griffiths and Martin McKee

Overview

This chapter will review what is known about climate change and its potential impact on health. It will explore the concepts of sustainable development, ecological public health, mitigation and adaptation in the context of climate change. The roles of all health professionals and of the public health specialist will be considered, including how best to harness involvement at a professional level. There will also be a challenge to the reader to take action at a personal level. The particular role of the health system in addressing climate change and sustainable development will be examined. Many of the examples will be taken from the UK and Europe, but consideration of global issues will be included.

Learning objectives

By the end of this chapter you should be able to:

- understand and explain to others our understanding of the impact of climate change on human health
- understand the links between sustainable development, climate change and health
- take appropriate steps in your working life to support activity to reduce the adverse impacts of climate change
- understand the role of health services in mitigating and adapting to the effects of climate change
- take action to minimize the impact of climate change on health inequalities
- consider your own actions in relation to climate change

Key terms

Adaptation Short term adjustment in natural or human systems in response to actual or expected climatic events, to reduce the impact of climate change.

Carbon footprint A measure of the impact of human activities on the environment, and in particular on climate change. It relates to the amount of greenhouse gases produced, measured in units of tonnes (or kg) of carbon dioxide equivalent.

Climate change Long-term (minimum one decade) change in the statistical distribution of weather patterns over periods of time; usually now refers to changes in modern climate due to human activities.

Co-benefits The results of action likely to impact favourably on climate change, which are also likely to reduce mortality or morbidity due to other causes, or to improve the health of a population.

Contraction and Convergence Model that sets out a global framework for reducing greenhouse gas emissions to safe levels in a socially just way.

Ecological public health Integration of ecological and environmental issues within public health research and practice to seek to benefit both human and environmental health.

Mitigation A human intervention over the longer term to reduce the concentrations of greenhouse gases, so reducing the severity of climate change.

Sustainable development Development that uses resources to meet present day needs, while not compromising the ability of future generations to meet their own needs.

Why is climate change happening?

Greenhouse gases, such as carbon dioxide (CO_2), methane and water vapour act like a blanket to trap the heat of the sun in the earth's atmosphere and warm our planet, making it habitable: this is often called the 'greenhouse effect' (The Royal Society 2010). Changes in the amount or characteristics of greenhouse gases, particles and clouds, or changes in the reflectivity of the Earth's surface, can initiate changes in global temperature. This is called 'radiative forcing': the effect greenhouse gases have on the net amount of incoming and outgoing radiation received at the tropopause, the atmospheric boundary below which all weather occurs. A positive change in radiative forcing usually results in more warming of the atmosphere, a net negative change results in cooling.

So we need greenhouse gases to live on the earth. It is also true that some variation in the earth's climate and average temperatures is natural: ice ages and warm periods have occurred at intervals, probably due to changes in the earth's orbit around the sun. But recent human activities, particularly the ubiquitous burning of fossil fuels for power and transport, together with the destruction of forests around the world, have led to substantial rises in the concentration of greenhouse gases, trapping more heat in the atmosphere. Although climate change is particularly linked to humanity's dependence on fossil fuels, the United Nations Environment Programme estimates that about 20 per cent of current global greenhouse gas emissions are linked with deforestation, because the global forest area has shrunk by approximately 40 per cent in the last 300 years. So the idea of a forest for the National Health Service in England is not as strange as it may initially appear: the project aims to plant a tree for each member of staff, 1.3 million in total (http://www.nhsforest.org).

Greenhouse gases are now at their highest level for 650,000 years. As Figure 12.1 shows, the speed of the rise in emissions is both sharp and accelerating. Over the last 650,000 years and until 50 years ago, the fastest rise was 30 parts per million over 1,000 years: that same level of increase has been achieved in the last 20 years. At the beginning of the industrial revolution, carbon dioxide concentrations were about 280 parts per million; by 1950 they were about 300 parts per million; they are now about 385 parts per million (Liggins 2009).

The increased heat leads to climate instability: extreme weather events such as floods, storms, heat waves and droughts have been recorded with increased frequency in recent decades. Loss of snow and ice cover due to warming, particularly at the poles, causes further changes in the climate. Soil acts as a net carbon sink, tying up CO_2 from the atmosphere as plants grow. The increase in temperature is already beginning to cause more respiration by living organisms in the soil, leading to more CO_2 being released into the atmosphere.

Relentless population growth will make climate change worse. In 1950, the world population was just over 2.5 billion; it is now 6.7 billion. The United Nations projects an increase to 9.2 billion by 2050. Clearly more people on the planet are likely to cause the emission of more carbon emissions, both directly by their own behaviour and through releasing the CO_2 in land cleared for crops and livestock.

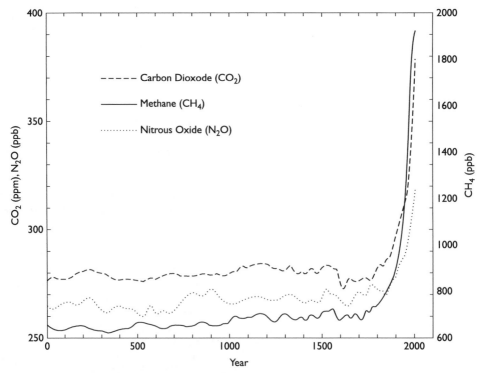

Figure 12.1 Increase in greenhouse gases to the twenty-first century

Source: IPCC (2007)

Why is climate change important for public health?

Climate change is already bringing about harm to human health. If not tackled effectively by the world's governments, this trend is projected to accelerate. We shall look at what is known, why this is happening and what actions are necessary to limit the impact now and in the future. It is worth noting that some health impacts of climate change may be for the better, but these are far outweighed by the negative effects. In some cases, climate change is already causing major changes to the lifestyle and health of whole populations, such as communities living in island locations affected by rising sea levels. In others, such as the UK, climate change is showing itself more subtly, through the increasing incidence of skin cancer, for example.

The Climate Vulnerable Forum (DARA 2010), a global partnership of leaders of countries most vulnerable to climate change, with links to the United Nations, has estimated that across the world, 350,000 deaths are now occurring each year due to climate change, nearly all in 'developing' countries in south Asia and sub-Saharan Africa, with many due to climate-driven desertification, that is the loss of cultivable soil due to drought and soil erosion. This number is set to escalate rapidly in the absence of an effective international response. The key areas of linkage between population health and climate change are summarized in Box 12.1.

Box 12.1 Areas of linkage between public health and climate change

Patterns of disease and mortality
Food security
Water and sanitation
Shelter and human settlements
Extreme climatic events [eg Tsunami]
Population migration

The evidence for climate change

There remains concern among some governments and individuals about the reality of climate change and whether it is anthropogenic (man-made). It is common to find denial of the evidence, usually by people for whom the actions required for mitigation are challenging or unpalatable.

However, the evidence for climate change is impressive. More than 2,500 scientific expert reviewers were involved in preparation of the Intergovernmental Panel on Climate Change (IPCC) 2007 report. The report concludes the following:

• Warming of the climate system is unequivocal.
• Greenhouse gas concentrations have increased as a result of human activities.
• There is **very high confidence** (9/10 probability) that the net effect of human activities since 1750 has been one of warming.

The evidence (Faculty of Public Health 2009) suggests that there is an increasing risk of abrupt or irreversible climatic shifts between 2012 and the mid-2030s.

As a result of this evidence, governments have made various commitments to mitigation of the effects of climate change. National targets are set in order to reduce global warming, but obviously require the majority of nations to act, especially those responsible for the greatest emissions. Paradoxically, many countries that contribute the least to climate change are likely to be worst affected by its harmful impacts. This is the case for most countries in Africa, whose energy consumption per capita is low in comparison to many 'developed' countries. However poor countries have limited capacity to adapt and so their populations are more likely to be among the worst affected by global climate change.

Internationally, a series of conferences under the auspices of the United Nations have recognized the need for deep cuts in emissions but have yet to reach a binding agreement, although efforts continue.

In the UK, legislation enacted in 2008 commits the government to reduce green-house gas emissions by 80 per cent by 2050 and 34 per cent by 2020. The Parliamentary Committee on Climate Change, in a report giving advice to the government on the fourth 'carbon budget' (2010), and recognizing the seriousness of the situation, now proposes an indicative 2030 target of 46 per cent in emissions relative to 2009 levels. The Committee emphasizes the need for new policies to drive a 'step change' in energy efficiency improvements in residential and non-residential buildings, accompanied by behaviour change in transport patterns, as well as carbon-efficient practices on farms.

The direct impact of climate change on health

Climate change brings about changes in the environment which directly impact on human health. These direct impacts include:

- infectious diseases, including insect-borne diseases, appearing in temperate regions, which were previously endemic only in subtropical or tropical regions;
- heatstroke occurring more commonly in temperate regions where it had previously been rare;
- mortality by drowning in floods or other freak weather phenomena;
- famine, as a result of failed crop harvests or floods;
- increasing prevalence of skin cancers and sunburn associated with exposure to UV rays; and
- increasing prevalence of eye cataracts due to greater exposure to UV rays from the sun.

The impact of climate change on the wider determinants of health

In addition to the direct effects of climate change on human health, it is now recognized that climate change affects many of the wider determinants of health. The determinants of health that are most affected by climate change are:

- access to food and clean water;
- living conditions and overcrowding;
- hygiene and sanitation;
- infectious disease and vaccinations;
- access to health services and essential medicines;
- economic instability;
- civil unrest;
- war.

The reasons for some of these are obvious. For example, if climate change adversely affects crop harvests, access to food is directly affected. Similarly, drought will affect the availability of sources of clean water in affected areas. More subtly, civil unrest is associated with poverty and lack of access to basic necessities, and the risk of war likewise when a neighbouring state or community may have better access to scarce resources.

It is very important to note that this is a two-way relationship. Addressing climate change often has a positive impact on health and conversely, addressing health – especially tackling health inequalities – often has a positive impact on climate change (Marmot 2005). Barton and Grant have adapted Dahlgren and Whitehead's well-known social model of health to take account of the importance of the global ecosystem (Dahlgren and Whitehead 1992) (Figure 12.2).

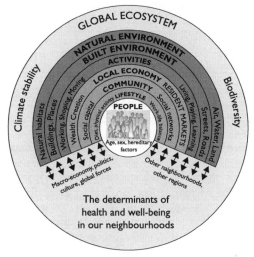

Figure 12.2 The Ecosystem Model of Settlements
Source: Barton and Grant (2006)

Box 12.2 shows an example of the impact of climate change in one country, India.

Box 12.2 How climate change is impacting on health in India

Climate change is already having severe impacts in India and risks widening health and social inequalities at a time when the country is attempting to improve the lives of its poor. India's poor people live mainly in rural areas and depend on climate-sensitive activities such as agriculture and fishing for their livelihoods.

Extreme weather events such as heat waves, tropical cyclones and floods are increasing in severity and frequency, causing many deaths and human misery and increasing poverty.

India's food security is closely linked to the monsoon, which is increasingly unpredictable due to climate instability.

The island of Lohachara in the Bay of Bengal, previously inhabited by 10,000 people, was the first island in the world to be submerged by rising sea levels in 2006.

Rising sea levels risk the infusion of salt water into fresh water sources, which are themselves seriously threatened as the severity and frequency of droughts and floods increase, and the pace of retreat of the Himalayan glaciers accelerates.

Climate change threatens to further widen gender inequalities in India. Women are the primary care-givers within the family and carry the responsibility for providing food and fetching drinking water. Shrinking water sources are resulting in women having to walk longer distances to collect water, reducing their availability for work and consequently, their family income.

Rao (2010)

Tackling climate change

There are two main strategies for tackling climate change, which are complementary. They are usually described as mitigation and adaptation. To place these terms in a public health context, mitigation comprises interventions for primary prevention and adaptation is secondary (or arguably tertiary) prevention.

Mitigation is defined in the IPCC 4th Report as 'a human intervention to reduce the sources or enhance the sinks of greenhouse gases'. Therefore mitigation reduces the *severity* of climate change. It requires reducing greenhouse gas concentrations and that requires long-term interventions. An example is reducing the amount of transport using fossil fuels.

Adaptation is defined in the IPCC report as 'any adjustment in natural or human systems in response to actual or expected climatic stimuli or their effects, which moderates harm or exploits beneficial opportunities'. Therefore adaptation reduces the *impact* of climate change. This requires changing systems in order to reduce the harm from climate effects. Adaptations are necessary short-term interventions. Examples include health warnings in heatwaves and building coastal defences to stop flooding.

A third term, resilience, has been introduced (Hopkins 2008) to describe 'the capacity of a system to absorb disturbance and reorganise while undergoing change, so as to still retain essentially the same function, structure, identity and feedbacks'. Through adaptation we develop resilience.

The developed world's dependence on carbon

The world's increasing dependence on carbon is a critical contributory factor to climate change and global warming. The most commonly cited example of our use of carbon is in relation to energy use, with the bulk of our energy coming from non-renewable carbon-based sources, chiefly coal and oil. Figure 12.3 shows how our use of fossil fuels has grown massively during the past 150 years.

Reduction in the world's reliance on fossil fuels must therefore be a key element of strategies to tackle climate change. While fossil fuels tend to be the focus of public attention to climate change, food production has only recently become a widespread concern. We now know that livestock farming remains the greatest contributor to methane and carbon dioxide production – even more than transport and other uses of

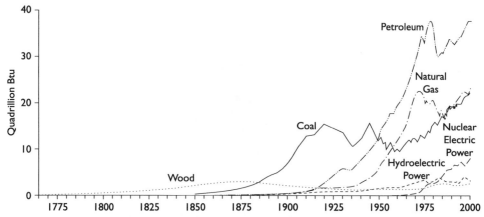

Figure 12.3 Changes in consumption of fossil fuels since the beginning of the Industrial Revolution

fossil fuels. The consumption of meat is a very important contributory factor to climate change and one which has only just begun to be considered by governments, but could readily be tackled by individuals aware of the issue and minded to make changes to their diet. It has been calculated that if everyone in the UK stopped eating meat for 1 day a week, the CO_2 savings would be equivalent to taking five million cars off the road.

Activity 12.1

Why do you think the consumption of meat is such a major cause of greenhouse gas emissions? What processes are responsible?

Feedback

Figure 12.4 summarizes the impact of food production on climate change (Roberts 2009):

- Providing pasture for grazing is a major reason for deforestation. About one third of the world's land surface is used for livestock, either to provide pasture for grazing or to grow grain for cattle feed.
- Grain production for feed also requires the use of energy-intensive nitrogenous fertilizers.
- Methane released from animal manure and from enteric fermentation is a powerful greenhouse gas with 34 times the global warming potential of carbon dioxide.
- Cattle manure also releases nitrous oxide, a greenhouse gas with nearly 300 times greater global warming potential than carbon dioxide.
- Global average meat consumption is currently about 100 grams per person per day, ranging from about 25 grams per person in low-income countries to as much as 250 grams per person in high-income countries.
- To benefit both health and the environment, it is suggested that each person eats no more than 100 grams of meat per day, and has at least one meat-free day per week.

In the developed world, we are all at risk of carbon dependence. See http://www. carbonaddict.org/ for a light-hearted take with serious undertones on this topic.

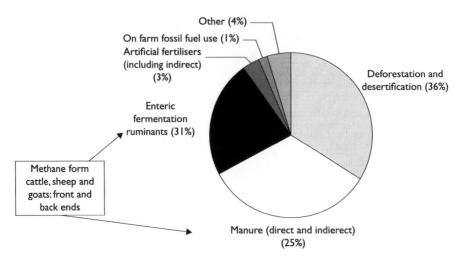

* includes feed production and associated land use changes

Figure 12.4 Greenhouse gas emissions from livestock production
Source: Based on FAO (2006)

The role of health care systems

As a major user of energy, health care clearly contributes to carbon emissions. For obvious reasons, no one is advocating the wholesale cessation of health care, merely the recognition that health care is in a good position to act as an exemplar in the areas of climate change and sustainable development. In England, the National Health Service (NHS) is the largest public sector contributor to climate change in Europe. Each year it emits 21 million tonnes of carbon dioxide equivalent (NHS Sustainable Development Unit 2009).

In England, the NHS Sustainable Development Unit (www.sdu.nhs.uk) was established in 2008 to encourage health care providers and commissioners to become good environmental citizens, emphasizing the benefits to the organizations themselves, to their patients and staff, and to the overall agenda of tackling climate change.

Health care organizations are responsible for standards of buildings and other hardware – transport, computers, technical equipment – all of which consume energy, as well as influencing the behaviour of their staff and, to some extent, of patients. The health service is also a major consumer of food for patients, staff and visitors, and an important contributor to travel-related greenhouse gas emissions from its 1.3 million staff and its patients. However, about 60 per cent of the NHS carbon footprint is associated with procurement, in particular pharmaceutical products.

The NHS East Midlands Carbon Reduction Project is a good example of NHS engagement.

Produced by the Nottingham Energy Partnership (you can read more at www.nottenergy.com/NHScarbonreduction). In summary, this project has identified baseline carbon footprints for the NHS in the East Midlands. It makes recommendations that link energy efficiency with financial savings, for example:

- savings of £13–14 million possible from energy bills;
- savings of £2.35 million from improved waste management and waste segregation;

- the need to think beyond estates and facilities management to organizational carbon management;
- a proposed regional scheme to get key NHS suppliers of goods and services to calculate and set targets for the reduction of their carbon footprints;
- the need for hands-on training for procurement staff;
- emphasis on the increasing cost of oil, water and waste management and the need therefore to take action now to avoid transfer of funds away from patient care and public health.

A nationwide network of health care organizations supporting standards in this area could be a powerful force for change, if there are governance arrangements in place to monitor compliance and progress and to levy sanctions on those who fail to adhere to the standards.

A route map for sustainable health care, published in 2011 by the Sustainable Development Unit, asks people and organizations within the NHS to be more efficient with their use of resources, which includes energy, carbon, water and people's time. It builds on the earlier NHS Carbon Reduction Strategy, published in 2009. A major thrust of the initiative is a drive to greater efficiency, which will have a favourable impact on climate change – examples include reducing hospital admissions of people with long-term conditions, reducing the use of pharmaceuticals (through regular review, reduced wastage and alternative forms of therapy), improved insulation, heating and cooling systems, action to reduce wasted energy (e.g. turning computers off overnight) and greater emphasis on preventive medicine. The route map depends upon adherence to standards, behaviours and innovation. It makes ambitious statements requiring intersectoral action, such as the NHS deciding to fund home insulation in order to reduce the number of winter hospital admissions attributable to hypothermia, which is particularly prevalent among elderly people living in older properties.

Engaging health care organizations is an example of a systems approach to tackling climate change. 'Systems thinking' was defined by the former Climate Connection as 'a framework that is based on the belief that the component parts of a system can best be understood in the context of relationships with each other and with other systems, rather than in isolation'.

When things go wrong

The following examples demonstrate what can (and have been known to) happen in the event of a heatwave in Britain (Centre for Sustainable Healthcare http://greener-healthcare.org/):

- Nurses and administrative staff walked out in protest at high temperatures in a brand-new privately financed hospital 'We can't work in this – we're suffering from heat exhaustion and everything'.
- Angry relatives claimed a hospital could not provide for its most vulnerable patients. People on strict nil by mouth diets were left to lie in pools of their own sweat without ice and proper air conditioning as their limbs swelled in the heat.
- A hospital was facing demands for an enquiry into how vital equipment was allowed to break down during a recent heatwave, forcing the cancellation of scores of operations.
- A public health (pathology) laboratory stopped work – machines failed in heat.

- Nurses on a cardiac ward were in tears at their inability to keep patients as cool as they should have been.
- Drugs may be vulnerable to extreme temperatures in summer, affecting their efficacy.

In order to address the problems brought about by the increased likelihood of heat-waves, the government in England has responded with its Heatwave Plan.

The Heatwave Plan for England was addressed primarily at the NHS and allied social care services. The 'Heat-Health Watch' system defines four levels of response:

- Level ONE: Summer preparedness and long-term planning
- Level TWO: Alert and readiness
- Level THREE: Heatwave action
- Level FOUR: Heatwave emergency

The Plan sets out responsibilities of organizations to raise awareness of risks relating to severe hot weather. It then sets out the responsibilities at national and local level of the health and social care sectors for alerting people once a heatwave is forecast and advising people what to do during a heatwave in order to minimize the risks to health, particularly of the most vulnerable. It raises awareness of risks relating to severe hot weather and what preparations both individuals and organizations should make to reduce those risks.

Co-benefits for health of tackling climate change

As we have seen, climate change is a difficult subject on which to achieve action for many reasons. One of these is the long-term nature of the adverse impact of climate change, when politicians the world over are interested in short-term impact and large corporations mainly interested in short-term profit and medium-term sustainability for their business. It may be easier to market the need for action in ways that demonstrate how addressing the long-term impacts of climate change can also be of benefit to people and organizations in the shorter term. The term 'co-benefit' has come into use to describe such features – i.e. not only is an action likely to impact favourably on climate change, it is also likely to reduce mortality or morbidity sooner due to other causes, or to contribute to improvement in the health of a population or of a particular group within a population. In this context it has been noted by Ian Roberts that 'Public policies that prevent additional climate change present unrivalled opportunities for improving public health'. Or as a simple slogan: 'What's good for the climate is good for health' (see www.climateandhealth.org).

The health co-benefits of mitigation might include the following examples:

1 As a consequence of increasing the price of petrol:
    - fewer petrol-fuelled cars on the roads;
    - streets becoming safer – fewer road accidents and associated injuries and deaths. Internationally, there are currently 3,000 road deaths daily and many more injuries. There is evidence to suggest that as petrol prices rise, the incidence of child road traffic injuries falls;
    - less congestion on roads and consequently less urban air pollution. There are an estimated 800k deaths per year globally from the consequences of air pollution.

2 Active travel comprises of means of transport that rely on human effort, chiefly walking and cycling. The co-benefits of active travel include:

- reducing obesity: risk of obesity correlates with a sedentary lifestyle and with time spent in a car. Walking or cycling to school or work is one of the most consistent ways to increase physical activity;
- cardiovascular disease: walking more than 1.5 miles per day is associated with a 50 per cent lower risk of myocardial infarction in older men;
- mental health: regular exercise is effective in the prevention and treatment of depression and anxiety, and may help to prevent the onset of dementia;
- maintaining regular exercise such as walking contributes to prevention of falls and osteoporosis in older people;
- noise reduction: road traffic noise is associated with hypertension;
- the impact on road deaths attributable to fewer motorized vehicles: e.g. accident rates are lower in the Netherlands where there are higher rates of walking and cycling;
- reduced air pollution: reducing emissions from car travel produces improved air quality, associated with major benefits to both cardiovascular and respiratory morbidity.

Box 12.3 is a practical example of action led by a Director of Public Health to put climate change and sustainable development on the local health agenda.

Box 12.3 NHS Bristol Annual Public Health Report 2010

Environment

Taking care of the environment is one of NHS Bristol's core values. All of the organisation's services must be delivered in a way that conserves natural resources and cuts carbon emissions.

Steps toward this have included changing insulation, thermostats and timer switches which have, so far, resulted in a 14 percent cut in energy use. NHS Bristol's travel footprint is shrinking thanks to new policies that support lower carbon emissions. NHS Bristol is improving the availability of healthy, sustainably produced food for local people, and links have been forged with the 'Joint Transport Executive' to support improvements in public transport, walking and cycling, so that these become first choice for most urban journeys.

Impact on health inequalities

Justice has been identified as one of the four main bioethical principles, alongside beneficence (doing good), non-maleficence (not doing harm) and autonomy. If we accept the relevance of justice in the context of public health, then we are obliged to seek equitable and just solutions to major issues that impact on public health, in this instance, climate change.

The impact of climate change on health inequalities may be considered at a number of levels. As mentioned earlier, among the poorest populations in the world are those that are already facing the adverse impacts of climate change, for instance, needing to migrate from islands affected by flooding and recurrent 'freak' weather conditions to safer land-masses. With migration come the recognized risks to physical and mental human health.

Within populations, at a local level, a similar pattern may be reflected. For instance, poorer communities often live in highly polluted urban areas compared with their more affluent neighbours, or have the most poorly insulated homes.

The impact of mitigation of climate change on health inequalities may be positive or negative. If we explore the positive, here are some examples of the impact on health inequalities of interventions to mitigate climate change:

• Insulation of homes reduces fuel poverty and expenditure on fuel; improves resilience to cold and hot weather; reduces excess seasonal deaths; and promotes health and wellbeing.
• Active transport, i.e. walking and cycling, reduce obesity and improve mental well-being and social cohesion.
• Green spaces improve air quality and mental wellbeing; they increase safety, social cohesion and activity levels.
• Breastfeeding carries a recognized health benefit to the infant and bonding with the parent.
• Reducing food waste means that more value is derived from food purchased.

Against these positive impacts, we must weigh the interventions to tackle climate change that might increase health inequalities:

• Energy or carbon pricing has the potential to harm the poorest in society, if safeguards are not in place to protect them (this is one of the reasons for the Climate and Health Council's support of a tradeable personal carbon quota, www.climateandhealth.org).
• Some energy efficiency measures can reduce ventilation, impacting on indoor air quality and radon exposure.
• Buying only local food will reduce the choice of fresh fruit and vegetables in winter. This may discourage an adequate intake and so impair nutritional status in some people.

Box 12.4 Sustainable Commissioning for Public Health

Example:

A County Council awarded a waste and recycling contract to a locally based charity rather than one of the multinational companies that had put in a bid.

This community recycling provider offers voluntary placements and employs people with disabilities. It helps people come off benefits and find work. This way it reduces the bills for financial support and for health and social care that would otherwise fall to central and local government.

Adapted from Arora (2009)

The Contraction and Convergence model and health inequalities

Contraction and Convergence is a framework for carbon reduction which also reduces inequalities. It is designed to keep health and justice at the heart of policy-making. It was developed by Aubrey Meyer. Governed by the principle of equity, it sets out a global framework for reducing greenhouse gas emissions to safe levels in a socially just way. Implementation of the model would result in a global 'carbon budget' with annual reduction targets based on levels considered safe to avert dangerous climate change (i.e. limit temperature rise from global warming to 2°C) and a shared commitment to continue to reduce or 'contract' global emissions year-on-year. In the long term every individual would have access to the same personal carbon 'budget' and the choices regarding how to use it. Under this model, developing countries would be allowed to increase initially their carbon usage, using cost- and carbon-efficiency lessons already learnt by developed countries (IPCC 2007). See also the Climate and Health Council's Charter at http://www.climateandhealth.org/charter, which has the contraction and convergence model as its central proposition.

The role of public health

Public health practitioners are active in the three domains of public health practice: health protection, health improvement and ensuring health services quality and access. Each of these has a part to play in tackling climate change. As we have seen, health care systems have a clear responsibility to address climate change by taking and promoting effective actions. The domain allied to health care is about improving health services: in the context of climate change, it is therefore incumbent on public health to ensure that health care has a favourable impact on climate change.

Health care planners and purchasers should be in a strong position to influence the providers of health care, since compliance with intervention that mitigates climate change can be included in contracts with providers and their progress with implementation monitored. We know that '... the procurement of goods, services and equipment ... is responsible for the largest proportion of carbon emissions from the NHS' (NHS SDU 2009), so commissioners should strive to ensure that procurement has the minimum impact on climate change. The sort of requirements that public health, in the *health services quality* domain, can seek to include in commissioning may include the following:

- It is expected that the amount of electricity used by the providers will fall by 10 per cent in the forthcoming year OR what reduction in electricity use will you need to achieve to keep our electricity bill constant?
- It is assumed that the amount of petrol used by Trusts will decrease by 5 per cent in the forthcoming year OR is the mileage driven by staff and patients increasing or decreasing?
- What is the electricity footprint of your building, namely how many kilowatts per hour per sq metre? How do you intend to reduce it?
- It is expected that water use will decrease by 5 per cent in the forthcoming year.
- Are you taking the carbon impact of change into account when redesigning care – e.g. use of telemedicine and email consultations?
- How much of the food that is bought is thrown out as waste? How will you reduce it? And how much of the food purchased is sourced locally?

Looking at the other domains of public health practice, the former Climate Connection suggested that everyone working in public health must be equipped to take action because *health protection* demands detailed understanding of climate impacts, and not only in emergency planning, i.e. how will the climate affect food and energy security, patterns of disease and health inequalities? Will the developed world be insulated from conflict over land, water and food elsewhere?

And as for health improvement, strategies to reduce greenhouse gas emissions are almost synonymous with *health improvement*, whether through improved housing, active transport, reduced meat consumption or economic localization.

Activity 12.2

Public health practitioners are respected advocates in society. Think about what they can do to ensure that the health arguments are deployed more effectively.

Feedback

- Health practitioners are well organized, through their professional associations and colleges. Most of these have some work underway on climate change and would welcome more involvement. The Climate and Health Council is a specific organization that works both within the UK and internationally to ensure that the health voice is heard (www.climateandhealth.org), and there are many other networks.
- Through daily communications with patients and the public, there is an opportunity to mention the benefits for the environment and climate change when engaging with health issues such as reducing obesity (walking and cycling more, healthier diets and so on).
- The power of leadership by example, through your own actions (see Activity 12.3) is not to be underestimated; maintaining the profile of climate change in professional media is also important, and health professionals can influence both local and national politicians.
- Though the challenge may appear daunting, success is possible: 12 per cent of the earth's surface is now within protected areas, such as nature reserves; and international agreement was reached which has reduced the production of ozone-damaging chemicals by 95 per cent in response to the identification of holes in the ozone layer.

Personal action

This might be contentious (since not all public health practitioners are non-smokers and some are obese, for example) but as a public health practitioner, it seems a reasonable expectation that you will strive to support the climate change agenda in an individual capacity as well as through your work. At a personal level, you need to understand about your own situation in order to make changes. A starting point is to become familiar with your carbon footprint.

Why should you care about your carbon footprint?

A person's carbon footprint is the amount of carbon emitted by an individual (or a family, town, country), usually measured as kg or tonnes of CO_2 equivalent (CO2e) released. So carbon is becoming a currency and the carbon costs of our activities are being identified.

The reason for knowing the carbon footprint of an activity is because the greater the release of carbon emissions, the greater the impact; conversely, activities resulting in fewer emissions are associated with less impact – so, for instance, travelling by foot clearly is associated with lower CO_2 emissions than travelling by car, which in turn causes fewer emissions than air travel. One person's carbon footprint may be argued to be irrelevant, but the footprint produced by a whole population comprises the actions of individuals. If you intend to practise public health, an interest in your own carbon footprint is as relevant to your practice as whether you smoke, are physically active or drink to excess: self-awareness is an important feature of ethical professional practice – and the awareness may help you decide to change your behaviour.

Activity 12.3

Draw up a list of the actions you have already taken to reduce your own greenhouse gas emissions (at home, in the community and at work) and a second list of actions you might be able to take over the next 12 months. You might like to decide on one new action that you can implement immediately.

Feedback

- The four main causes of individual carbon emissions (each of which account for about a quarter of emissions in the United Kingdom) are: consumption of food and drink; energy to heat and light homes and workplaces; transport, mainly cars and planes; and emissions from the consumption of other goods and services (from public services to clothes and consumer goods). It is possible to have an action plan to reduce gradually your carbon emissions in each of these areas.
- A reduction of 5 per cent a year will accumulate over time to meet the necessary targets. Many countries have had a year of action to reduce emissions by 10 per cent in the year 2010, and this type of campaign breaks down the substantial reductions required (e.g. 80 per cent by 2050) into manageable fractions.
- 'I will if you will …': people are more likely to change their behaviour if they see others are doing it too, making them feel that their efforts are worthwhile. And by taking action ourselves, we are, in effect, demonstrating our willingness for government to take action.

Community action

Rob Hopkins (2008) has expressed the view that governments will take too little action, too late and that if we act as individuals – as we must – it will be too little. But if we act as communities, it might just be enough, just in time. Hopkins started the Transition movement in Kinsale, Ireland in 2005, promoting a community response to the twin threats of peak oil (i.e. the belief that oil supplies have reached their peak, are set to decline rapidly and that we need to wean ourselves off oil dependence) and climate change. There are now over 150 Transition Initiatives in the UK and an equivalent number in continental Europe, North America, Australia and New Zealand. Transition initiatives are also beginning to appear in South American and Africa. They vary in scale and scope from villages to islands to cities, and from churches to universities. The movement is based on the following ideas:

(a) A reduction in energy consumption is not only required because of climate change but inevitable because of peak oil.
(b) This will require developing more local economic self-sufficiency and building resilience at the local level.
(d) More resilient and self-sufficient local communities could offer us a future better than the present.
(e) It is more inspiring and effective to work together towards making a positive vision the reality than to protest against the current situation.

The approach is community based. Interested individuals come together to create an umbrella grouping – a Transition Initiative – that aims to act as a catalyst for people in the area to create local projects.

Activity 12.4

What types of projects do citizens involved in Transition Initiatives typically instigate, and what might be their links to health? You might want to look on the Internet for a Transition initiative near where you live or work (go to www.transitionnetwork.org/).

Feedback

The most common Transition projects are:

• local food projects, e.g. garden-sharing, food-buying groups, community orchards, farmers markets;
• local energy projects, e.g. household energy audits, local renewable energy generation, energy fairs and advice;
• local transport projects, e.g. car-sharing schemes, bicycle repair workshops;
• local economy projects, e.g. local social enterprises (such as eco-building).

It is evident that the types of projects listed above, although developed from the starting point of local resilience, in fact relate closely to the areas of possible co-benefit to health of tackling climate change described earlier in this chapter.

For public health practitioners working in the domain of *health improvement*, the empowerment of individuals and communities through participation has been an important strategy since the 1990s at least. Empowerment has been defined as: 'A social process that promotes the participation of individuals, organisations and communities in actions with the goal of increased individual and community control, political efficacy, improved quality of life and social justice' (Handsley 2007: 200). The Transition movement offers tremendous opportunities to public health practitioners to build bridges with active local communities to improve health, reduce health inequalities and promote a low-carbon, sustainable society. Most importantly, it creates a positive vision of a better society and enables people to have fun.

Climate change and sustainable development

The now-classic definition of sustainable development – meeting the needs of the present without compromising the ability of future generations to meet their needs – was first fully articulated in 1987 by Dr Gro Harlem Brundtland, as Chair of the World Commission on Environment and Development which produced the seminal report, *Our Common Future* (Brundtland 1987). Social and economic development that is sustainable safeguards supplies of natural resources (water, cultivable soil, biodiversity) for future generations. Sustainable development is concerned with notions of social justice, both over time and between and within societies.

The principles of sustainable development offer a guiding framework for government and social action, consistent with the 'social model' of health and highly relevant to tackling differences in health status between different socioeconomic groups. Key principles include (Sustainable Development Commission 2010):

- a long-term perspective, drawing attention to the needs of future generations and inter-generational equity;
- a focus on the environmental determinants of health and health inequalities, including – but not only – the effects of climate change;
- a concern to reduce the dominance of economic growth as the only model for social development, in order to improve well-being and to ensure that sufficient natural resources remain for future generations (see for example, the New Economic Foundation's *Green, Well, Fair* which makes the case for a new social settlement);
- policies and actions that improve life for the poorest people in the global population.

In the business world, and indeed in the world of health care providers, sustainable development is often embedded in 'corporate social responsibility', the use of corporate powers and resources in ways that benefit the social, economic and physical environment in which we all live. Recognizing that their customers increasingly expect them to be reducing their environmental impact and make a contribution to the sustainability of local communities, many businesses now implement – and publicize – corporate social responsibility strategies. Lloyd's, the international insurance underwriter, concluded in its 360 Risk Insight report on Sustainable Energy Security that surging energy consumption, constraints on conventional fuel production and international recognition of the impact of carbon dioxide on the climate 'mean[s] businesses need to adapt to a new local carbon world' (Lloyd's 2010). Compared with the public sector, the business sector has accepted the reality of anthropogenic climate change and is getting on with mitigation and adaptation.

Nature, biodiversity, green space and health

Evidence has accumulated that living or working near to, and time spent in, the natural environment has a strong positive impact on perceived general health, stress, mental health and also physical health indicators such as blood pressure and speed of recovery from illness. The presence of green space also encourages physical activity, social contact and integration, including children's play. Green spaces are unequally distributed across socioeconomic groups, with poorer social groups having, in general, lower access. Research suggests that across England, income-related inequality in health is less pronounced in populations with greater exposure to green spaces (SDC 2010).

However, the work of the United Nations Environment Programme reminds us that climate change is taking place against a background of major global threats to this health-promoting natural environment, partly due to the need for water and land to feed a growing population. The last UNEP *Global Environment Outlook: Environment for Development* (GEO-4) report was published in 2007. Some of the major areas of global environmental damage – which, like climate change, are at risk of passing the point of no return – highlighted in the GEO-4 report include the following:

- There are oxygen 'dead zones' in the seas and oceans, caused by acidification from CO_2 emissions. The seas and oceans absorb about one quarter of the carbon dioxide emitted to the atmosphere, reducing the effects of climate change. However, the absorption of atmospheric CO_2 has resulted in changes to the chemical balance of the oceans, causing them to become more acidic. It is predicted that by 2050, ocean acidity could increase by 150 per cent, 100 times faster than any change in acidity experienced in the marine environment over the last 20 million years. Acidification contributes to the decline of fish stocks and the destruction of coral reefs (20 per cent of which have been lost already).
- Fish stocks are in decline: fish consumption more than tripled from 1961 to 2001. Fishing capacity is estimated at 250 per cent more than is needed to catch the oceans' sustainable production.
- The sixth major extinction of life on earth is underway – the last one was when the dinosaurs were wiped out – and this extinction is anthropogenic. Current biodiversity changes are the fastest in human history. Species are becoming extinct a hundred times more quickly than the rate shown in the fossil record – it is estimated that we are losing three species *an hour*. Of the major vertebrate groups that have been assessed comprehensively, over 30 per cent of amphibians, 23 per cent of mammals and 12 per cent of birds are threatened.
- Loss of fertile land through degradation, especially in Africa, is a threat as serious as climate change and biodiversity loss. It affects up to a third of the world's people, through pollution, soil erosion, nutrient depletion, water scarcity and salinity.
- A dwindling amount of fresh water is available for humans and other creatures to share.

The combination of climate change with these other environmental threats means that we are destroying the context in which the human species evolved and to which we are adapted.

Ecological public health

Ecology is the study of the interactions between plants, animals, people and their environments within ecosystems, which are dynamic complexes of different forms of life interacting with their nonliving environments (such as water and rock). The integration of ecological and environmental issues and concerns within public health has led some to use the label 'ecological public health' for research and practice that seek to benefit

both human and environmental health simultaneously. Ecological public health may use existing policies and targets (for example, to reduce obesity) to support wider ecological goals and mitigation and adaptation to climate change. Ecological approaches, drawing on our understanding of how healthy ecosystems function, emphasize:

* networks – drawing out interconnections and common solutions;
* partnerships – environmental and wider determinants;
* cycles – life course and systems approaches;
* balance – health, environmental and inequalities impact assessments.

Ecological public health draws on systems thinking (see above) and emphasizes the need to grapple with complexity, emphasizing that health and health inequality are never solely about behaviour change and that working in silos, independently, is very unlikely to achieve lasting progress. A good example is the English Government's Foresight work – *Tackling Obesity: Future Choices* (Foresight 2007) which applies modelling and systems thinking. Issues are mapped, and solutions proposed, as systemic, that is interdependent and interconnected. In their complexity and opportunities for synergy, climate change and health, particularly the health co-benefits of action to create a lower-carbon society, are an excellent illustration of the characteristics of ecological public health.

The ecological paradigm enables public health practitioners to look for common causes and risks across policy and practice and work through partnerships and networks, to promote short-term opportunities to improve wellbeing and longer-term opportunities to improve the environment that sustains health.

Summary

This chapter has introduced you to the evidence behind climate change and the impact of climate change on the health of populations. It has proposed reasons why public health practitioners should be at the forefront of tackling climate change for the benefit of mankind, whether through personal action, or by seizing the opportunities that present during their day-to-day working lives or through a wider advocacy role in society: hopefully all of these.

References

Annett H (2010) *Annual Public Health Report*. Bristol: Bristol City Council and NHS Bristol. (available at http://www.bristol.nhs.uk/about-us/publications/public-health-report.aspx).

Arora S (2009) *Commissioning Sustainable Healthcare*. Gloucestershire: NHS.

Brundtland GH (1987) *Our Common Future: The World Commission on Environment and Development*. Oxford: Oxford University Press.

Committee on Climate Change (2010) *The Fourth Carbon Budget: Reducing Emissions Through the 2020s* (available at http://www.theccc.org.uk/reports/fourth-carbon-budget).

Dahlgren G and Whitehead M (1992) *Policies and Strategies to Promote Equity in Health*. Copenhagen: WHO Regional Office for Europe (document number: EUR/ICP/RPD 414 (2); http://whqlibdoc.who.int/euro/-1993/EUR_ICP_RPD414(2).pdf).

DARA Climate Vulnerability Monitor (2010) (available at http://daraint.org/climate-vulnerability-monitor/climate-vulnerability-monitor-2010/).

Faculty of Public Health (2009) *Sustaining a Healthy Future: Taking Action on Climate Change*, 2nd edn (available at http://www.fph.org.uk/resources/sustainable_development/Default.asp).

FAO (2006) *The State of Food Insecurity in the World*. Rome: Food and Agriculture Organization of the United Nations (available at http://www.fao.org/docrep/009/a0750e/a0750e00.htm).

Foresight (2007) *Tackling Obesity: Future Choices* (available at http://webarchive.nationalarchives.gov.uk/+/www.dh.gov.uk/en/Publichealth/Healthimprovement/Obesity/DH_079713).

Handsley S (2007) The potential for promoting public health at a local level: community strategies and health improvement, in C Lloyd, S Handsley et al. (eds) *Policy and Practice in Promoting Public Health*. London: Sage Publications (in association with the Open University).

Hopkins R (2008) *The Transition Handbook: From Oil Dependency to Local Resilience*. Chelsea Green publishing (available free at http://transitionus.org/sites/default/files/TransitionHandbook_freedit Version.pdf).

IPCC (2007) Summary for Policymakers. In: *Climate Change 2007: The Physical Science Basis*. Contribution of Working Group I to the Fourth Assessment Report of the Intergovernmental Panel on Climate Change (S Solomon, D Qin, M Manning, Z Chen, M Marquis, KB Averyt, M Tignor and HL Miller (eds)). Cambridge and New York: Cambridge University Press (available at http://www.ipcc.ch/pdf/assessment-report/ar4/wg1/ar4-wg1-spm.pdf).

Liggins F (2009) Greenhouse gas emissions: the hard facts, in J Griffiths, M Rao, F Adshead, and A Thorpe (eds) *The Health Practitioner's Guide to Climate Change: Diagnosis and Cure*. London: Earthscan.

Lloyd's (2010) http://www.lloyds.com/News-and-Insight/360-Risk-Insight/Research-and-Reports/Energy-Security/Energy-Security

Marmot M (2005) Social determinants of health inequalities. *The Lancet* **365** (9464): 1099–104. doi:10.1016/S0140-6736(05)71146-6.

NHS Sustainable Development Unit (2009) *NHS Carbon Reduction Strategy for England: Saving Carbon, Improving Health, 2009*. Cambridge: NHS Sustainable Development Unit.

Rao M (2010) The impact of climate change on health in India. *Perspectives in Public Health* **130** (1): 15–17.

Roberts I (2009) The health benefits of action on climate change, in J Griffiths, M Rao, F Adshead, and A Thorpe (eds) *The Health Practitioner's Guide to Climate Change: Diagnosis and Cure*. London: Earthscan.

Sustainable Development Commission (2010) *Sustainable Development: The Key to Tackling Health Inequalities*. London: Sustainable Development Commission.

The Royal Society (2010) *Climate Change: A Summary of the Science*. London: The Royal Society.

United Nations Environment Programme (UNEP) (2007) *Global Environment Outlook: Environment for Development (GEO-4)* (available at www.unep.org/geo/geo4/).

Further reading

Carbon Addict. Visit: http://www.carbonaddict.org

Centers for Disease Prevention and Control. Syndemics Prevention Network. Visit http://www.cdc.gov/syndemics/. For work on understanding and preventing major, simultaneously occurring, events which have negative impacts on population health.

Climate and Health. Visit: www.climateandhealth.org

Griffiths G, Rao M, Adshead F and Thorpe A (2009) *The Health Practitioner's Guide to Climate Change: Diagnosis and cure*. London: Earthscan.

The Campaign for Greeneer Healthcare. Visit: http://greenerhealthcare.org/public-health-climate-connection

Glossary

Addiction Dependence on something that is psychologically or physically habit-forming.

Age-standardization Way of controlling for age so that we can compare rates of deaths or disease in populations with different age structures.

Allele One member of two or more alternative genes that occupy a specific position on a specific chromosome.

Avoidable mortality Premature deaths that should not occur in the presence of timely and effective health care.

Blue-ribbon panels An expert committee appointed to investigate particularly complex or important matters; can be used (sceptically) to describe any government-appointed group [originates from UK Order of the Garter, who wore a blue ribbon to denote their rank].

Burden of disease A measure of the physical, emotional, social and financial impact that a particular disease has on the health and functioning of the population.

Community development A long-term value-based process which aims to bring about change founded on social justice, equality and inclusion. The process enables people to organize and work together to identify their own needs and aspirations, to be empowered to take action regarding decisions which affect their lines and improve the quality of their own lives, the communities in which they live and societies of which they are part.

Community regeneration The aim of regeneration is to enable communities that have suffered from economic, social and environmental decline to 'work' again. Regeneration is usually applied primarily to improvements in the physical environment in which people live.

Discrimination Direct discrimination occurs where one person is treated less favourably than another is, has been, or would be treated in a comparable situation on grounds of race, ethnic origin or other factor; indirect discrimination occurs where an apparently neutral provision, criterion or practice would put persons with a given trait (for example racial or ethnic origin) at a particular disadvantage compared with other persons, unless that provision, criterion or practice is objectively justified by a legitimate aim and the means of achieving that aim are appropriate and necessary.

Ecological footprint Accounting tool for ecological resources developed by the Task Force on Healthy and Sustainable Communities at the University of British Columbia (Canada). It corresponds to the area of productive land and aquatic ecosystems required to produce the resources used, and to assimilate the wastes produced, by a defined population at a specified material standard of living, wherever on Earth that land may be located.

Environmental or occupational exposure Any contact between a substance in an environmental medium (for example water, air, soil) and the surface of the human body (for example skin, respiratory tract); after uptake into the body it is referred to as dose.

Exposure assessment Is the study of distribution and determinants of substances or factors affecting human health.

Food miles Distance that foods travel from where they are grown to where they are ultimately purchased or consumed by the end user.

Food security Physical and economic access for everyone and at all times to enough foods that are nutritious, safe, personally acceptable and culturally appropriate, produced and distributed in ways that are environmentally sound and just.

Gentrification The restoration of run-down urban areas, usually by and for the middle class – which may result in the displacement of the area's original low-income residents.

Germ theory The theory that all contagious diseases are caused by microorganisms.

Globalization A set of processes that are changing the nature of human interaction by intensifying interactions across certain boundaries that have hitherto served to separate individuals and population groups. These spatial, temporal and cognitive boundaries have been increasingly eroded, resulting in new forms of social organization and interaction across these boundaries.

Health expectancy Summary measure of population health that estimates the expectation of years of life lived in various health states.

Health gap Summary measure of population health that estimates the gap between the current population health and a normative goal for population health.

Health inequalities Differences in health experience and health status between countries, regions and socioeconomic groups.

Health system A health system includes all the activities whose primary purpose is to promote, restore or maintain health.

Health system goals Improving the health of the population they serve, responding to people's expectations, providing financial protection against the cost of ill health.

International Refers to cross-border flows that are, in principle, possible to regulate by national governments.

Intersectoral action for health The promotion of health through the involvement of actors in other sectors, such as transport, housing, or education.

Inverse care law Those who need care most are least likely to receive it.

Libertarianism Philosophical approach that favours individualism, with a free-market economic policy and non-intervention by government.

Life course epidemiology Study of the long-term effects on later health or disease risk of physical or social exposures during gestation, childhood, adolescence, young adulthood or later adult life.

Life expectancy The average number of years a person can expect to live on average in a given population.

Nosologic Deals with the classification of diseases.

Nutrition transition Process of change in which populations shift their diet from a restricted diet to one higher in saturated fat, sugar and refined foods, and low in fibre; as a result, diet-related ill health previously associated with affluent Western societies takes root in developing countries.

Precautionary principle This principle states that when there is reasonable suspicion of harm, lack of scientific certainty or consensus must not be used to postpone preventative action to avoid serious or irreversible harm.

'Prevention Paradox' Using a population approach (as distinct from a targeted approach targeting only individuals at high risk, there will be only a small benefit for the majority of individuals, but large potential for whole population improvement. Term coined by leading epidemiologist, Geoffrey Rose, in the 1970s.

Prolegomena A preliminary discussion, often an introduction to a work of considerable length or complexity.

Public health The science and art of promoting health and preventing disease through the organized efforts of society.

Regeneration Reviving run-down or deprived areas, for example by providing employment and training schemes, improving housing, developing transport links, offering local health services, landscaping and creating green spaces from derelict areas etc.

Reticulated Forming a net or network, so in the context of health inequalities, the linkages between social inequalities and emerging disease.

Social model of health The social model of health carefully considers how wider determinants, and not just the presence or absence of disease, have an impact on people's health. The wider determinants include cultures and belief systems, relative income, access to housing, education attainment, and the wider environmental, political and socioeconomic conditions and community in which people live.

Summary measures of population health Indicators that combine information about mortality and health states to summarize the health of a population into a single number.

Tort Legal term used to describe a wrongful act, resulting in harm or loss to another person or their property, on which a civil action for damages may be brought.

Transnational (as opposed to international) Refers to transborder flows that largely circumvent national borders and can thus be beyond the control of national governments alone.

Zoonotic infections [zoonoses] Human diseases acquired from a vertebrate animal. They include many common infectious diseases transmitted to man via an animal host.

Index

Page numbers in *italics* refer to figures and tables.

PUBLIC HEALTH IN HISTORY

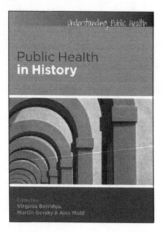

Virginia Berridge, Martin Gorsky
and Alex Mold

9780335242641 (Paperback)
2011

eBook also available

This fascinating book offers a wide ranging exploration of the history of
public health and the development of health services over the past two
centuries. The book surveys the rise and redefinition of public health
since the sanitary revolution of the mid-nineteenth century, assessing
the reforms in the post World War II years and the coming of welfare
states.

Written by experts from the London School of Hygiene and Tropical
Medicine, this is the definitive history of public health.

Key features:

- Case studies on malaria, sexual health, alcohol and substance
  abuse
- A comparative examination of why healthcare has taken such
  different trajectories in different countries
- Exercises enabling readers to easily interact with and critically
  assess historical source material

www.openup.co.uk

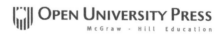

OPEN UNIVERSITY PRESS
McGraw · Hill Education

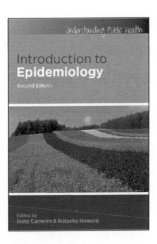

INTRODUCTION TO EPIDEMIOLOGY
Second Edition

Ilona Carneiro and Natasha Howard

9780335244614 (Paperback)
September 2011

eBook also available

This popular book introduces the principles, methods and application of epidemiology for improving health and survival. It assists readers in applying basic epidemiological methods to measure health outcomes, identifying risk factors for a negative outcome, and evaluating health interventions and health services.

The book also helps to distinguish between strong and poor epidemiological evidence; an ability that is fundamental to promoting evidence-based health care.

Key features:

- A broad range of examples and activities covering a range of contemporary health issues including obesity, mental health and cervical cancer
- New chapter on study design and data handling
- Updated and additional exercises for self-testing

www.openup.co.uk

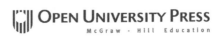

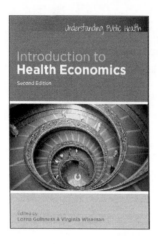

**INTRODUCTION TO HEALTH
ECONOMICS
Second Edition**

Lorna Guinness and Virginia Wiseman

9780335243563 (Paperback)
September 2011

eBook also available

This practical text offers the ideal introduction to the economic
techniques used in public health and is accessible enough for those
who have no or limited knowledge of economics. Written in a user-
friendly manner, the book covers key economic principles, such as
supply and demand, healthcare markets, healthcare finance and
economic evaluation.

Key features:

- Extensive use of global examples from low, middle and high
  income countries, real case studies and exercises to facilitate the
  understanding of economic concepts
- A greater emphasis on the practical application of economic
  theories and concepts to the formulation of health policy
- New chapters on macroeconomics, globalization and health and
  provider payments

www.openup.co.uk

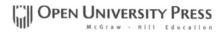
OPEN UNIVERSITY PRESS
McGraw · Hill Education